Evidence Synthesis
Number 113

Behavioral Counseling to Promote a Healthy Lifestyle for Cardiovascular Disease Prevention in Persons With Cardiovascular Risk Factors: An Updated Systematic Evidence Review for the U.S. Preventive Services Task Force

Prepared for:
Agency for Healthcare Research and Quality
U.S. Department of Health and Human Services
540 Gaither Road
Rockville, MD 20850
www.ahrq.gov

Contract No. HHS-290-2007-10057-I-EPC3, Task Order No. 13

Prepared by:
Kaiser Permanente Research Affiliates Evidence-based Practice Center
Kaiser Permanente Center for Health Research
Portland, OR

Investigators:
Jennifer S. Lin, MD, MCR
Elizabeth A. O'Connor, PhD
Corinne V. Evans, MPP
Caitlyn A. Senger, MPH
Maya G. Rowland, MPH
Holly C. Groom, MPH

AHRQ Publication No. 13-05179-EF-1
August 2014

This report is based on research conducted by the Kaiser Permanente Research Affiliates Evidence-based Practice Center (EPC) under contract to the Agency for Healthcare Research and Quality (AHRQ), Rockville, MD (Contract No. HHS-290-2007-10057-I-EPC3, Task Order No. 13). The findings and conclusions in this document are those of the authors, who are responsible for its contents, and do not necessarily represent the views of AHRQ. Therefore, no statement in this report should be construed as an official position of AHRQ or of the U.S. Department of Health and Human Services.

The information in this report is intended to help health care decisionmakers—patients and clinicians, health system leaders, and policymakers, among others—make well-informed decisions and thereby improve the quality of health care services. This report is not intended to be a substitute for the application of clinical judgment.

This report may be used, in whole or in part, as the basis for development of clinical practice guidelines and other quality enhancement tools, or as a basis for reimbursement and coverage policies. AHRQ or U.S. Department of Health and Human Services endorsement of such derivative products may not be stated or implied.

This document is in the public domain and may be used and reprinted without permission except those copyrighted materials that are clearly noted in the document. Further reproduction of those copyrighted materials is prohibited without the specific permission of copyright holders.

None of the investigators has any affiliations or financial involvement that conflicts with the material presented in this report.

Acknowledgments

The authors gratefully acknowledge the following individuals for their contributions to this project: Daphne Plaut, MLS, and Smyth Lai, MLS, for creating and conducting the literature searches; Kevin Lutz, MFA, for his editorial assistance; David Brown, PhD, Janet de Jesus, MS, RD, David Hopkins, MD, MPH, Abby King, PhD, Penny Kris-Etherton, PhD, RD, and Laura Svetkey, MD, MHS, who provided expert review of the report; Lawrence Fine, MD, Linda Kinsinger, MD, MPH, Charlotte Pratt, PhD, RD, Wendy B. Smith, OBSSR, OD, and Catherine Witkop, MD, MPH, who provided federal partner review of this report; Robert McNellis, PA, at AHRQ; and Sue Curry, PhD, Mark Ebell, MD, MS, and Michael LeFevre, MD, MSPH, on behalf of the U.S. Preventive Services Task Force.

Suggested Citation

Lin JS, O'Connor EA, Evans CV, Senger CA, Rowland MG, Groom HC. Behavioral Counseling to Promote a Healthy Lifestyle for Cardiovascular Disease Prevention in Persons With Cardiovascular Risk Factors: An Evidence Update for the U.S. Preventive Services Task Force. Evidence Report No. 113. AHRQ Publication No. 13-05179-EF-1. Rockville, MD: Agency for Healthcare Research and Quality; 2014.

Structured Abstract

Purpose: We conducted a systematic evidence review of the benefits and harms of behavioral counseling interventions to prevent cardiovascular disease (CVD) in persons with established risk factors to assist the U.S. Preventive Services Task Force (USPSTF) in updating its previous recommendation statements.

Data Sources: We searched MEDLINE, PsycInfo, the Database of Abstracts of Reviews of Effects, and the Cochrane Central Register of Controlled Trials from 2001 through October 2013 to locate relevant trials for all key questions published since the previous reviews in support of prior recommendations. We supplemented our searches with reference lists from relevant existing systematic reviews, suggestions from experts, and information from Clinicaltrials.gov to identify ongoing trials.

Study Selection: Two investigators independently reviewed 7,218 abstracts and 553 articles against a set of a priori inclusion criteria. Investigators also independently critically appraised each study using design-specific quality criteria based on USPSTF methods. We included fair- or good-quality trials evaluating behavioral counseling interventions to promote a healthy diet, physical activity, or both in persons with CVD risk factors, including hypertension, dyslipidemia, metabolic syndrome, and impaired fasting glucose or glucose tolerance. We resolved discrepancies by consensus.

Data Extraction and Analysis: One investigator abstracted data from 74 included studies into evidence tables and a second reviewer checked these data. We conducted meta-analyses on 57 of the 71 trials that provided necessary data to estimate the effect size of counseling on intermediate health outcomes (lipids, blood pressure, weight measures, and glucose measures). We qualitatively summarized the evidence for effects on health outcomes, behavioral outcomes, and harms.

Data Synthesis: *Key Question 1. Do healthy lifestyle counseling interventions improve CVD health outcomes in adults with known CVD risk factors?* Only a subset of trials (k=16) reported measures of patient health outcomes, including CVD events (k=5) and self-reported measures of quality of life (QOL) or depression symptoms (k=11). In general, intensive interventions that combined lifestyle interventions did not reduce CVD events or mortality at up to 10 years of followup, although event rates were generally low. In one early good-quality trial, a high-intensity behavioral counseling intervention in conjunction with a protocol to start medication reduced CVD events at 6.6 years compared with usual care (relative risk [RR], 0.71 [95% CI, 0.51 to 0.99]). This study was conducted in Swedish men at high risk for CVD (which included persons with diabetes and known CVD). Overall, combined lifestyle interventions did not appear to improve self-reported depression symptoms (k=4) in persons with impaired fasting glucose or glucose tolerance at 6 to 12 months. Findings that showed a benefit on self-reported QOL measures were mixed. While three combined lifestyle counseling trials showed improvement on selected QOL measures, two combined lifestyle counseling trials and two physical activity–only counseling trials showed no benefit on self-reported QOL at 6 to 12 months.

Key Question 2. Do healthy lifestyle counseling interventions improve intermediate CVD outcomes in adults with known CVD risk factors? Medium- (31 to 360 minutes) to high-intensity (>360 minutes) combined lifestyle counseling in persons selected for CVD risk factors reduces total cholesterol, low-density lipoprotein (LDL) cholesterol, blood pressure, fasting glucose, diabetes incidence, and weight outcomes. Overall, at 12 to 24 months, behavioral counseling appears to reduce total cholesterol (k=34) by an average of 4.48 mg/dL (95% CI, 6.36 to 2.59), LDL cholesterol (k=25) by 3.43 mg/dL (95% CI, 5.37 to 1.49), systolic blood pressure (k=31) by 2.03 mm Hg (95% CI, 2.91 to 1.15), diastolic blood pressure (k=24) by 1.38 mm Hg (95% CI, 1.92 to 0.84), fasting glucose (k=22) by 2.08 mg/dL (95% CI, 3.29 to 0.88), diabetes incidence (k=8) by an RR of 0.58 (95% CI, 0.37 to 0.89), and weight outcomes (k=34) by a pooled mean difference of 0.26, using standardized units (95% CI, 0.35 to 0.16). There was substantial statistical heterogeneity for weight outcomes. High-intensity combined lifestyle counseling in persons with impaired fasting glucose or glucose tolerance (k=5) can reduce diabetes incidence in the long term (RR, 0.55 [95% CI, 0.45 to 0.67]). Intensive diet-only counseling interventions primarily in persons with dyslipidemia who are not yet taking medications can also modestly lower total (k=8) and LDL (k=7) cholesterol at 12 to 24 months. In contrast, medium-intensity (k=8) physical activity–only counseling interventions (k=10) did not appear to improve intermediate CVD outcomes at 12 to 24 months. Findings from trials that could not be included in quantitative analyses were generally consistent with pooled findings.

Key Question 3. Do healthy lifestyle counseling interventions improve diet and physical activity behavioral outcomes in adults with known CVD risk factors? Overall, objectively measured and self-reported changes in dietary intake and physical activity were concordant with intermediate outcome findings. Only three of the 61 trials that reported behavioral outcomes did not also report intermediate health outcomes. In selected trials conducted in persons who were already taking medications to lower cholesterol or blood pressure, counseling interventions appeared to improve dietary intake and physical activity despite a lack of benefit on lipid or blood pressure outcomes. Many physical activity–only counseling trials (k=9) had less than 12 months of followup. Four of five trials reporting behavioral outcomes at 12 to 24 months found statistically significant improvements in self-reported physical activity (i.e., number of persons meeting the recommended 150 minutes of moderate activity per week, minutes per week of total or moderate physical activity).

Key Question 4. What are the adverse effects of healthy lifestyle counseling in adults with known CVD risk factors? We examined all included counseling trials for harms, including any paradoxical change in outcomes. While we searched for additional studies examining harms of healthy lifestyle counseling interventions, we did not find any. Overall, harms (or lack thereof) were not commonly reported (k=10). In general, included interventions did not have significant adverse effects, except for two persons who had serious events resulting from physical activity in one trial targeting older adults. Reported increases in carbohydrate intake (k=8) were accompanied by dietary improvements in fat, saturated fat, fiber, or fruits and vegetables, without an overall increase in sugar or total calories consumed.

Limitations: Only a small subset of trials reported patient health outcomes, longer-term followup of intermediate and behavioral outcomes, and harms. We were unable to identify important contributors to statistical heterogeneity other than gross categorizations of type of population or intervention.

Conclusions: Medium- and high-intensity diet and physical activity behavioral counseling in overweight or obese persons with CVD risk factors resulted in consistent improvements across a variety of important cardiovascular intermediate health outcomes up to 2 years. High-intensity combined lifestyle counseling reduced diabetes incidence in the longer term. The applicability of these findings depends largely on the availability of intensive counseling in practice and real-world fidelity and adherence to these interventions.

Table of Contents

Chapter 1. Introduction 1
   Purpose 1
   Definitions 1
      Healthy Diet 1
      Physical Activity 1
      Cardiovascular Risk Factors 2
   Prevalence and Burden of Preventable Illness 2
   Dietary and Physical Activity Behaviors in the United States 3
   Current Clinical Practice in the United States 4
   Previous USPSTF Recommendations 4

Chapter 2. Methods 6
   Scope and Purpose 6
   Analytic Framework and Key Questions 6
   Data Sources and Searches 6
   Study Selection 7
   Data Extraction and Quality Assessment 9
   Data Synthesis and Analysis 9
   Expert Review and Public Comment 11
   USPSTF Involvement 11

Chapter 3. Results 12
   Description of Included Studies 12
      Included Populations 12
      Included Interventions 13
      Quality 14
   KQ 1. Do Primary Care–Relevant Behavioral Counseling Interventions for Healthy Diet and/or Physical Activity Improve CVD-Related Health Outcomes in Adults With Known CVD Risk Factors? 14
      Overall Results 14
      Detailed Results for CVD Events and/or Mortality 15
      Detailed Results for Self-Reported Patient Health Outcomes 16
   KQ 2. Do Primary Care–Relevant Behavioral Counseling Interventions for Healthy Diet and/or Physical Activity Improve CVD-Related Intermediate Outcomes in Adults With Known CVD Risk Factors? 17
      Overall Results 17
      Results in Persons With Dyslipidemia 18
      Results in Persons With Hypertension 20
      Results in Persons With Impaired Fasting Glucose or Glucose Tolerance 22
      Results in Persons With Mixed Cardiovascular Risk Factors. 23
      Results by Intervention Type 24
      Exploration of Heterogeneity 25
      Publication Bias 27

KQ 3. Do Primary Care–Relevant Behavioral Counseling Interventions for Healthy Diet and/or Physical Activity Improve Diet and Physical Activity Behavioral Outcomes in Adults With Known CVD Risk Factors? 27
    Overall Results 28
    Detailed Results for Behavioral Outcomes 28
KQ 4. What Are the Adverse Effects of Healthy Diet and/or Physical Activity Behavioral Counseling Interventions in Adults With Known CVD Risk Factors? 31
    Overall Results 31
    Detailed Results for Harms 31

Chapter 4. Discussion 33
Summary of Evidence 33
Clinical Interpretation of Benefit and Harms Given Paucity of Direct Health Outcome Data. 34
    Effects on Lipids and Blood Pressure 34
    Effects on Glucose and Diabetes Incidence 34
    Effects on Weight Outcomes 35
    Effects on Increases in Self-Reported Physical Activity 35
    Adverse Effects 36
Considerations for Applicability of Findings 36
    Population Considerations 36
    Intervention Considerations 37
Review Limitations 38
Study Limitations and Future Research Needs 40
Conclusions 41

References 43

Figures
Figure 1. Analytic Framework: Behavioral Counseling to Promote a Healthy Lifestyle for Cardiovascular Disease Prevention in Persons With Cardiovascular Risk Factors
Figure 2. Pooled Analysis of Total Cholesterol in Persons With Dyslipidemia, Sorted by Length of Followup Time
Figure 3. Pooled Analysis of Low-Density Lipoprotein Cholesterol in Persons With Dyslipidemia, Sorted by Length of Followup Time
Figure 4. Pooled Analysis of Total Cholesterol in Persons With Dyslipidemia or Multiple Risk Factors, Sorted by Length of Followup Time
Figure 5. Pooled Analysis of Low-Density Lipoprotein Cholesterol in Persons With Dyslipidemia or Multiple Risk Factors, Sorted by Length of Followup Time
Figure 6. Pooled Analysis of Weight in Persons With Dyslipidemia or Multiple Risk Factors, Sorted by Length of Followup Time
Figure 7. Pooled Analysis of Systolic Blood Pressure in Persons With Hypertension, Sorted by Length of Followup Time
Figure 8. Pooled Analysis of Diastolic Blood Pressure in Persons With Hypertension, Sorted by Length of Followup Time
Figure 9. Pooled Analysis of Systolic Blood Pressure in Persons With Hypertension or Multiple Risk Factors, Sorted by Length of Followup Time
Figure 10. Pooled Analysis of Diastolic Blood Pressure in Persons With Hypertension or Multiple Risk Factors, Sorted by Length of Followup Time

Figure 11. Pooled Analysis of Weight in Persons With Hypertension or Multiple Risk Factors, Sorted by Length of Followup Time
Figure 12. Pooled Analysis of Diabetes Incidence in Persons With Impaired Fasting Glucose or Impaired Glucose Tolerance, Sorted by Length of Followup Time
Figure 13. Pooled Analysis of Diabetes Incidence in Persons With Impaired Fasting Glucose, Impaired Glucose Tolerance, or Multiple Risk Factors, Sorted by Length of Followup Time
Figure 14. Pooled Analysis of Fasting Glucose in Persons With Impaired Fasting Glucose or Impaired Glucose Tolerance, Sorted by Length of Followup Time
Figure 15. Pooled Analysis of Weight in Persons With Impaired Fasting Glucose, Impaired Glucose Tolerance, or Multiple Risk Factors, Sorted by Length of Followup Time
Figure 16. Pooled Analysis of Total Cholesterol for Combined Healthy Diet and Physical Activity Interventions in All Risk Groups, Sorted by Length of Followup Time
Figure 17. Pooled Analysis of Low-Density Lipoprotein Cholesterol for Combined Healthy Diet and Physical Activity Interventions in All Risk Groups, Sorted by Length of Followup Time
Figure 18. Pooled Analysis of Systolic Blood Pressure for Combined Healthy Diet and Physical Activity Interventions in All Risk Groups, Sorted by Length of Followup Time
Figure 19. Pooled Analysis of Diastolic Blood Pressure for Combined Healthy Diet and Physical Activity Interventions in All Risk Groups, Sorted by Length of Followup Time
Figure 20. Pooled Analysis of Fasting Glucose for Combined Healthy Diet and Physical Activity Interventions in All Risk Groups, Sorted by Length of Followup Time
Figure 21. Pooled Analysis of Diabetes Incidence for Combined Healthy Diet and Physical Activity Interventions in All Risk Groups, Sorted by Length of Followup Time

Tables
Table 1. Included Studies by Population and Key Question
Table 2. Included Studies by Intervention Focus and Key Question
Table 3. Behavioral Counseling Trials in Persons With Dyslipidemia or Elevated Cholesterol: Study and Population Characteristics
Table 4. Behavioral Counseling Trials in Persons With Hypertension: Study and Population Characteristics
Table 5. Behavioral Counseling Trials in Persons With Impaired Fasting Glucose or Impaired Glucose Tolerance: Study and Population Characteristics
Table 6. Behavioral Counseling Trials in Persons With Mixed Cardiovascular Risk Factors: Study and Population Characteristics
Table 7. Behavioral Counseling Trials in Persons With Dyslipidemia or Elevated Cholesterol: Intervention Characteristics
Table 8. Behavioral Counseling Trials in Persons With Hypertension: Intervention Characteristics
Table 9. Behavioral Counseling Trials in Persons With Impaired Fasting Glucose or Impaired Glucose Tolerance: Intervention Characteristics
Table 10. Behavioral Counseling Trials in Persons With Mixed Cardiovascular Risk Factors: Intervention Characteristics
Table 11. Behavioral Counseling Trials: Key Question 1 Outcomes
Table 12. Behavioral Counseling Trials in Persons With Dyslipidemia or Elevated Cholesterol: Key Question 2 Outcomes

Table 13. Behavioral Counseling Trials in Persons With Hypertension: Key Question 2 Outcomes
Table 14. Behavioral Counseling Trials in Persons With Impaired Fasting Glucose or Impaired Glucose Tolerance: Key Question 2 Outcomes
Table 15. Behavioral Counseling Trials in Persons With Mixed Cardiovascular Risk Factors: Key Question 2 Outcomes
Table 16. Pooled Effect Sizes for Intermediate Outcomes in Persons With Dyslipidemia
Table 17. Pooled Effect Sizes for Intermediate Outcomes in Persons With Hypertension
Table 18. Pooled Effect Sizes for Intermediate Outcomes in Persons With Impaired Fasting Glucose or Impaired Glucose Tolerance
Table 19. Pooled Effect Sizes for Intermediate Outcomes in Persons in All Risk Groups
Table 20. Pooled Effect Sizes for Intermediate Outcomes by Intervention Type
Table 21. Behavioral Counseling Trials in Persons With Dyslipidemia or Elevated Cholesterol: Key Question 3 Outcomes
Table 22. Behavioral Counseling Trials in Persons With Hypertension: Key Question 3 Outcomes
Table 23. Behavioral Counseling Trials in Persons With Impaired Fasting Glucose or Impaired Glucose Tolerance: Key Question 3 Outcomes
Table 24. Behavioral Counseling Trials in Persons With Mixed Cardiovascular Risk Factors: Key Question 3 Outcomes
Table 25. Overall Summary of Evidence by Key Question

Appendixes
Appendix A. Detailed Methods
Appendix B. Ongoing Studies
Appendix C. Excluded Studies
Appendix D. Detailed Results of Intermediate Outcomes
Appendix E. Intervention Descriptions of Included Studies
Appendix F. Additional Meta-Analysis Figures
Appendix G. Detailed Results of Final Health Outcomes and Behavioral Outcomes

Chapter 1. Introduction

Purpose

The U.S. Preventive Services Task Force (USPSTF) will use this report to update its 2002 and 2003 recommendations on primary care–relevant behavioral counseling to promote a healthy diet and physical activity in adults with traditional risk factors for cardiovascular disease (CVD).

Definitions

Healthy Diet

A healthy diet promotes health and reduces an individual's risk for chronic disease through nutritious eating patterns. For the purposes of this review, we will include any dietary counseling interventions that promote a balanced diet (e.g., appropriate energy content); balance of fats (e.g., consumption of mono and poly unsaturated fats, omega-3 fats, avoidance of excess saturated fat, avoidance of trans fat); increased consumption of fruits and vegetables; increased consumption of legumes; increased consumption of lean proteins; increased consumption of nonfat or low-fat dairy; balance of carbohydrates (e.g., consumption of whole grain and fiber; avoidance of excess refined carbohydrates, including excess sweetened beverages); and avoidance of excess sodium. This guidance is generally consistent with dietary recommendations of a number of groups, including the Institute of Medicine, the World Health Organization, the U.S. Department of Health and Human Services (DHHS), the U.S. Department of Agriculture, the Academy of Nutrition and Dietetics (previously the American Dietetic Association), the Centers for Disease Control and Prevention (CDC), the American Heart Association (AHA) and American College of Cardiology (ACC), the American Cancer Society, and the American Diabetes Association. We did not review dietary counseling interventions that only focused on micronutrient intake, vitamin and/or antioxidant supplementation, or alcohol moderation.

Physical Activity

Although no internationally accepted definition of physical activity exists, American researchers have defined physical activity as "bodily movement produced by the contraction of skeletal muscle that increases energy expenditure above the basal level."[1] DHHS and other organizations[2-4] recommend that adults age 18 years and older should engage in at least 150 minutes of moderate-intensity or 75 minutes of vigorous-intensity aerobic physical activity per week, in addition to engaging in strengthening activities at least twice per week. Based on these definitions, this review focused on counseling interventions promoting aerobic- or strength-related physical activity. We did not review counseling that focused primarily on flexibility or balance.

Cardiovascular Risk Factors

Risk factors for CVD are well established and include both modifiable and nonmodifiable components. Modifiable risk factors include: dyslipidemia or hyperlipidemia (referred to as dyslipidemia in this report), hypertension, diabetes, overweight and obesity, smoking, lack of physical activity, and unhealthy diet.[5-7] Nonmodifiable risk factors include: age, sex, and family history.[5,6]

This review focuses on patients who are at high risk for CVD, which we defined as having one or more of the following risk factors: dyslipidemia, hypertension, impaired fasting glucose/impaired glucose tolerance, and/or metabolic syndrome. Metabolic syndrome is a clustering of metabolic risk factors that include abdominal obesity, dyslipidemia, increased blood pressure, insulin resistance, or glucose intolerance. While diabetes is a strong risk factor for CVD,[8,9] we considered existing diabetes to be a CVD risk equivalent. As such, we did not review studies primarily aimed at patients with diabetes or pre-existing coronary heart disease, cerebrovascular disease, peripheral artery disease, or severe chronic kidney disease.

Prevalence and Burden of Preventable Illness

Diseases associated with modifiable risk factors are the leading causes of illness and death in the United States.[10] CVD is the leading cause of death in the United States and nearly a quarter of CVD deaths are considered avoidable.[11,12] Declines in cardiovascular mortality in recent decades have been attributed to improvements in modifiable risk factors, including reductions in blood pressure, cholesterol, and physical inactivity.[13]

A substantial portion of the U.S. population has at least one modifiable risk factor for CVD. In 2009–2010, for example, the overall age-adjusted prevalence of hypertension among U.S. adults was approximately 29 percent.[14] During this same time period, an estimated 13 percent of adults had high total cholesterol and 21 percent had low high-density lipoprotein (HDL) cholesterol.[15] In 2007–2010, the overall prevalence of high low-density lipoprotein (LDL) cholesterol was 27 percent in the United States.[16] National Health and Nutrition Examination Survey (NHANES) data from 2005–2006 indicate that about 30 percent of U.S. adults have impaired fasting glucose or impaired glucose tolerance.[17] Likewise, 2003–2006 NHANES data show a 34 percent prevalence of metabolic syndrome.[18] In 2011, 19 percent of U.S. adults smoked cigarettes.[19] While the prevalence of hypertension and dyslipidemia has declined in the United States, these conditions are still very common, and adequate control of these risk factors remains suboptimal.[14,20,21]

Cardiovascular risk factors and CVD burden is not equally distributed across the U.S. population. Certain groups experience a higher prevalence of risk factors and rates of avoidable death from CVD, including older adults, men, persons with low income, and some racial/ethnic groups.[12,14,15,17,22] Selected examples of the large variation in the distribution of risk factors include: the prevalence of hypertension is approximately 67 percent in adults age 60 years and older and just 7 percent in younger adults ages 18 to 39 years,[14] and the prevalence of hypertension is 40 percent in blacks compared with 26 percent in Hispanics and 27 percent in nonHispanic whites.[14] Similarly, poor Americans are nearly twice as likely to smoke as the nonpoor (28% vs. 16%).[19] Finally, the avoidable death rate for CVD among blacks is almost twice that of whites.[12]

Dietary and Physical Activity Behaviors in the United States

Observational research consistently shows that a healthy diet and physical activity are associated with benefits in important health outcomes, including reductions in cardiovascular events and all-cause mortality.[23-31] Despite this convincing evidence, however, U.S. adults do not comply with healthy diet and physical activity recommendations.[32,33] According to NHANES data from 2005–2006, greater than 30 percent of men and 32 percent of women do not engage in any leisure time physical activity. Previous years of NHANES data reveal that rates of physical activity did not significantly improve from 1999 to 2006 for men or women.[34] Similarly, greater than 81 percent of men and 70 percent of women eat a poor diet, which is defined by inadequate consumption of fruits/vegetables, fish, and whole grains and excess intake of sodium and sweets/sugar-sweetened beverages.[34] Adherence to an ideal diet has improved only minimally from 1999 to 2008 (0.3% to 0.6% for men and 0.9% to 1.4% for women).[34] Some research shows that high-risk adults are even less likely to adhere to healthy lifestyle behaviors than their lower-risk counterparts. An analysis of NHANES data from 2001 to 2006 found that adults with hypertension or dyslipidemia were less likely to adhere to five healthy lifestyle habits (including consuming five or more fruits/vegetables per day, regular exercise, maintaining a healthy weight, moderate alcohol consumption, and not smoking) than adults with no CVD or its risk factors (5% and 8%, respectively, vs. 11%).[35] Secondary analysis of 1999–2004 NHANES data for adults with hypertension found that 20 percent of individuals adhered to DASH (Dietary Approaches to Stop Hypertension) dietary recommendations, which emphasize fruits, vegetables, whole grains, and low-fat dairy consumption while limiting sugar-sweetened foods and beverages, reducing red meat consumption, and avoiding added fats.[36]

There is also a marked disparity in healthy diet and physical activity behaviors by important subpopulations. Persons of lower socioeconomic status or those with lower educational attainment tend to exercise less, eat fewer fruits and vegetables, and eat fewer foods rich in dietary fiber compared with those in a higher socioeconomic position or with higher educational attainment.[37-39] Nonwhites tend to exercise less than whites,[39,40] and blacks consume fewer servings of fruits and vegetables than whites.[37,41,42] Physical activity rates are lower in older persons and women than in younger persons and men.[39,43] Major barriers to healthy eating include: low income, food marketing, lack of accessible and accurate information on what constitutes a healthy diet, poor accessibility to affordable healthy foods, lack of opportunity to experiment and to develop cooking skills (e.g., poor literacy, reduced access to well-equipped kitchens, homelessness, poor educational attainment), and sociocultural factors (e.g., family or cultural food norms, family resistance, lack of support, and child care demands can all inhibit dietary change). Major barriers to physical activity in adults include: high costs of exercise facilities, exercise equipment, and sports teams; poor access to facilities; and unsafe or unsupportive environments.[39,44] Psychosocial barriers to physical activity include: anxiety about unfamiliar settings for exercise, poor body image, lack of social support for exercise, low self-efficacy for maintaining an exercise program, and lack of belief in the benefits of exercise.[39]

Current Clinical Practice in the United States

Consistent with the 2002 USPSTF recommendation, the American Academy of Family Physicians recommends that primary care physicians or other qualified professionals provide intensive behavioral dietary counseling for adults with dyslipidemia and other known risk factors for cardiovascular and diet-related chronic disease.[45] The American College of Physicians has endorsed the USPSTF recommendation and other organizations, including the AHA and Academy of Nutrition and Dietetics, have produced similar guidance.[46-49]

Although patients perceive family doctors as one of the most reliable sources of information on food and nutrition,[50] dietary counseling practices of primary care clinicians fall short of recommendations, even for patients at high risk for CVD. A 2002 survey showed that among adults with hypertension, just 21 percent reported being advised by a physician or other health professional to start a diet or change their eating habits and 22 percent reported receiving advice to reduce their sodium intake.[51] A direct observation study of family medicine visits found that although diet was discussed in 31 percent of visits, offers of assistance and followup were infrequent (17% and 10% of visits, respectively).[52]

Despite improvements in physician advice to encourage physical activity over the past decade, the prevalence of physical activity counseling remains low. The 2010 National Health Interview Survey, for example, showed that approximately 44 percent of adults with hypertension reported that their physician recommended they exercise (up from 34% in 2000).[53] This survey found a higher proportion of physical activity advice among adults with chronic conditions, including CVD and diabetes, compared with the overall population (32%). A recent systematic review of providers' attitudes toward physical activity counseling found that most primary care providers agree that such counseling is important and that they have a role in promoting physical activity to their patients.[54] Barriers to physical activity counseling cited by providers, however, are substantial and include: lack of time, lack of knowledge or training about physical activity counseling, and lack of success with changing patient behavior.[54]

Previous USPSTF Recommendations

In 2012, the USPSTF updated the recommendation for adults without pre-existing CVD or its risk factors, concluding that the average benefit of behavioral counseling interventions in primary care to promote a healthy diet and/or physical activity for CVD prevention is small, and that clinicians may consider selectively providing or referring individual patients for medium- or high-intensity behavioral counseling interventions (C recommendation).

The 2012 recommendation did not address counseling in persons with known traditional CVD risk factors. In 2002, the USPSTF issued separate recommendations for healthy diet and physical activity counseling, both of which included persons with cardiovascular risk factors (as well as unselected persons). In 2002, the USPSTF recommended intensive behavioral dietary counseling for adult patients with hyperlipidemia and other known risk factors for cardiovascular and diet-related chronic disease (B recommendation). It concluded, however, that the evidence was insufficient to recommend for or against behavioral counseling in primary care settings to promote physical activity (I statement).

In 2012, the USPSTF issued a related recommendation on screening for and management of adult obesity. It recommended screening all adults for obesity, and that clinicians should offer or refer obese patients to intensive, multicomponent behavioral interventions (B recommendation).

As a result, we conducted this systematic review to support the USPSTF in updating its 2002 recommendations on primary care–relevant behavioral counseling to promote a healthy diet and physical activity in patients with known CVD risk factors. This review was designed to complement the existing systematic reviews that supported the 2012 USPSTF recommendations and, therefore, does not include healthy lifestyle interventions aimed at persons without CVD risk factors or interventions primarily aimed at weight loss or weight management.

Chapter 2. Methods

Scope and Purpose

This systematic review was designed to complement the systematic review supporting the 2012 USPSTF recommendation that focused on healthy lifestyle counseling for individuals without pre-existing CVD or its risk factors.[55] For this review, we adapted our previous analytic framework and key questions to address the benefits and harms of primary care–relevant counseling interventions to improve diet and physical activity in adults with known cardiovascular risk factors (e.g., hypertension, dyslipidemia, impaired fasting glucose or glucose tolerance, metabolic syndrome), but without pre-existing CVD.

Analytic Framework and Key Questions

Using the USPSTF's methods (detailed in **Appendix A**),[56] we developed an analytic framework (**Figure 1**) and four key questions (KQs):

1. Do primary care–relevant behavioral counseling interventions for healthy diet and/or physical activity improve CVD health outcomes (e.g., prevent morbidity and mortality) in adults with known CVD risk factors (e.g., hypertension, dyslipidemia, impaired fasting glucose, metabolic syndrome)?
    a. Are there population or intervention characteristics that influence the effectiveness of the interventions?
2. Do primary care–relevant behavioral counseling interventions for physical activity and/or healthy diet improve intermediate outcomes associated with CVD (e.g., blood pressure, lipids, glucose, weight) in adults with known CVD risk factors (e.g., hypertension, dyslipidemia, impaired fasting glucose, metabolic syndrome)?
    a. Are there population or intervention characteristics that influence the effectiveness of the interventions?
3. Do primary care–relevant behavioral counseling interventions for physical activity and/or healthy diet change associated health behaviors in adults with known CVD risk factors (e.g., hypertension, dyslipidemia, impaired fasting glucose, metabolic syndrome)?
    a. Are there population or intervention characteristics that influence the effectiveness of the interventions?
4. What are the adverse effects of primary care–relevant behavioral counseling interventions for physical activity and/or healthy diet in adults with known CVD risk factors (e.g., hypertension, dyslipidemia, impaired fasting glucose, metabolic syndrome)?

Data Sources and Searches

We designed this review to serve as an extension of our prior systematic review that was completed in 2009.[55] As such, we examined all included and excluded studies from that systematic review, paying particular attention to excluded studies in persons with CVD risk factors. The literature search for this systematic review includes searches from MEDLINE, PubMed, PsycInfo, the Database of Abstracts of Reviews of Effects, and the Cochrane Central Register of Controlled Trials from January 2001 through October 2013. We also searched for recent relevant existing systematic reviews on healthy lifestyle counseling in persons with CVD risk factors from January 2008 through January 2013 in MEDLINE, the Cochrane Database of Systematic Reviews, and the Database of Abstracts of Reviews of Effects, and publications from the Institute of Medicine, the Agency for Healthcare Research and Quality (AHRQ), and the National Institute of Health and Clinical Excellence. We worked with a medical librarian to develop our search strategy (**Appendix A Table 1**) and all searches were limited to articles published in the English language. We managed the literature search results using version 12.0 of Reference Manager® (Thomson Reuters, New York, NY), a bibliographic management software database.

To ensure the comprehensiveness of our search strategy, we reviewed the reference lists of included studies and relevant systematic reviews and meta-analyses to identify relevant articles that were published before the timeframe of or not identified in our literature searches. We also supplemented our database searches with suggestions from experts and searched Clinicaltrials.gov to identify relevant ongoing trials (**Appendix B**).

Study Selection

Two investigators independently reviewed the titles and abstracts of 7,218 identified articles to determine if the study met the inclusion and exclusion criteria for design, population, intervention, and outcomes (**Appendix A Figure 1**). Two reviewers then independently evaluated 553 full-text articles of potentially included studies against the complete inclusion and exclusion criteria (**Appendix A Table 1**). We resolved disagreements by discussion and consultation with a third reviewer, if necessary. Excluded studies and reasons for their exclusion are listed in **Appendix C**.

We developed an a priori set of inclusion and exclusion criteria (**Appendix A Table 1**). We included studies in adults who had at least one cardiovascular risk factor, including hypertension, dyslipidemia, impaired fasting glucose or glucose tolerance, and metabolic syndrome. We excluded trials in persons with known CVD (i.e., coronary artery disease [CAD], cerebrovascular disease, peripheral artery disease), severe chronic kidney disease, and diabetes. While diabetes is a strong risk factor for CVD,[8,9] we considered existing diabetes to be a CVD risk equivalent. As such, we excluded trials evaluating lifestyle counseling interventions for the management of diabetes. While many included trials targeted persons with a combination of risk factors, including smoking and obesity, we did not find any diet and/or exercise counseling trials that selected persons exclusively based on smoking history. We excluded populations in which obesity was the only CVD risk factor, as these trials recruited persons exclusively for obesity with a primary aim of weight loss or weight management. These trials were excluded because this evidence base is covered by a separate systematic review conducted for the USPSTF;[57] the USPSTF issued a separate recommendation statement in 2012 for the management of obesity in adults.[58] We also excluded populations with increased risk for CVD (e.g., due to physical inactivity, prehypertension), but without traditional CVD risk factors. Again, these trials were covered by a separate systematic review[55] and are addressed in the 2012 USPSTF recommendation on healthy lifestyle behavioral counseling.[59]

We included behaviorally-based counseling interventions to promote a healthy diet, physical activity, or both. Counseling interventions could be delivered alone or as part of a multicomponent intervention. Interventions had to be either conducted in primary care or judged to be feasible for delivery or referral from primary care. Therefore, we excluded interventions delivered through nonreferable community settings (e.g., work sites, churches). We included physical activity interventions that incorporated activities such as walking, cycling, swimming, or resistance training. We included healthy diet interventions aiming to change dietary behavior or improve or maintain cardiovascular health through a balanced diet (e.g., appropriate calorie intake; increased fruits and vegetables, whole grains, and fiber; balanced fats intake; and decreased sodium). We excluded interventions that were primarily aimed at evaluating if behavior change (i.e., improved diet or increased physical activity) resulted in physiologic or health benefits, as opposed to including interventions aimed at evaluating if counseling could change behavior. Therefore, we generally excluded interventions that focused on providing controlled diets or supervised physical activity. However, we included counseling interventions if they provided limited samples of foods or access to (optional) guided physical activity. We excluded counseling interventions primarily aimed at weight loss, falls or fracture prevention, or cognitive functioning, rather than CVD prevention.

Given the maturity and volume of literature, we focused on the most rigorous and most applicable evidence. Therefore, we limited studies of efficacy or effectiveness to fair- to good-quality randomized, controlled trials or controlled clinical trials that were conducted in developed countries and whose results were published in 1990 or later. Included trials had to compare an active intervention with usual care, a minimal intervention, or an attention control group. Because usual care for persons with known cardiovascular risk factors includes lifestyle counseling, we allowed included trials to use comparator groups that received nontailored printed materials, a single annual session (limited to 45 to 60 minutes), or two to three brief sessions annually (limited to 15 minutes each). We required that included trials have a followup duration of 6 months or greater. We examined health outcomes, including morbidity or mortality related to CVD. Intermediate health outcomes, or physiologic outcomes, included blood pressure, total cholesterol, LDL cholesterol, HDL cholesterol, fasting serum glucose, glucose tolerance, hemoglobin A1c, weight, and body mass index (BMI). Consistent with current USPSTF methods, true health outcomes (KQ 1) are those that are experienced by the patient. Therefore, we considered disease incidence (e.g., diabetes) and changes in CVD risk score as intermediate outcomes (KQ 2), as opposed to health outcomes (KQ 1), for this review. We accepted a number of behavioral outcomes, including self-reported dietary intake, self-reported physical activity, or objectively measured markers of behavior change, such as VO_2max and urinary sodium. We also included observational studies that reported serious harms (i.e., adverse events resulting in unexpected or unwanted medical attention), but did not include case series or case reports.

Data Extraction and Quality Assessment

One reviewer extracted data from all included studies rated as fair or good quality into a standard evidence table. A second reviewer checked the data for accuracy. The reviewers abstracted population characteristics (e.g., details about baseline demographics and baseline CVD risk), study design elements (e.g., recruitment procedures, inclusion/exclusion criteria, duration of followup and attrition), intervention and control characteristics (e.g., content, format, setting, number and length of sessions, duration, provider), any behavioral outcomes related to healthy diet and physical activity, and intermediate health outcomes (e.g., blood pressure, lipids, glucose tolerance, measures of weight, medication use, diabetes incidence, composite CVD risk), as well as patient health outcomes (e.g., mortality, CVD events, quality of life [QOL]) and harms (**Appendix D Tables 1–9; Appendix E Table 1**).

Two reviewers independently appraised all articles that met inclusion criteria using the USPSTF's design-specific quality criteria,[60] which we supplemented with the National Institute for Health and Clinical Excellence methodology checklists (**Appendix A Table 2**).[61] We rated articles as good, fair, or poor quality. In general, a good-quality study met all criteria well. A fair-quality study did not meet, or it was unclear if it met, at least one criterion, but also had no known important limitation that could invalidate its results. A poor-quality study had important limitations, or a fatal flaw, that would invalidate results. We excluded poor-quality studies from this review. Poor-quality studies had important limitations, including one or more of the following risks for bias: very high attrition (>40%), with or without differential attrition between intervention arms; lack of randomization, with biased assignment of participants to intervention arms, often with differences in or no reporting of baseline characteristics, per protocol analyses only; and poor description of methods that did not allow for adequate quality assessment.

Data Synthesis and Analysis

Because of the clinical heterogeneity across this body of evidence, we separately analyzed identified evidence according to how populations were targeted or defined (i.e., dyslipidemia, hypertension, impaired fasting glucose or glucose tolerance, or mixed risk factors), as well as according to type of intervention evaluated (i.e., focus on dietary counseling alone, physical activity alone, or both diet and physical activity counseling). We used summary tables to describe key characteristics of trials capturing the major sources of heterogeneity among included trials and results for the multiple outcomes reported for each trial.

We conducted random-effects meta-analyses using the DerSimonian and Laird method to estimate the effect size of counseling on intermediate health outcomes (KQ 2) (i.e., weight or BMI; systolic and diastolic blood pressure; total, HDL, or LDL cholesterol; triglycerides; fasting blood glucose; and diabetes incidence).[62] Other measures of adiposity (i.e., waist circumference) and glucose (i.e., hemoglobin A1c, 1- or 2-hour glucose tolerance) were not as commonly reported. We conducted qualitative synthesis of health outcomes (KQ 1) and harms (KQ 4) given the sparse reporting of these outcomes. We also conducted qualitative syntheses of behavioral outcomes (KQ 3) (e.g., self-reported physical activity; objectively measured fitness; intake of total energy, fat, saturated fat, fiber, fruits and vegetables; and urinary sodium as a measure of sodium intake) because of the wide variation in reporting of these outcome measures across included trials. Outcome analyses were also stratified by length of followup after randomization. Short-term followup included outcome measurements from 6 to less than 12 months. Intermediate-term followup included outcome measurements from 12 to 24 months. Long-term followup included outcome measurements after 24 months. Because the interventions were quite variable in their duration, the length of followup does not reflect duration of effect postintervention. We also used intervention intensity as a key characteristic of heterogeneity. Low-intensity interventions were estimated to include 30 minutes or less of contact with providers. These trials generally included only a single contact, two very brief contacts, or mail-only interventions. Medium-intensity interventions were estimated to involve greater than 30 minutes, but less than 6 hours, of contact with providers (e.g., 1-hour group meeting monthly for up to 6 months). High-intensity interventions were estimated to involve greater than 6 hours of contact. Because many articles did not report detailed information about the duration of contact, these categorizations often involved some reviewer judgment. As such, at least one other team member reviewed the studies' categorizations, and we resolved discrepancies through discussion.

For all intermediate health outcomes, we pooled the difference in change from baseline to followup between groups. We converted all outcomes to a common metric (e.g., mg/dL, mm Hg, lb) using standard conversion factors.[63] We calculated the pooled weighted mean difference separately for short-, intermediate-, and long-term followup. For weight outcomes, we estimated a standardized mean difference because measures could be either weight (lb) or BMI (kg/m^2). If there were multiple intervention arms, we selected the most intensive or comprehensive arm to include in the meta-analysis. If the active intervention arms were of similar intensity and comprehensiveness, we calculated combined means and standard deviations using standard formulas. We adjusted results for cluster-randomized trials, but did not report adjusting for the clustering effect.

We assessed the presence of statistical heterogeneity among the studies using standard chi-squared tests and the magnitude of heterogeneity was estimated using the I^2 statistic.[64] In instances of 10 or more studies, we formally assessed for publication bias, whether the distribution of the effect sizes was symmetric with respect to the precision measure, using funnel plots and Egger's linear regression method.[65,66]

We used stratified analyses and visual inspection of forest plots arranged by effect size and/or meta-regressions (combining all studies included for KQ 2) to examine the effect of a priori–specified primary sources of heterogeneity on effect size: study population, intervention type, intervention intensity (including number of contacts and duration of intervention), length of followup, overall methodologic quality of study, year of publication, country setting (United States vs. other), type of control group, and population risk (including average age, percent smokers, percent with hypertension, percent with dyslipidemia, percent with diabetes, average systolic blood pressure [SBP], average LDL cholesterol, average BMI, medication use). For each of the intermediate health outcomes, we also used meta-regressions to examine whether population, intervention focus, intervention intensity (high vs. not high), publication year, study quality (rated on a 4-point scale), and mean age of the study sample were associated with effect size. We conducted two sets of models when examining intervention by intensity, year, study quality, and age—one controlling for population (using the multiple risk factors population as the reference group) and one controlling for intervention focus (using the combined healthy diet plus physical activity interventions as the reference group). We performed all analyses using Stata 11.2 (StataCorp, College Station, TX).

Expert Review and Public Comment

A draft research plan was available for public comment from January 29 to February 25, 2013 that included the analytic framework, KQs, and inclusion criteria. We made no substantive changes to our review methods based on comments received. A draft version of this report was reviewed by six invited content experts as well as federal partners from the CDC, Centers for Medicare & Medicaid Services, National Institutes of Health, U.S. Department of Veterans Affairs (VA), and the Military Health Service. Comments received during this process were presented to the USPSTF during its deliberation of the evidence and subsequently addressed, as appropriate, in this final version of the report. Additionally, a full draft report was posted for public comment on the USPSTF's Web site from May 13 to June 9, 2014. We received comments from five unique individuals or organizations. All comments were reviewed and considered. No new substantive issues were brought up during the public comment periods that were not previously considered. No major changes were made to the text in the final report. Minor editorial suggestions/corrections were addressed as appropriate.

USPSTF Involvement

The authors worked with three USPSTF liaisons at key points throughout the review process to refine the inclusion criteria, address methodological decisions on applicable evidence, and resolve issues around the scope of the final evidence synthesis. AHRQ funded this research under a contract to support the work of the USPSTF. AHRQ staff provided oversight for the project and assisted in external review of the draft evidence synthesis.

Chapter 3. Results

Description of Included Studies

We included 74 fair- to good-quality healthy lifestyle counseling trials in persons with cardiovascular risk factors that met our inclusion criteria (**Tables 1** and **2**). Of these 74 included trials, only 16 trials reported health outcomes (KQ 1) (e.g., CVD events, self-reported QOL), 71 trials reported intermediate health outcomes (KQ 2) (e.g., lipid measures, blood pressure, glucose, diabetes incidence, weight measures), 61 trials reported behavioral outcomes (KQ 3) (e.g., objective or self-reported measures of change in diet or physical activity), and 10 trials explicitly reported on harms (or lack thereof) of counseling interventions (KQ 4). We did not identify any additional studies that addressed harms of counseling interventions other than the trials included for KQs 1–3.

Included Populations

We included 17 trials conducted exclusively in persons with dyslipidemia or that included an intervention aim that was primarily focused on reducing cholesterol (**Table 3**).[67-83] We included 15 trials conducted exclusively in persons with hypertension (**Table 4**).[67,69-87] We included 16 trials aimed at preventing diabetes in persons with impaired fasting glucose or glucose tolerance (**Table 5**).[88-103] We included 26 trials in persons selected for any one or a combination of CVD risk factors, most commonly including dyslipidemia, hypertension, elevated glucose (including diabetes), metabolic syndrome, obesity, and smoking (**Table 6**). Most trials ranged from 50 to 1,000 participants. Only one trial had fewer than 50 participants.[104] Seven trials had more than 1,000 participants, including Vitalum,[105] Diabetes Prevention Program (DPP),[89] Euroaction,[106] Inter99,[107] WISEWOMAN California,[108] Rural Health Promotion Project (RHPP), and the National Exercise Referral Scheme (NERS) trial.[109] The mean age in populations studied ranged from 40.5 to 71 years (interquartile range [IQR], 52.0 to 59.4 years). Nine trials specifically targeted older adults. The mean age in these trials ranged from 64.5 to 71 years. Both men and women were well represented in included trials, most of which included both sexes. Four trials included only women[82,104,108,110] and five trials included only men.[75,93,97,111,112] About one third (k=28) of included trials were conducted in the United States. The remaining trials were conducted in western Europe (k=33), Australia (k=6), Japan (k=3), Canada (k=2), and New Zealand (k=2). Of the trials conducted in the United States, 23 trials reported including nonwhite populations that ranged from 4 to 100 percent. More than one third of participants were nonwhite in 12 of the U.S.-based trials.

The proportion of participants with dyslipidemia at baseline ranged from 5.5 to 100 percent for included trials, where reported, with a range of baseline LDL cholesterol from 105.7 to 202.7 mg/dL. The proportion with hypertension ranged from 0 to 100 percent, with a range of SBP from 123 to 162 mm Hg. In trials including persons with impaired fasting glucose or glucose intolerance, fasting blood glucose at baseline ranged from 93.2 to 110.6 mg/dL. When reported, the proportion of smokers in included trials ranged from 0 to 100 percent. The average BMI in all but two trials[93,97] ranged from overweight to obese. The median BMI was 29.8 kg/m^2 (IQR,

28.4 to 31.2 kg/m^2). While we excluded trials conducted exclusively in persons with diabetes, many trials included some persons with diabetes, ranging from 3.6 to 45.4 percent.

Trials did not generally restrict or require the use of lipid-, blood pressure-, or glucose-lowering medications. In nine of the 17 trials conducted exclusively in persons with dyslipidemia, however, participants were not allowed to be taking lipid-lowering medications. Three of the 15 trials were conducted exclusively in persons with hypertension who were not allowed to be taking antihypertension medication, while five trials explicitly selected for persons taking them. None of the trials in persons with impaired fasting glucose or glucose tolerance included participants taking medications for glycemic control.

Included Interventions

The 74 trials included 49 diet and exercise counseling intervention arms, 18 diet-only intervention arms, and 10 physical activity intervention arms (**Table 2**). Of the interventions evaluated, only two were low-intensity, 48 were medium-intensity, and 37 were high-intensity interventions (**Tables 7–10**). Medium-intensity interventions had a median number of five contacts (IQR, 3 to 8 contacts), with a median duration of 9 months (IQR, 4 to 11 months). High-intensity interventions had a median number of 16 contacts (IQR, 9 to 31 contacts), with a median duration of 12 months (IQR, 8 to 18 months). The vast majority of interventions relied on face-to-face sessions, either in individual or group sessions (**Appendix E**). Although many interventions used adjunctive telephone contacts, five medium-intensity trials relied solely on telephone and mail contacts to deliver the behavioral counseling.[67,84,105,113,114] Given the intensity and expertise needed for these interventions, the counseling interventions evaluated are primarily referable from primary care, as opposed to delivered in primary care. Counseling interventions were delivered by dieticians or nutritionists, physiotherapists or exercise professionals/consultants, and/or trained interventionists (e.g., health educators, psychologists, nurses, case managers, life coaches).

Counseling interventions were aimed at promoting knowledge, motivation, and skills for healthy diet and/or increased physical activity (**Appendix E**). Individually-tailored healthy diet counseling included at least one, but most often a combination of messages, including: decreased portion sizes/calories; decreased fat, saturated fat, and cholesterol; decreased salt; increased fruits and vegetables; increased complex carbohydrates and/or fiber; decreased refined sugar; and alcohol in moderation. Individually-tailored physical activity counseling focused on increasing physical activity, some of which included optional supervised exercise sessions, pedometers, and diaries. Counseling interventions, regardless of focus on diet, physical activity, or combined lifestyle messages, included didactic education (i.e., with limited patient interaction) as well as individualized care plans, problem solving skills, and audit and feedback. A few interventions also included financial incentives (including low-cost exercise options) and family/spouse support. Although our review excluded interventions solely aimed at weight loss or weight management, many included trials involved weight loss or weight goals for participants who were overweight. Similarly, although our review excluded interventions solely aimed at smoking cessation, some counseling interventions included smoking cessation counseling when applicable. Some counseling interventions were paired with management algorithms to adjust medications (start, stop, change dosage). The vast majority of trials (k=47) used usual care as a comparator. Therefore, while we assume that persons in the control group received some sort of counseling, it was not well described in the majority of articles. Twelve trials used a wait-list control, in which participants in the control group likely did not receive active counseling during the trial period. Fourteen trials used minimal intervention as a control, and these trials included counseling that may not be provided as standard of care in most primary care settings (e.g., reminder email prompts to primary care clinicians, substantive nontailored written patient education materials, pedometers, brief annual counseling).

Quality

All trials were rated as fair to good quality. Thirteen trials were excluded for poor quality (**Appendix C**). We included 11 good-quality and 63 fair-quality trials. We rated one trial as good quality for health outcomes (KQ 1), but only fair quality for intermediate health outcomes (KQ 2) because of higher attrition for measurement of intermediate outcomes. In general, the limitations for these fair-quality studies included: lack of reporting of details about randomization; small differences in baseline characteristics between intervention arms; lack of blinding of outcomes assessment (for nonobjective measures); attrition greater than 20 percent, but less than 40 percent; differential attrition between study arms; evidence of attrition bias or lack of details to assess for attrition bias; and lack of reporting on how missing data were handled or having completers-only analyses. Fidelity of, and adherence to, the intervention was not commonly reported.

KQ 1. Do Primary Care–Relevant Behavioral Counseling Interventions for Healthy Diet and/or Physical Activity Improve CVD-Related Health Outcomes in Adults With Known CVD Risk Factors?

Overall Results

Only 16 included trials reported measures of patient health outcomes (**Table 11**). Five of these trials reported CVD events, including mortality.[89,115-118] Nine of these trials combined lifestyle interventions[85,86,92,94,95,110,119-121] and two of the physical activity–only trials[98,122] reported self-reported QOL or depression symptom outcomes. One additional physical activity counseling trial used QOL outcomes (the 36-Item Short-Form Health Survey [SF-36]), but only reported results for selected domains (subscores).[123] Overall, there was no reduction in CVD events or mortality at 6 to 79 months across four of five trials reporting these outcomes. Event rates, however, were generally low. One good-quality trial, the Finnish Diabetes Prevention Study, found no difference in CVD events or mortality at the 10-year observational followup from the original trial.[124] One early good-quality trial, the Risk Factor Intervention Study, was a high-intensity behavioral counseling intervention in conjunction with a protocol to start medication for dyslipidemia or elevated glucose or nicotine replacement therapy for tobacco smoking among Swedish men. This intervention reduced a composite measure of all CVD events compared with usual care at 6.6. years (relative risk [RR], 0.71 [95% CI, 0.51 to 0.99]).[112] Overall, combined lifestyle interventions do not appear to improve self-reported depression symptoms (k=4) in persons with impaired fasting glucose or glucose tolerance at 6 to 12 months.[85,92,94,95] Findings of benefit on self-reported QOL measures were mixed. While three combined lifestyle counseling interventions appeared to improve selected measures of QOL,[86,110,119] two combined lifestyle counseling interventions[120,121] and two physical activity–only counseling interventions[98,122] showed no benefit on self-reported QOL at 6 to 12 months.

Sparse reporting of both CVD events and self-reported measures of depression symptoms or QOL do not allow for definitive conclusions as to whether or not behavioral counseling interventions can improve patient health outcomes. We did not consider diabetes incidence or changes in CVD risk score as health outcomes. We discuss these outcomes with intermediate health outcomes in KQ 2.

Detailed Results for CVD Events and/or Mortality

Four good-quality trials (n=3,962) of high-intensity combined lifestyle behavioral counseling interventions did not reduce CVD outcomes or mortality (**Table 11**; **Appendix G Table 1**).[89,116-118] These event rates were very low, however. DPP (n=2,161) was aimed at preventing diabetes in overweight persons with impaired fasting glucose.[89] The mean age of participants was 51 years and about one quarter to one third of participants had hypertension or dyslipidemia, respectively. PREMIER (n=304, hypertension subgroup only) was aimed at lowering blood pressure in persons who were not yet taking medications.[116] The mean age of participants was 52 years and the mean SBP at baseline was 144 mm Hg. The Trial of Non-pharmacologic Intervention in the Elderly (TONE) (n=975) was aimed at lowering blood pressure in persons who were already taking antihypertension medications; participants were older, with a mean age of 67 years, and the mean SBP at baseline was 128 mm Hg.[117] None of these studies included persons with diabetes. PREMIER only had 6 months of followup. While DPP and TONE reported longer-term followup (up to 36 months), they had low CVD event rates at approximately 6 to 15 CVD events per 1,000 person-years. One good-quality trial, the Finnish Diabetes Prevention Study (n=522), was conducted in Finland and evaluated a high-intensity combined lifestyle counseling intervention to prevent diabetes. This trial reported long-term observational followup on mortality and CVD events from the original trial.[124] At approximately 10 years, the study reported no statistically significant difference in mortality (hazard ratio [HR], 0.57 [95% CI, 0.21 to 1.58]) (2.2 vs. 3.8 deaths per 1,000 person-years in the intervention and control groups, respectively) or CVD events (HR, 1.04 [95% CI, 0.72 to 1.51]) (22.9 vs. 22.0 events per 1,000 person-years in the intervention and control groups, respectively) between the group originally assigned to a high-intensity combined lifestyle intervention to prevent diabetes and the usual care control group.

The Risk Factor Intervention Study (n=508) was also a good-quality trial that evaluated a high-intensity behavioral counseling intervention that reported CVD outcomes, including mortality.[112] This trial, however, was conducted in Sweden in the late 1980s and only included men. The mean age of participants was 66 years, all participants had hypertension, the mean SBP was 155 mm Hg, and three quarters of participants also had dyslipidemia (mean LDL cholesterol, 178 mg/dL). Notably, 29 percent of participants were current smokers and 22 percent had diabetes. Eight percent of participants had a previous myocardial infarction (MI). In addition to this population being at much higher risk for CVD events than those in the other four trials, the intervention included a protocol to start medication for dyslipidemia or elevated glucose or nicotine replacement therapy if counseling was not sufficient. At 6.6 years, 41 persons had died in the intervention group compared with 64 persons in the usual care group (RR, 0.62 [95% CI, 0.42 to 0.92]). The trial reported 63 CVD events (fatal or nonfatal MI or cerebrovascular accident) in the intervention group compared with 84 CVD events in the usual care group (RR, 0.71 [95% CI, 0.51 to 0.99]).[112] It is unclear if the higher event rate (presumably due to a sicker population and inclusion of persons with diabetes and prior MI), the addition of medication adjustment to behavioral counseling, or the difference in standard of care for CVD risk reduction in the 1980s led to the difference in beneficial effect on health outcomes seen in this trial.

Detailed Results for Self-Reported Patient Health Outcomes

Four trials (n=893), three fair-quality trials conducted in Australia and Germany and one good-quality trial conducted in the United States, evaluated high-intensity combined lifestyle behavioral interventions (**Table 11**).[85,92,94,95] These trials reported that the interventions did not reduce self-reported depression symptoms as measured by the Depression Anxiety Stress Scale, Hospital Anxiety and Depression Scale, or Center for Epidemiologic Studies Depression Scale at 6 to 12 months. Although conducted in different countries, all trials included similar populations: middle-aged adults (mean age range, 52 to 65 years) at risk for developing diabetes (mean fasting blood glucose range, 93 to 106 mg/dL). The U.S. trial was conducted in mostly Latina women with a mean BMI of 34 kg/m^2, which was somewhat higher than in the other three trials.[94]

Five fair-quality trials (n=1,268) evaluated combined lifestyle counseling interventions and showed mixed findings of benefit on self-reported QOL measures, two of which were conducted in the United States.[86,110,119-121] While PREMIER also reported self-reported QOL measures, these results were not reported for the hypertension subgroup and are not discussed further.[125] The three fair-quality trials (n=529) evaluating medium- to high-intensity counseling interventions showed greater improvement in self-reported QOL compared with usual care at 6 to 12 months.[119,120] A small trial (n=63) conducted in Sweden showed a statistically significant difference in health status as measured on a 100-mm Visual Analogue Scale (72.8 vs. 54.5 in the intervention and usual care groups, respectively; p<0.001 at 12 months). This study was conducted by Nilsson and colleagues in 1992 among mostly men with hypertension and a mean age of 56 years.[119] A more recent, and much larger, trial (n=640) conducted in France, the Pan European Grid Advanced Stimulation and State Examination, included both men and women with a mean age of 57 years and a mixture of CVD risk factors. This trial showed a small, but statistically significant, change in the physical component score (PCS) of the SF-36: an increase of 2.57 in the intervention group versus a decline of 0.5 in the usual care group at 6 months.[120] This trial found no difference in results for the mental component score (MCS) of the SF-36. Finally, a recent trial, Live Well Be Well (n=230), evaluated a high-intensity diabetes prevention intervention in a racially diverse U.S. population with impaired fasting glucose.[86] This trial showed a small, but statistically significant, improvement in QOL as measured by the Psychological Well-Being II scale at 6 and 12 months. However, there were no statistically significant differences between groups at 12 months in other measures, including self-rated health and the Psychological Distress II scale.

Two fair-quality trials (n=739) that evaluated medium- to high-intensity counseling interventions did not show any difference in self-reported QOL measures compared with usual care at 6 to 12 months. A small trial (n=99), the Patient-motivated Health Promotion Program, was conducted in Japanese men and women with a mean age of 64 years. Participants had hypertension or impaired fasting glucose and showed no change in General Health Questionnaire-30 scores at 12 months.[121] A larger trial (n=236), WISEWOMAN North Carolina, was conducted in poor underinsured and uninsured American women. Participants had a mean age of 53 years and a mixture of hypertension, dyslipidemia, diabetes, and obesity. This trial reported no changes in the MCS or PCS of the SF-8 at 6 or 12 months.[110]

Two fair-quality trials (n=422) evaluated physical activity–only counseling interventions and showed no benefit on self-reported QOL measures.[98,122] One U.S.-based trial (n=302), the Enhanced Fitness Trial, included men attending a VA hospital center with a mean age of 67 years and impaired fasting glucose. This trial found no improvements in SF-36 scores at 12 months between participants receiving a high-intensity counseling intervention to increase physical activity and those receiving a minimal intervention that included a referral to a physical activity and nutrition program.[98] A Canadian trial (n=120), the Physical Activity Counseling trial, targeted inactive adults who had CVD risk factors, including hypertension, diabetes, and obesity. The mean age of participants was 47 years. This trial found no improvement in the MCS or PCS of the SF-12 at 6 months between participants receiving a medium-intensity counseling intervention to increase physical activity and those receiving a minimal intervention of a tailored physical activity prescription.[122]

KQ 2. Do Primary Care–Relevant Behavioral Counseling Interventions for Healthy Diet and/or Physical Activity Improve CVD-Related Intermediate Outcomes in Adults With Known CVD Risk Factors?

Overall Results

Seventy-one of the 74 included trials evaluating diet and/or physical activity counseling interventions reported intermediate health outcomes (**Tables 1** and **2**). Commonly reported intermediate outcomes included: objective lipid measures, blood pressure, glucose, weight, composite cardiovascular risk scores, medication use, and diabetes incidence (**Appendix D Tables 1–9**). Of the 71 trials, only 14 trials could not be included in meta-analyses of intermediate health outcomes, primarily because of limitations in data reporting at the primary study level (e.g., no measure of dispersion).[69,76,77,97,108,117,120,126-132] Therefore, we focus primarily on results of meta-analyses and discuss discrepancies between meta-analysis findings and trial results that we did not include in quantitative analyses. In a handful of instances, there were minor discrepancies in results presented in the meta-analyses and summary tables because unadjusted values were used in the meta-analyses (if adjusted values could not be used in quantitative pooling) and adjusted results were presented in the summary tables. These differences are noted in the summary tables (**Tables 12–15**).

Medium- to high-intensity diet and physical activity counseling interventions in persons selected for CVD risk factors (dyslipidemia, hypertension, and/or impaired fasting glucose or glucose intolerance) can decrease total cholesterol, LDL cholesterol, blood pressure, fasting glucose, diabetes incidence, and measures of weight (**Appendix D Tables 1–9**). Overall, benefits in these intermediate health outcomes appear to be most robust at 12 to 24 months. The limited number of trials that included longer-term followup limits interpretation of the benefit of findings to after 24 months. Across all trials that reported each specific outcome at 12 to 24 months, behavioral counseling appears to reduce total cholesterol (k=34) by an average of 4.48 mg/dL (95% CI, 6.36 to 2.59), LDL cholesterol (k=25) by 3.43 mg/dL (95% CI, 5.37 to 1.49), SBP (k=31) by 2.03 mm Hg (95% CI, 2.91 to 1.15), diastolic blood pressure (DBP) (k=24) by 1.38 mm Hg (95% CI, 1.92 to 0.84), fasting glucose (k=22) by 2.08 mg/dL (95% CI, 3.29 to 0.88), diabetes incidence (k=8) by an RR of 0.58 (95% CI, 0.37 to 0.89), and measures of weight (k=34) by a pooled mean difference of 0.26, using standardized units (standardized mean difference [SMD], 0.26 [95% CI, 0.35 to 0.16]). However, statistical heterogeneity across all trials for fasting glucose and weight outcomes was very high. Pooled effect sizes were generally similar for medium- versus high-intensity counseling interventions (**Appendix F Figures 1–12**). High-intensity combined lifestyle counseling in persons with impaired fasting glucose or glucose tolerance (k=5) reduces diabetes incidence in the longer term (RR, 0.55 [95% CI, 0.45 to 0.67]; I^2=27%). Medium- to high-intensity counseling interventions focusing on dietary changes alone, primarily in persons with dyslipidemia who are not yet taking medications to lower cholesterol, can modestly lower total cholesterol (k=9) by 3.75 mg/dL (95% CI, 6.50 to 1.01; I^2=24%) and LDL cholesterol (k=7) by 4.27 mg/dL (95% CI, 7.84 to 0.70; I^2=40%) at 12 to 24 months. Both medium- and high-intensity interventions were effective. While high-intensity counseling resulted in slightly larger pooled estimates of total and LDL cholesterol and fasting glucose, the confidence interval estimates for medium- and high-intensity interventions overlapped (**Appendix F Figure 3**). Most physical activity–only counseling interventions were of medium intensity (k=8), although two were of high intensity. While our ability to draw definitive conclusions is limited by the small number of physical activity only–counseling trials (k=10) and heterogeneity (e.g., in populations studied, outcomes measured) among the trials, these types of interventions do not appear to improve intermediate CVD-related outcomes at 12 to 24 months.

The populations targeted and the types of counseling interventions evaluated were the two main a priori–specified explanatory factors for clinical (and statistical) heterogeneity in this body of literature. Populations were defined as selected primarily for having: 1) dyslipidemia, 2) hypertension, 3) impaired fasting glucose or glucose tolerance, or 4) a mixture of CVD risk factors, including dyslipidemia, hypertension, elevated glucose (including diabetes), metabolic syndrome, smoking, and obesity. We categorized interventions as focusing on: 1) both diet and physical activity counseling, 2) diet-only counseling, or 3) physical activity–only counseling. Therefore, we present our results stratified by population (**Tables 16–19**) and intervention type (**Table 20**).

Results in Persons With Dyslipidemia

Seventeen fair- to good-quality counseling trials (n=4,963) selected primarily for persons with dyslipidemia.[67-83] An additional 24 fair- to good-quality trials (n=15,997) selected participants for a mixture of risk factors, including dyslipidemia, and reported intermediate outcome measures (**Table 12**). Of the 17 trials in persons with dyslipidemia, we rated only one trial[72] as good quality and all the others as fair quality. For limitations in fair-quality trials, please see the "Quality" section under "Description of Included Studies." All but three trials conducted in persons selected primarily for dyslipidemia evaluated diet-only counseling. One of these trials was conducted in persons with familial hyperlipidemia (PRO-FIT), one evaluated a telephone counseling intervention (CouPLES [Couples Partnering for Lipid Enhancing Strategies]), and one was an older trial from 1993 (RHPP) that included both diet and physical activity counseling.[67-69] The mean age in these trials ranged from 40.5 to 71 years (**Table 3**). Most trials included a fair representation of both men and women, except for three trials in mostly (or entirely) men[67,75,80] and one trial in entirely women.[82] Average baseline total and LDL cholesterol ranged from 233 to 282 mg/dL and from 156 to 200 mg/dL, respectively, in persons who were not taking lipid-lowering medications. The majority of trials (k=13) evaluated medium-intensity interventions. All but one trial used a usual care, wait list, or attention control.[67] In this trial, CouPLES, the control group physicians received email reminders emphasizing the use of lipid-lowering medications. All but three trials (earlier trials from the 1990s) were included in the meta-analyses.[69,76,77] For a similar description of trials in populations with mixed risk factors, please see the section below, "Results in Persons With Mixed CVD Risk Factors."

The majority of trials conducted in persons selected primarily for dyslipidemia reported outcome measures of total (k=9) and LDL cholesterol (k=8) at 12 to 24 months (**Table 16**). Fewer trials (k=5) reported outcomes at less than 12 months. No trials reported longer-term outcomes (>24 months). At 12 to 24 months, medium- to high-intensity diet-only counseling trials reduced total (k=9) and LDL cholesterol (k=8) by 3.31 mg/dL (95% CI, 5.98 to 0.64) and 3.93 mg/dL (95% CI, 7.23 to 0.62), respectively (**Figures 2** and **3**). Because most trials included persons who had not yet started medications, these results are most applicable to persons who are not yet taking lipid-lowering medication. Looking more broadly across all types of medium- to high-intensity interventions in persons selected for dyslipidemia or a mixture of CVD risk factors, counseling interventions reduced total (k=22) and LDL cholesterol (k=17) by 5.11 mg/dL (95% CI, 7.77 to 2.45) and 3.74 mg/dL (95% CI, 6.39 to 1.09), respectively (**Figures 4** and **5**), at 12 to 24 months. The statistical heterogeneity is much higher in these combined pooled analyses, which reflects the greater clinical heterogeneity in population and intervention characteristics. High-intensity counseling resulted in slightly larger pooled estimates of total and LDL cholesterol, but results were not statistically significantly different from effects of medium-intensity counseling (**Appendix F Figures 1** and **3**). Two trials in persons explicitly with dyslipidemia[76,77] and three trials in mixed CVD risk populations reporting lipid outcomes[120,129,130] that could not be included in the meta-analyses only reported short-term (<12 months) outcomes. We could not include one fair-quality trial in the meta-analyses, WISEWOMAN California (n=1,093), because of data limitations. This study found no statistically significant reduction in total cholesterol between persons receiving a high-intensity combined lifestyle counseling intervention and usual care at 12 months. The baseline total cholesterol in this population, however, was not elevated (mean, 198.1 mg/dL).[108] We could not include one fair-quality trial in the meta-analyses, RHPP (n=1,197), because of data limitations. This study, however, found no statistically significant difference in total cholesterol between persons receiving a medium-intensity combined lifestyle counseling intervention and usual care at 30 months.[69] Limited available data prevent any definitive conclusions about the efficacy of lifestyle counseling interventions beyond 24 months.

Fewer trials reported HDL cholesterol and triglycerides as outcome measures (**Table 16**). The trials that did report HDL cholesterol found no statistically significant effects. While there were statistically significant reductions in triglycerides, there was evidence of publication bias due to small-study effects. Many studies also reported weight measures (i.e., weight and/or BMI) as an outcome. Across all trials in persons with dyslipidemia or a mixture of CVD risk factors, medium- to high-intensity counseling can reduce measures of weight (k=18) by an SMD of 0.22 (95% CI, 0.35 to 0.10) (**Figure 6**). The statistical heterogeneity of this pooled analysis, however, was very high. Two earlier trials from the 1990s appear to be outliers, which contributes to the statistical heterogeneity.[71,80]

Results in Persons With Hypertension

Fourteen (n=4,990) of 15 fair- to good-quality trials[67,69-87] in persons selected primarily for hypertension and 24 fair- to good-quality trials (n=15,997) in persons selected for a mixture of risk factors, including hypertension, reported intermediate outcome measures (**Table 13**). Of the 13 trials in persons with hypertension, only two trials were of good quality[116,117] and the others were fair-quality. For limitations in fair-quality trials, please see the "Quality" section under "Description of Included Studies." Two trials had multiple intervention arms evaluating diet or physical activity only versus combined lifestyle counseling.[117,128] Therefore, we included a total of 13 combined diet and physical activity counseling interventions, three diet-only counseling interventions, and two physical activity–only counseling interventions. The mean age in these trials ranged from 51 to 67 years and most included an even representation of both men and women, except for two trials in mostly (or entirely) men[111,113] and one trial in entirely women.[104] The majority of trials included persons who were taking antihypertension medications. Only three trials explicitly targeted persons who were not yet taking medications.[111,116,127] Average baseline SBP and DBP ranged from 127 to 162 mm Hg and from 71 to 96 mm Hg, respectively, in persons taking medications and averaged approximately 144/87 mm Hg in persons not yet taking them (**Table 4**). Nine trials evaluated medium-intensity[84,104,105,111,113,128,133-135] and six trials evaluated high-intensity[116,117,126,127,136,137] counseling interventions. Most trials used a usual care or wait list control in which participants were assumed to receive usual care as a comparator group, except for four trials in which the control group received minimal interventions.[76,113,126,134] Four trials could not be included in the meta-analyses because of limitations in how data were reported in the primary studies.[117,126-128] For a similar description of trials in populations with mixed risk factors, please see the section below, "Results in Persons With Mixed CVD Risk Factors."

Medium- to high-intensity diet and physical activity counseling interventions resulted in reductions in blood pressure up to 12 to 24 months. Only three trials (two included in the meta-analyses) reported outcomes beyond 24 months. At 12 to 24 months, counseling trials conducted exclusively in persons with hypertension reduced SBP (k=6) and DBP (k=6) by 2.29 mm Hg (95% CI, 3.82 to 0.76) and 1.22 mm Hg (95% CI, 2.53 to -0.08), respectively (**Figures 7–8**). While point estimates of reductions in SBP were greatest in the short term (<12 months), the confidence intervals overlap with estimates at 12 to 24 months. Trials included a range of participants who were and were not taking medications. Therefore, these findings are applicable to both persons who are and are not yet taking medication. Looking more broadly across persons selected explicitly for hypertension and a mixture of CVD risk factors, medium- to high-intensity counseling interventions reduced SBP (k=20) and DBP (k=16) by 1.99 mm Hg (95% CI, 3.15 to 0.83) and 1.23 mm Hg (95% CI, 1.91 to 0.56), respectively (**Figures 9–10**), at 12 to 24 months. Pooled effect sizes were similar for medium- and high-intensity counseling interventions (**Appendix F Figures 5** and **7**).

Of the seven trials that were not included in the meta-analyses (k=4 for hypertension, k=3 for mixed CVD risk factors), four trials only reported outcomes at 6 months.[120,127,128,130] One fair-quality trial, WISEWOMAN California (n=1,093), could not be included in the meta-analyses because of data limitations. This trial found a statistically significant reduction in SBP between persons receiving a high-intensity combined lifestyle counseling intervention and usual care at 12 months. These findings are consistent with findings from meta-analyses.[108] One fair-quality trial (n=337) conducted by Migneault and colleagues found no statistically significant reduction in SBP or DBP between a high-intensity combined lifestyle counseling intervention group and a minimal intervention control group (who received a 75-page resource manual in addition to a pedometer and scale) at 8 to 12 months.[126] The nonstatistically significant reduction in SBP and DBP in this trial was consistent with the magnitude of results of trials included in the meta-analyses. Another good-quality trial, TONE (n=975), did not report SBP or DBP. Instead, this trial used a composite measure (proportion of participants free of CVD events, hypertension, or medications)[117] and found that a high-intensity diet and physical activity counseling intervention increased the proportion of persons free of CVD events, hypertension, or medications compared with a usual care control group at 30 months (HR, 0.69 [95% CI, 0.59 to 0.81]). Limited available data prevent us from drawing definitive conclusions about the efficacy of lifestyle counseling interventions beyond 24 months.

Fewer trials reported lipid or glucose outcome measures (**Table 17**). Mostly combined diet and physical activity counseling interventions found reduced total (k=4) and LDL cholesterol (k=2) in persons with hypertension, as well as total (k=17) and LDL cholesterol (k=11) in persons with hypertension or a mixture of CVD risk factors. The magnitude of effect on lipid reduction was similar to that seen in persons who explicitly had dyslipidemia. Many studies also reported weight measures as an outcome. Across all trials in persons with hypertension or a mixture of CVD risk factors, medium- to high-intensity counseling can reduce measures of weight (k=16) by an SMD of 0.21 (95% CI, 0.34 to 0.08) (**Figure 11**). The statistical heterogeneity of this pooled analysis, however, is very high. Again, the effect size of the reduction in weight measures is similar to that seen in persons explicitly with dyslipidemia. One trial in particular, the Activity Diet and Blood Pressure Trial (ADAPT) (n=241), appears to be an outlier that contributes to the statistical heterogeneity.[138]

Other outcomes that were not included in meta-analyses were medication use and composite CVD risk scores (**Tables 13** and **15**). Three trials conducted exclusively in persons with hypertension (n=1,520) sought to reduce the use of antihypertension medication.[116,117,138] Two good-quality trials conducted in the United States, PREMIER (n=304, hypertension subgroup only) and TONE (n=975), showed a statistically significant increase in the proportion of persons who were free of medication at 18 to 36 months.[116,117] Participants in the PREMIER trial were not taking antihypertension medications and all participants in the TONE trial were taking them. In PREMIER, 21 percent of persons in the high-intensity counseling intervention group versus 41 percent of persons in the usual care control group were taking antihypertension medications at

18 months.[116] In TONE, the mean interval from intervention start to withdrawal of medications was about 3 months. At 36 months, 93.2 percent of persons in the high-intensity combined diet and physical activity counseling intervention group versus 86.8 percent of persons in the control group had stopped taking antihypertension medications. One fair-quality trial, ADAPT (n=241), included participants who were taking antihypertension medications and found no difference in medication use requirement between the medium-intensity counseling intervention group and usual care control group at 36 months.[138]

Twelve of the included trials (n=6,781) used a composite CVD risk score as an outcome measure.[100,102,103,108,116,120,123,132,133,138-140] Two of these trials were conducted exclusively in hypertensive populations[116,138] and 10 were conducted in populations selected for a mixture of CVD risk factors.[100,102,103,108,120,123,132,133,139,140] Overall, there was generally no difference in 10-year CVD risk as measured by the Framingham Risk Score or Systematic Coronary Risk Evaluation at 6 to 36 months. Two trials found a very small, albeit statistically significant, change in 10-year risk at 12 months.[133,140] One trial, Improving Patient Adherence to Lifestyle Advice (n=615), was conducted in the Netherlands. This trial found a difference of 0.9 percent (p=0.023) in 10-year risk using the Systematic Coronary Risk Evaluation between a medium-intensity combined lifestyle counseling intervention group and usual care group.[133] The baseline 10-year CVD risk was low in this population at approximately 5 percent. One good-quality trial (n=315) conducted by Wister and colleagues in Canada found a 1.8 percent difference (p<0.05) in 10-year risk using the Framingham Risk Score between a medium-intensity combined lifestyle counseling intervention group and usual care group.[140] The baseline 10-year CVD risk was slightly higher in this trial population at 11 percent.

Results in Persons With Impaired Fasting Glucose or Glucose Tolerance

Sixteen fair- to good-quality counseling trials (n=5,883) in persons selected primarily for impaired fasting glucose or glucose intolerance[88-103] and an additional 24 fair- to good-quality trials (n=15,997) in persons selected for a mixture of risk factors, including elevated glucose or metabolic syndrome, reported intermediate outcome measures (**Table 14**). Of the 16 trials in persons with impaired fasting glucose or glucose intolerance, five trials were good-quality,[86,87,89,94,118] and the others were all rated as fair quality. For limitations in fair-quality trials, please see the "Quality" section under "Description of Included Studies." The majority of trials (k=13) were combined diet and physical activity counseling trials; only one trial was diet-only counseling and two trials were physical activity–only counseling. The mean age in these trials ranged from 51 to 67 years (**Table 5**). Most trials had an even representation of both men and women, except for three trials in mostly (or entirely) men.[93,97,98] Average baseline fasting blood glucose ranged from approximately 94 to 111 mg/dL. Measures of glucose tolerance (1- or 2-hour) and hemoglobin A1c were less commonly reported. None of the trials included participants who were taking glucose-lowering medications at trial entry. In general, the mean BMI ranged from 29 to 34 kg/m^2. Both trials conducted in Japanese men had a mean baseline BMI of 24 kg/m^2.[93,97] The majority of trials (k=13) evaluated high-intensity interventions, two trials evaluated medium-intensity interventions, and one trial evaluated a low-intensity intervention. The medium-intensity combined lifestyle counseling intervention had 12 contacts over 24 months. The other medium-intensity intervention was a physical activity–only counseling intervention with only three contacts over 6 months. All trials used a usual care or wait list control in which participants were assumed to receive usual care as a comparator group, except for three trials that used minimal intervention control groups.[89,93,98] All but one trial was included in the meta-analyses.[97] This trial was quite different from the others in that it was the only low-intensity trial included and the only diet-only counseling intervention in this population. In addition, this trial was conducted in persons who were not overweight. For a similar description of trials in populations with mixed risk factors, please see the section below, "Results in Persons With Mixed CVD Risk Factors."

The majority of trials in persons with impaired fasting glucose or glucose tolerance reported outcome measures of diabetes incidence (k=11) and fasting blood glucose (k=13) at 12 months or greater (**Table 14**). At 12 to 24 months, medium- to high-intensity (mostly high-intensity) counseling trials (k=6) reduced diabetes incidence by an average of 35 percent (RR, 0.65 [95% CI, 0.42 to 1.02]), albeit not statistically significant (**Table 18**). At longer-term followup greater than 24 months, high-intensity combined lifestyle interventions (k=5) reduced diabetes incidence by an average of 65 percent (RR, 0.55 [95% CI, 0.46 to 0.67]) (**Figure 12**). These findings were similar when the three trials in populations selected for mixed CVD risk factors that also reported diabetes incidence as an outcome were added, and results were statistically significant at both intermediate and long-term followup, with a reduction of diabetes incidence by an RR of 0.58 (95% CI, 0.37 to 0.89) at 12 to 24 months (k=8) and 0.61 (95% CI, 0.46 to 0.79) at greater than 24 months (k=6) (**Figure 13**). Meta-analyses for fasting glucose outcomes support the findings of a reduction in progression to diabetes. While medium- to high-intensity counseling interventions in persons with impaired fasting glucose or glucose tolerance (k=11) reduced fasting glucose by 2.05 mg/dL (95% CI, 3.86 to 0.24) at 12 to 24 months (**Figure 14**), the statistical heterogeneity is very high. In addition, there are a limited number of trials that report fasting glucose outcomes at greater than 24 months (**Table 18**).

Lipid and blood pressure outcomes were not as commonly reported (**Table 18**). Nonetheless, pooled results for these outcomes are generally consistent with findings in other populations. Many studies, however, also reported weight measures as an outcome. Across all trials in persons with impaired fasting glucose or glucose tolerance or a mixture of CVD risk factors, medium- to high-intensity counseling reduced measures of weight (k=24) by an SMD of 0.21 (95% CI, 0.29 to 0.13), similar to the magnitude of reduction seen in other included populations (**Table 18**). The statistical heterogeneity of this pooled analysis, however, is very high.

Results in Persons With Mixed Cardiovascular Risk Factors

Of the total 26 trials conducted in populations that were selected for a mixture of cardiovascular risk factors, 24 fair- to good-quality trials (n=15,997) reported intermediate outcome measures (**Table 15**). Only three of these trials were of good quality,[139-141] however, and the remaining trials were all rated as fair quality. The majority of these trials (k=20) evaluated combined diet and physical activity counseling interventions, although six trials evaluated physical activity–only counseling interventions. The mean age in these trials ranged from 47 to 68 years and most trials included a fair representation of both men and women, except for one early trial exclusively in men[112] and two trials entirely in women (**Table 6**).[108,110] The proportion of persons with hypertension ranged from 9 to 100 percent, with an average SBP of 125 to 158 mm Hg and

DBP of 73 to 91 mm Hg. The proportion of persons with dyslipidemia ranged from 13 to 88 percent, with an average baseline total cholesterol of 185 to 259 mg/dL and LDL cholesterol of 112 to 178 mg/dL. The proportion of persons with impaired fasting glucose or glucose tolerance was not commonly reported. The proportion of persons with diabetes ranged from 0 to 45 percent. The baseline fasting glucose ranged from 93 to 148 mg/dL. The majority of persons in all trials had an average BMI that identified them as overweight to obese. The majority of trials (k=17) evaluated medium-intensity interventions. While most trials used usual care or a wait list control as a comparator group, five trials used a minimal intervention as the control group.[100,102,107,114,122] Five trials were not included in the meta-analyses because of limitations in reporting of outcome data in the primary studies.[108,120,129-131]

Outcomes in trials that selected persons based on any number of CVD risk factors are discussed in conjunction with other populations. Please see the above sections, "Results in Persons With Dyslipidemia," "Results in Persons With Hypertension," and "Results in Persons With Impaired Fasting Glucose or Glucose Tolerance."

Results by Intervention Type

The majority of included trials evaluated combined lifestyle interventions with messages to improve diet and increase physical activity (49 intervention arms). Eighteen trials included counseling interventions that focused on diet alone, 14 of which were conducted in persons primarily selected for dyslipidemia, three in persons selected for hypertension, and only one in persons selected for impaired fasting glucose. Only 10 trials evaluated interventions that focused on increasing physical activity alone (**Table 2**). As a result, the findings of benefit on intermediate health outcomes are most robust for combined lifestyle counseling (**Table 20**). Medium- to high-intensity combined lifestyle counseling interventions reduced total cholesterol (k=22) (5.43 mg/dL [95% CI, 7.97 to 2.89]), LDL cholesterol (k=17) (3.69 mg/dL [95% CI, 5.98 to 1.40]), and triglycerides (k=10) (8.33 mg/dL [95% CI, 13.80 to 2.86]) and increased HDL cholesterol (k=14) (0.98 mg/dL [95% CI, 0.25 to 1.70]) at 12 to 24 months in persons selected for dyslipidemia or any number of CVD risk factors (**Figures 16** and **17**; **Table 20**). Very few trials, however, reported followup after 24 months and the reported effects generally did not seem to last at longer-term followup. Medium- to high-intensity diet-only counseling interventions also reduced total cholesterol (k=9) (3.75 mg/dL [95% CI, 6.50 to 1.01]), LDL cholesterol (k=7) (4.27 mg/dL [95% CI, 7.84 to 0.70]), and triglycerides (k=3) (17.86 mg/dL [95% CI, 33.10 to 2.62]). While the reduction in total cholesterol for diet-only counseling interventions may be smaller than for combined lifestyle interventions, the reduction in LDL cholesterol for these interventions appeared to be the same as for combined lifestyle interventions. None of these trials reported longer-term followup. Overall, while high-intensity counseling resulted in slightly larger pooled estimates of total and LDL cholesterol, confidence interval estimates were overlapping (**Appendix F Figures 1** and **3**).

Combined lifestyle interventions also reduced blood pressure, glucose, diabetes incidence, and measures of weight at both intermediate and longer-term followup. Medium- to high-intensity combined lifestyle counseling interventions reduced SBP (k=27) (2.06 mm Hg [95% CI, 3.03 to 1.08]) and DBP (k=21) (1.30 mm Hg [95% CI, 1.93 to 0.68]). These trials also reduced fasting glucose (k=18) (1.86 mg/dL [95% CI, 3.24 to 0.49]), diabetes incidence (k=6) (RR, 0.54 [95%

CI, 0.34 to 0.88]), and measures of weight (k=25) (SMD, 0.24 [95% CI, 0.35 to 0.14]) at 12 to 24 months in persons selected for CVD risk factors (**Figures 18–21**). Pooled effect sizes for blood pressure, glucose, and measures of weight were similar for medium- versus high-intensity counseling interventions (**Appendix F**). Trials reporting a reduction in diabetes incidence were mostly high-intensity counseling interventions. While fewer trials reported followup after 24 months, reductions in these outcomes persisted at longer-term followup. Trials evaluating diet-only counseling interventions did not commonly measure other intermediate health outcomes.

The included evidence base (k=10) for physical activity–only counseling interventions is much more sparse and less convincing. The majority of these interventions were medium-intensity (k=8), as opposed to high-intensity (k=2) interventions. Four trials were designed to specifically target older adults.[98,104,123,130] Six of the 10 trials were conducted in populations with mixed CVD risk factors, two were conducted in persons explicitly with impaired fasting glucose, and two were conducted in persons with hypertension. Therefore, the reported outcome measures varied across these trials and pooled analyses for each outcome included few studies, in general. Two fair-quality trials (n=232) only reported short-term outcomes at 6 months and both trials evaluated medium-intensity counseling interventions in persons selected for hypertension.[104,128] One very small trial (n=24) in women showed a small, but statistically significant, improvement in SBP.[104] Another trial (n=208) conducted in both men and women, however, found no change in SBP or DBP (**Table 13**).[128] Two fair-quality trials (n=400) were conducted in older adults with impaired fasting glucose.[98,99] Neither of these trials found a benefit in lipids, glucose, or measures of weight at 12 to 24 months. Finally, six trials were conducted in persons selected for a mixture of CVD risk factors, five of which reported intermediate outcome measures.[122,123,130,131,141] Four fair-quality trials (n=1,955) reported no changes in short-term (6 to 12 months) intermediate health outcomes (including lipids, glucose, and measures of weight).[122,123,130,131] One good-quality trial (n=101) conducted by Kallings and colleagues that evaluated a medium-intensity counseling intervention aimed at Swedish older adults found a very small, but statistically significant, benefit on total cholesterol, hemoglobin A1c, and measures of weight. However, this trial did not find an effect on measures of blood pressure or LDL cholesterol.[141] Given the limited number of trials and clinical heterogeneity among populations, interventions, and outcomes measured, it is still unclear if medium- or high-intensity counseling interventions aimed at increasing physical activity alone can improve lipids, blood pressure, glucose, and measures of weight in persons with CVD risk factors.

Exploration of Heterogeneity

Our review purposefully includes a wide range of healthy lifestyle counseling trials to improve cardiovascular health published over the past two decades. The main dimensions of clinical heterogeneity included variation in populations studied, interventions evaluated, and study characteristics (including outcomes measured). We a priori specified the major dimensions of heterogeneity and present results stratified by populations targeted and outcomes measured (e.g., trials targeting persons with dyslipidemia generally measured lipid outcomes), as well as stratified by intervention type (i.e., combined lifestyle, diet only, physical activity only). We used exploratory meta-regressions and visual inspection of forest plots to examine if other important a priori–specified variables influenced study effects. Based on this preliminary exploration of heterogeneity, we performed meta-regressions on lipids (total and LDL cholesterol, triglycerides), blood pressure (SBP and DBP), fasting glucose, and measures of weight outcomes using all data available from the 57 trials included in the meta-analyses. None of the factors we examined appeared to consistently influence effect size across all outcomes. Year of publication appeared to explain some statistical heterogeneity for effects on LDL cholesterol, blood pressure (SBP and DBP), and weight, such that more recent studies had smaller effects on LDL, blood pressure, and weight reduction than earlier studies. High-intensity interventions appeared to explain some statistical heterogeneity for effects on LDL cholesterol (but not on other outcomes), such that higher-intensity interventions had greater LDL cholesterol reduction compared with less intensive interventions. Finally, study quality appeared to explain some statistical heterogeneity for effects on SBP and triglycerides, but not for other outcomes. That is, better-quality studies had smaller effects than studies with more risk for bias. Overall, the differences in effect sizes, as modified by these variables, were very small and likely not clinically significant.

We also assessed if trials targeting specific a priori subpopulations or that included subgroup analyses of these populations showed similar or differential findings of benefit on intermediate health outcomes. In general, there were a limited number of trials that included subgroup analyses by sex, age, or race/ethnicity. Nonetheless, we believe our findings are broadly applicable to men and women, middle- and older-aged adults, as well as nonwhite persons, based on available evidence and a body of evidence that includes an adequate representation of these populations. Nine trials were conducted in men only (or nearly all men)[67,75,80,93,97,98,111-113] and four trials were conducted in women only.[82,104,108,110] Direct comparisons of results among these trials are difficult because of the differences in population characteristics (other than sex), interventions, outcomes, and lengths of followup across these studies. Only five of the included studies reported results for intermediate health outcomes stratified by sex.[71,87,89,142,143] There was no difference in benefit on reduction of cholesterol or diabetes incidence between men and women in the Diet and Exercise for Elevated Risk trial (n=189), which evaluated a high-intensity diet-only counseling intervention to reduce cholesterol, or in DPP (n=2,161), which evaluated a high-intensity combined lifestyle counseling intervention to prevent diabetes.[71,89] ADAPT (n=241) evaluated a medium-intensity combined lifestyle counseling intervention to reduce blood pressure and demonstrated some differences between sexes at 4 months. These differences, however, did not persist at 12 months. Additionally, there was no statistically significant benefit in blood pressure reduction in the intervention group compared with the control group for either men or women at 36 months.[142] One good-quality trial, E-LITE (Evaluation of Lifestyle Interventions to Treat Elevated Cardiometabolic Risk in Primary Care) (n=241), which evaluated a high-intensity combined lifestyle intervention in persons with impaired fasting glucose or metabolic syndrome, found statistically significant weight loss for men, but not women, at 15 months.[87] Subgroup analyses by sex for other measured intermediate health outcomes (i.e., blood pressure, lipids, fasting blood glucose) were not reported. PREMIER (n=810) evaluated a high-intensity combined lifestyle intervention in persons with prehypertension and hypertension. Subgroup analyses for PREMIER did not report findings separately for persons with hypertension only. Nonetheless, blood pressure reductions at 6 months were greater for black men compared with black women, but no sex differences were noted for whites.[143]

Included trials generally included populations of middle-aged adults that accurately reflect the distribution of CVD risk factors in the general population. Overall, we did not find a large variation in mean ages across studies, which ranged from 40 to 71 years. Nine trials specifically targeted older adults or the average mean age of the population was 65 years or older.[69,98,99,112,113,117,127,130,141] Although direct comparison across trials targeting older adults and those with younger mean ages is difficult because of clinical heterogeneity among trials, the high-intensity combined lifestyle counseling interventions in older adults did improve intermediate health outcomes similar to those in middle-aged adults. Physical activity–only counseling interventions targeting older adults generally (except for one trial conducted by Kallings and colleagues) did not improve intermediate health outcomes, similar to the results of studies conducted in middle-aged adults. Two trials included subgroup analyses that compared older adults with middle-aged adults.[89,123] DPP, for example, evaluated a high-intensity combined lifestyle intervention to prevent diabetes and found no statistically significant interaction for age (25 to 44 years, 45 to 59 years, and 60 years or older) on reduction of diabetes incidence between the intervention and control groups.[89] The Green Prescription Programme, which evaluated a medium-intensity physical activity–only counseling intervention, found no significant difference between younger and older participants (ages 65 to 79 years) and generally found no statistically significant differences between intervention and control groups for blood pressure outcomes.[123]

Of the trials conducted in the United States, 20 trials were conducted in populations that included between 4.4 and 100 percent nonwhite persons.[67,72-74,81,82,89,98,108,110,113,117,123,126,127,129,135,136] Two trials explicitly targeted Latino Americans[94,108] and two trials explicitly targeted black Americans.[126,135] DPP (45% nonwhite participants) conducted post-hoc subgroup analyses by race/ethnicity and found no statistically significant interaction on diabetes incidence.[89] PREMIER (34% black participants) also conducted subgroup analyses, although they were performed on the entire trial population (including persons with prehypertension). Nonetheless, subgroup analyses showed the greatest blood pressure reductions at 6 months for black men, followed by whites (men and women), and the smallest blood pressure reductions for black women.[143]

Publication Bias

For quantitative analyses, we assessed for publication bias using funnel plots and Egger's test. We found no evidence for significant publication bias except for triglyceride outcomes (Egger's test p=0.02). Therefore, the findings of benefit on reductions in triglycerides for counseling interventions should be interpreted with caution, as the true effects are likely less optimistic than our estimated effects. In general, one should interpret any findings for outcomes with only a very limited number of trials (i.e., only a small representation of included studies reported a certain outcome), with caution because of possible selective reporting of that outcome and limited reproduction of the specific outcome effect across trials.

KQ 3. Do Primary Care–Relevant Behavioral Counseling Interventions for Healthy Diet and/or Physical Activity Improve Diet and Physical Activity Behavioral Outcomes in Adults With Known CVD Risk Factors?

Overall Results

Sixty-one of the included trials reported behavioral outcomes (**Tables 1** and **2**). Three of these trials reported only behavioral outcomes (KQ 3) and did not report intermediate health outcomes (KQ 2).[105,109,114] Overall, objectively measured and self-reported changes in dietary intake and physical activity were concordant with intermediate outcome findings (**Tables 16–19**). In several instances in which trials did not find any benefit in intermediate health outcomes, trials demonstrated statistically significant improvements in dietary intake (e.g., fat, saturated fat, fruit and vegetable, total energy) and various measures of self-reported physical activity in the short and intermediate term. In selected trials conducted in persons who were already taking medications to lower cholesterol or blood pressure, counseling interventions appeared to improve dietary intake (e.g., sodium, fat, saturated fat, fruit and vegetable, total energy) and various measures of self-reported physical activity despite a lack of benefit on lipid measures or blood pressure. Many physical activity–only counseling trials only reported short-term outcomes. Four of five trials that reported behavioral outcomes at 12 to 24 months found statistically significant improvements in self-reported physical activity. We did not conduct quantitative pooled analyses because of sparse reporting of objectively measured behavior change (e.g., urinary sodium, VO_2max) and the heterogeneity in self-reported measures of behavior change. Given the robust and consistent findings of benefit on intermediate health outcomes, our summary of results for this question focuses on discrepant or added information that behavioral outcomes provided.

Detailed Results for Behavioral Outcomes

In trials targeting persons with dyslipidemia, all but two trials[68,76] that reported on dietary intake of fat and/or saturated fat found a statistically significant decrease in consumption at 6 to 24 months, even in trials that did not find a statistically significant benefit on total or LDL cholesterol (**Table 21**; **Appendix G Table 2**). Only two trials targeting persons with dyslipidemia included those who were already taking lipid-lowering medications,[67,68] which may make it more difficult to detect an improvement in serum lipid measurements (e.g., total or LDL cholesterol). One fair-quality trial, CouPLES (n=255), was conducted in a VA population in which approximately 46 percent were already taking lipid-lowering medications, and evaluated a medium-intensity combined lifestyle telephone counseling intervention.[67] At 11 months, although there were no statistically significant differences in medication use or LDL cholesterol, the intervention group reported statistically significant improvements in fat (approximately 11 g fewer per day) and saturated fat (approximately 4 g fewer per day) intake, as well as total energy intake (approximately 200 kcal fewer per day). In another fair-quality trial, PRO-FIT (n=340), Dutch persons with confirmed familial hyperlipidemia, 69 percent of whom were taking lipid-lowering medications, were randomized to receive a medium-intensity combined lifestyle intervention.[68] At 12 months, there were no statistically significant differences in saturated fat, fruit, or vegetable intake, as well as no statistically significant differences in intermediate health outcomes between those who received counseling and those who received usual care. The findings of improvement in dietary and physical activity outcomes were consistent with intermediate health outcomes in trials targeting persons with hypertension. In trials with no statistically significant benefit on blood pressure outcomes, these trials still found improvements in urinary sodium and self-reported dietary intake (including fat, saturated fat, and fruit/vegetable) and self-reported physical activity at 6 to 24 months (**Table 22**; **Appendix G**

Table 2). Five of these trials (n=2,335) evaluated medium- to high-intensity counseling interventions exclusively in persons taking antihypertension medications.[117,126,128,136,138] Four of the five trials reported no difference in blood pressure and one trial did not report blood pressure outcomes.[117] All of the four trials (n=1,698) that reported urinary sodium found a statistically significant decrease in urinary sodium at 6 to 36 months.[117,128,136,138] Two (n=449) of the four trials that reported physical activity change showed a small, but statistically significant, increase in physical activity (approximately 40 minutes more per week) at 6 and 36 months.[128,138] Two trials (n=515) also reported other measures of dietary intake and found small, but statistically significant, improvements in saturated fat and fruit and/or vegetable intake at 18 and 36 months.[136,138] One trial only reported behavioral outcomes.[105] This fair-quality trial conducted in the Netherlands (n=1,629) evaluated low- and medium-intensity mailed and/or telephone interventions with diet and physical activity counseling. This trial found that the medium-intensity telephone intervention (with or without mailed component) improved both physical activity (approximately 50 minutes more per week) and fruit/vegetable (approximately 0.25 more servings per day) intake at 18 months.

Trials targeting persons with impaired fasting glucose or glucose tolerance found improvements in behavioral change, which is consistent with findings of benefit on intermediate health outcomes (**Table 23**; **Appendix G Table 2**). Seven trials (n=2,127) without consistent statistically significant improvements in intermediate outcomes show that counseling interventions of any intensity could improve self-reported behavioral outcomes.[85,86,88,92,97,99] All of the five trials (n=1,727) that reported dietary intake showed a small, but statistically significant, improvement in diet (using different measures, including fat, saturated fat, fiber, energy, and a composite score) at 6 to 18 months.[85,86,88,92,97] Three (n=1,325) of the six trials that reported physical activity showed a statistically significant improvement in physical activity (using different measures, including total physical activity [minutes/week], percent meeting physical activity goal of 150 minutes per week, and moderate to vigorous physical activity [MET/minutes-week]).[88,98,99]

In trials in persons selected for a combination of risk factors, findings of behavioral change were again consistent with findings of benefit on intermediate health outcomes (**Table 24**; **Appendix G Table 2**). Eight medium- to high-intensity counseling trials found no consistent statistically significant benefit on intermediate or behavioral outcomes. Five of these trials evaluated a combined lifestyle counseling intervention (n=1,829) and three were physical activity–only counseling trials (n=1,077).[86,100,102,122,130,131,139,144] Six medium- to high-intensity counseling trials, five combined lifestyle trials (n=6,681), and one physical activity–only counseling trial (n=878) found no consistent statistically significant benefit on intermediate health outcomes, but demonstrated improvement in self-reported diet and/or physical activity behaviors. The physical activity–only trial, the Green Prescription Programme, reported improvement in diet (e.g., total energy, unsaturated fat to fat ratio, fish intake, meals per day with a serving of vegetables, and a composite diet score) and physical activity (e.g., total energy expenditure, leisure time physical activity, minutes per week of moderate to vigorous activity, meeting recommended physical activity levels, and steps per day) behaviors.[123] In the five trials (n=6,681) reporting dietary outcomes, medium- to high-intensity combined lifestyle counseling improved selected dietary outcome measures (including saturated fat to fat ratio, meeting fruit and vegetable intake recommendations, portions of fruits and vegetables per day, vegetables per day, and composite dietary measures) at 12 and 60 months.[103,107,110,121,132] In five (n=3,506) of the six trials that reported physical activity outcomes, medium- to high-intensity counseling interventions improved selected physical activity outcomes (including steps per day, minutes per week of moderate to vigorous physical activity, percent meeting physical activity goal of 150 minutes per week, physical activity assessment score) at 6 and 12 months.[103,110,121,123,132]

Two trials (n=2,594) reported only behavioral outcomes.[109,114] One fair-quality trial, Logan Healthy Living (n=434), evaluated a medium-intensity telephone-only combined lifestyle counseling intervention and found statistically significant improvements in fat, saturated fat, fiber, and fruit/vegetable intake at up to 18 months. This trial, however, did not find a statistically significant improvement in physical activity behaviors.[114] The other fair-quality trial, NERS (n=2,160), evaluated a medium-intensity physical activity–only counseling intervention and found an improvement in total physical activity (approximately 35 minutes more per week) at 12 months.[109]

Ten trials evaluated medium- to high-intensity physical activity–only counseling interventions.[98,99,104,109,122,123,128,130,131,141] Overall, while there was no consistent benefit observed for intermediate health outcomes, the limited number of trials and heterogeneity among these trials did not allow for any definitive conclusion of lack of benefit on intermediate outcomes for physical activity–only counseling interventions. Findings for behavioral outcomes in these trials are generally consistent with the findings for intermediate health outcomes (**Tables 21–24; Appendix G Table 2**). The two trials (n=125) that demonstrated a benefit on intermediate health outcomes showed an increase in self-reported physical activity outcomes.[104,141] Trials that found no benefit on intermediate outcomes found no statistically significant benefit on self-reported physical activity outcomes (including total or leisure physical activity, percent meeting physical activity guidelines). Five of the 10 trials only reported short-term outcomes (<12 months).[104,122,128,130,141] Three of these counseling trials (n=608) used objective measures of cardiorespiratory fitness and found no statistically significant benefit at 6 to 12 months.[98,122,130] Self-reported measures of physical activity varied across trials—the most commonly reported measures included total energy expenditure, steps per day, minutes per week of total or moderate to vigorous physical activity, and percent meeting physical activity goal (150 minutes/week). Five (n=4,209) of 10 trials reported outcomes at 12 months or greater.[98,99,109,123,131] Four (n=3,439) of these five trials found statistically significant improvements in self-reported physical activity outcomes at 12 to 24 months.[98,99,109,123] One of these trials, NERS (n=2,160), only reported behavioral outcomes.[109] This trial was conducted in the United Kingdom and evaluated a medium-intensity physical activity–only counseling intervention that also offered access to low-cost exercise classes. This trial found an improvement in total physical activity (approximately 35 minutes more per week) at 12 months.

Four trials reported subgroup analyses for behavioral outcomes that allow for direct comparisons of findings between men and women, as well as older and middle-aged adults.[107,109,123,145] While two of these trials (n=5,381) suggest that men had greater improvement in self-reported physical activity change at 12 months,[107,123] two trials (n=2,401) found no difference by sex in physical activity outcomes at 12 or 36 months.[109,145] Two trials (n=3,038) suggest no statistically significant differences in behavioral outcomes by age, such that older adults also appear to benefit from counseling aimed at improving physical activity levels.[109,123]

KQ 4. What Are the Adverse Effects of Healthy Diet and/or Physical Activity Behavioral Counseling Interventions in Adults With Known CVD Risk Factors?

Overall Results

We narrowly focused this question on harms of counseling interventions, rather than broadly on harms of dietary or physical activity changes themselves. We examined the 74 trials included for KQs 1 through 3 for harms, as defined by the study authors, or any paradoxical change in outcomes (e.g., worsening of blood pressure, lipids, glucose, measures of weight, dietary intake, physical activity) (**Tables 1** and **2**). While we searched for additional studies examining harms of healthy lifestyle counseling interventions, we did not find any such studies.

Overall, the harms of included counseling interventions were very sparsely reported, although we did not a priori hypothesize that these counseling interventions would result in serious harms (i.e., unexpected or unwanted medical attention). Only 10 of the included trials explicitly mentioned harms or lack of harms (**Tables 1** and **2**). In general, the included interventions did not have significant adverse effects. While four trials reported increased complaints in persons receiving behavioral counseling attributed to an increase in physical activity,[89,98,123,130] there were generally no serious injuries, except for one trial targeting older adults.[98] We found no consistent evidence for paradoxical changes in intermediate or behavioral outcomes. While nine of the 13 trials that reported carbohydrate intake reported an increase in carbohydrate intake, this increase was generally accompanied by dietary improvements in fat, saturated fat, fiber, and fruits and vegetables, without an overall increase in sugar or total calories consumed.[71,75,80,89,96,118,138,146,147]

Detailed Results for Harms

Six fair- to good-quality trials (n=2,420) that evaluated medium- to high-intensity combined diet and physical activity counseling interventions specifically reported no adverse events during the trial.[92,94,96,116,117,146] The mean age of participants in these trials ranged from 52 to 66 years. While four trials report "no adverse events," they did not offer any additional details.[92,94,96,146] The PREMIER (n=304, hypertension subgroup only) trial was aimed at lowering blood pressure in persons (mean age, 52 years) who were not yet taking medications and reported no differences between intervention arms in serious adverse events, including cardiovascular or musculoskeletal events, at 6 months.[116] TONE (n=975) was aimed at lowering blood pressure in persons (mean age, 66 years) who were already taking antihypertension medications; it reported no differences between intervention arms in "excessive" weight loss, physical injury, palpitations, chest pain, dizziness, edema, headaches, and "any" adverse events at 36 months.[117]

Six fair- to good-quality trials (n=3,961) that evaluated different medium- to high-intensity counseling interventions specifically reported adverse events during the trial.[89,98,113,114,123,130] The Logan Healthy Living trial (n=434) was aimed at persons with hypertension or diabetes in Australia with a mean age of 58 years. This trial reported that three persons allocated to the intervention arm, a medium-intensity telephone-counseling intervention, died of unknown causes during the 18-month trial.[114] No additional details are reported. Another trial conducted by Rodriguez and colleagues (n=533) evaluated a medium-intensity combined lifestyle counseling intervention in persons with hypertension (mean age, 67 years). The authors reported that nine participants were withdrawn during the 12-month trial by research staff because of an adverse event that would affect study participation, but no additional details (including how many participants in each arm) are given.[113] DPP (n=2,161), a high-intensity combined lifestyle counseling intervention aimed at preventing diabetes in overweight persons with impaired fasting glucose (mean age, 51 years), reported slightly more musculoskeletal complaints (i.e., myalgia, arthritis, arthralgia) in the intervention group receiving a high-intensity counseling intervention at 2.8 years (24.1 vs. 21.1 events per 100 person-years in the intervention and control groups, respectively; p<0.02).[89] Gastrointestinal symptoms (diarrhea, flatulence, nausea, vomiting) were more common in the control group. The trial reported no differences in hospitalizations between the intervention arms. Three trials evaluating physical activity–only counseling interventions reported complaints due to increased exercise.[98,123,130] The Lifestyle Intervention and Independence for Elders trial (n=186) was aimed at older adults with a mean age of 67 years. This trial reported that one participant in the high-intensity counseling group withdrew because of fatigue attributed to exercise at 11 months.[130] The Enhanced Fitness Trial (n=302), which was also aimed at older adults at the VA with a mean age of 67 years, reported a total of 691 adverse events during the 12-month trial, 650 (94%) of which were classified as nonserious (e.g., aches, pain, sore muscles, headaches, minor injuries).[98] Of the 64 (6%) events classified as serious (life threatening or requiring hospitalization), two events were attributed to physical activity. Both of these events occurred in the intervention group receiving a high-intensity counseling intervention—one person had angina while on a treadmill requiring hospitalization and the other person fell from the treadmill and broke his femur. A third physical activity counseling trial (n=878), the Green Prescription Programme, with a mean age of 58 years, reported increased "bodily pain" at 12 months (p=0.02) as measured by the SF-36 in the medium-intensity counseling intervention group compared with the wait list control group.[123] The authors stated, however, that there was no difference between the trial arms in falls, injuries, or hospital admissions at 12 months.

In examining the included trials, we found no consistent evidence that behavioral counseling resulted in unwanted paradoxical effects in intermediate or behavioral outcomes. Two fair-quality trials with a number of methodological limitations had paradoxical findings in intermediate health outcomes.[83,92] One small trial (n=92) conducted in Sweden in participants with a mean age of 42 years found lower HDL cholesterol at 12 months in the intervention group receiving a medium-intensity dietary counseling intervention compared with the usual care control group.[83] The authors note, however, that more women were included in the control group (accounting for higher HDL cholesterol in the control group) and results were not adjusted for sex differences. Another trial (n=307), Healthy Living Course, aimed at persons with impaired fasting glucose, reported a greater incidence of diabetes in the high-intensity counseling intervention group (n=24) than the control group (n=7) at 6 months (p=not reported).[92] We found no evidence that medium- or high-intensity counseling interventions negatively affected dietary intake or physical activity. Thirteen trials reported carbohydrate intake as a self-reported dietary outcome.[70,71,75,89,91,94,118,119,138,146-149] Four trials (n=654) reported no change in carbohydrate intake,[70,90,94,119] while nine (n=4,387) of the 13 trials reported an increase in consumption of carbohydrates in the intervention group compared with the control group at 6 to 36 months.[71,75,]

[80,89,96,118,138,146,147] The increased consumption of carbohydrates was generally accompanied by corresponding dietary improvements in decreased consumption of fat and saturated fats and increased consumption of fiber and fruits and vegetables. None of these trials reported an overall increase in total calories consumed. In fact, most often an increased consumption of carbohydrates was accompanied by a decrease in total calories consumed. Therefore, we did not consider the increase in carbohydrate consumption in the intervention group to represent a harm. In ADAPT (n=241), the authors suggest that a decrease in high-fat dairy products in the intervention group that was not replaced with low-fat dairy products could potentially result in a decrease in calcium consumption.[138]

Chapter 4. Discussion

Summary of Evidence

We conducted this systematic review to assist the USPSTF in updating its previous recommendations on physical activity and healthy diet counseling.[55,150,151] This review focused on the effectiveness and harms of primary care–relevant diet and physical activity counseling interventions in persons with CVD risk factors. We included 74 unique trials that met our inclusion criteria, the vast majority of which (k=51) were published since the previous USPSTF recommendations in 2002.

Based on a large body of evidence (k=71), we found that intensive combined lifestyle counseling in persons with CVD risk factors reduced cholesterol, blood pressure, measures of weight, glucose, and diabetes incidence at 12 to 24 months (**Table 25**). Effects of counseling interventions (k=61) on objectively measured or self-reported behavioral outcomes were generally consistent with findings on intermediate health outcomes. We found more limited information about longer-term benefits. Benefits on blood pressure, measures of weight, and glucose reduction appear to persist after 24 months, but are based on only a small subset of trials with longer-term followup. Reduction in diabetes incidence appears to persist for 3 to 4 years. Several trials evaluated a diet-only counseling message. Intensive diet-only counseling in persons with dyslipidemia also reduced cholesterol. Both medium- and high-intensity interventions reduced lipids, blood pressure, and measures of weight. High-intensity interventions reduced glucose and diabetes incidence. In general, effective counseling interventions were intensive and involved several hours (median, 13 hours [IQR, 9 to 19 hours]), over several contacts (median, 8 contacts [IQR, 5 to 16 contacts]), over several months duration (median, 12 months [IQR, 6 to 12 months]). We found more limited information about physical activity–only counseling interventions. Mostly medium-intensity physical activity–only counseling in persons with CVD risk factors did not appear to have consistent benefits on intermediate health outcomes, but trials were quite heterogeneous in populations studied, interventions evaluated, and outcomes measured. While findings were mixed for physical activity–only counseling interventions, the limited number of studies and heterogeneity across trials limits our ability to make any definitive conclusions about the benefits, or lack thereof, of these types of counseling interventions. Four of the five physical activity–only counseling trials that reported outcomes at 12 to 24 months, however, found statistically significant improvements in self-reported measures of physical activity.[98,99,109,123]

Only a small subset of trials (k=16) reported patient health outcomes, which prevented us from drawing any definitive conclusions as to whether these types of interventions can decrease CVD events or improve QOL.[85,86,89,92,94,95,98,110,115-122] Overall, there does not appear to be a significant reduction in CVD events in the long term, but event rates in these trials, even after 10 years of followup, are generally quite low. Findings of benefit on self-reported QOL measures were mixed. Likewise, only a small subset of trials (k=10) reported on harms of counseling interventions, but overall we found no serious harms, with the exception of two adverse events in one physical activity counseling intervention aimed at older adults.[89,94,98,113,114,116,117,123,130,138,146]

There are surprisingly few current existing systematic reviews addressing the effectiveness or harms of lifestyle behavioral counseling in persons with traditional CVD risk factors. Most recent reviews of lifestyle counseling interventions focus on obesity management or CVD prevention in populations with known diabetes and/or coronary heart disease. Our review found a similar reduction in progression to diabetes as in existing systematic reviews examining the effectiveness of these types of interventions to prevent diabetes in persons with impaired fasting glucose or glucose intolerance.[152-155] Our review found a similar reduction in blood pressure and cholesterol as a Cochrane review of multiple risk factor interventions for the primary prevention of CVD by Ebrahim and colleagues.[156] The Cochrane review, however, also found a decrease in mortality, primarily due to the inclusion of trials of early CVD prevention. Given the applicability of many earlier trials to current understanding and management of CVD risk, as well as trends in the distribution of CVD and its risk factors over time, our review was restricted to trials published after 1990.

Clinical Interpretation of Benefit and Harms Given Paucity of Direct Health Outcome Data

Effects on Lipids and Blood Pressure

Medium- to high-intensity combined lifestyle or diet-only counseling interventions decreased total cholesterol by approximately 3 to 8 mg/dL and decreased LDL cholesterol by approximately 1.5 to 6 mg/dL at 12 to 24 months. Based on observational data, a 10 percent reduction (approximately 20 mg/dL) in total cholesterol is associated with a decreased incidence of CAD by approximately 54 percent at age 40 years, 39 percent at age 50 years, and 27 percent at age 60 years.[157] Although plausible, it is still unclear if smaller reductions in cholesterol can also translate into reductions in CAD or CVD events.

Medium- to high-intensity combined lifestyle interventions can decrease SBP and DBP by approximately 1 to 3 and 1 to 2 mm Hg, respectively, at 12 to 24 months. Long-term observational followup of Trials of Hypertension Prevention I and II (n=3,126) showed that persons with prehypertension who were initially randomized to receive intensive lifestyle counseling had decreased composite CVD events over 10 to 15 years (HR, 0.70 [95% CI, 0.53 to 0.94]), suggesting that small reductions in blood pressure (i.e., approximately 2 mm Hg reduction in SBP and 1 mm Hg reduction in DBP) seen in the original Trials of Hypertension Prevention may result in longer-term reduction in CVD morbidity and mortality.[158] Epidemiologic data also suggest that small changes in blood pressure (i.e., 2 mm Hg reduction in SBP) are associated with a decreased risk for CAD by 6 percent or cerebrovascular accident by 16 percent.[159]

Effects on Glucose and Diabetes Incidence

Medium- to high-intensity combined lifestyle counseling interventions decreased fasting glucose and diabetes incidence. The reduction in fasting glucose across all 18 trials reporting this outcome was approximately 0.5 to 3.5 mg/dL at 12 to 24 months. Fewer trials (k=8) reported diabetes incidence at 12 to 24 months; these trials were generally high-intensity combined lifestyle counseling interventions aimed at persons with impaired fasting glucose or glucose tolerance. In the long term (>24 months), the overall pooled estimate of RR for high-intensity combined lifestyle counseling was 0.61 (95% CI, 0.46 to 0.79). In DPP, for example, fasting blood glucose was approximately 4 mg/dL lower in the intensive lifestyle counseling group than the control group at 3 years, which corresponded to 14.4 percent of persons developing diabetes in the intervention group compared with 28.9 percent in the control group (number needed to treat [NNT], about 7 [95% CI, 5 to 10]). The lifestyle intervention was more effective than metformin alone in reducing diabetes incidence (results were 39% lower [95% CI, 24 to 51]). Even in populations with lower rates of progression to diabetes than DPP, one would not have to intensively counsel many individuals to prevent a single case of diabetes mellitus. If only 10 percent of persons in the control group progress to diabetes over 3 to 6 years, for example, then the NNT would be 26 (95% CI, 19 to 48); if 20 percent of persons progress to diabetes, then the NNT would be 13 (95% CI, 9 to 24); if 25 percent of persons progress to diabetes, then the NNT would be 10 (95% CI, 7 to 19); and if 33 percent of persons progress to diabetes, then the NNT would be 8 (95% CI, 6 to 14).

Effects on Weight Outcomes

Medium- to high-intensity combined lifestyle counseling interventions also decreased weight outcomes by a standardized effect size of 0.24 (95% CI, 0.35 to 0.14) at 12 to 24 months. The statistical heterogeneity for this pooled effect was very high, however, and therefore should be interpreted with caution. Overall, this represents a small effect in weight reduction. When this effect size is back translated into individual trials, the effect is approximately equivalent to a 2- to 3-kg weight loss or 0.5- to 1.5-kg/m^2 decrease in BMI. These results are generally consistent with the small effects found in a recent systematic review of behavioral treatment of adult obesity. This review found that behavioral treatment resulted in an average of 3 kg of weight loss in the intervention versus control groups.[57] Our findings are also consistent with the 2013 AHA/ACC/Obesity Society Guideline for the Management of Overweight and Obesity in Adults, which found strong evidence to support the association of sustained weight loss of 3 to 5 percent and clinically meaningful reductions in triglycerides and glucose outcomes.[160] Epidemiological data also suggest that the risk for both CVD and diabetes increases with each kg/m^2 unit change in BMI.[161] However, it is still unclear if small sustained reductions in weight or BMI after the intervention's conclusion translate into better cardiovascular patient health outcomes (i.e., decreased CVD events and/or mortality from CVD or diabetes). The clinical significance of changes in weight measures should therefore primarily be based on accompanying changes in lipid, blood pressure, and glucose outcomes.

Effects on Increases in Self-Reported Physical Activity

Medium-intensity physical activity–only counseling trials generally found no effect on intermediate health outcomes at 12 to 24 months. Four of the five counseling trials that reported behavioral outcomes at 12 to 24 months found statistically significant improvements in physical activity in the intervention versus control groups.[98,99,109,123] These trials used different measures of physical activity and found a 10 to 25 percent increase in the percentage of persons who met the recommended 150 minutes per week of moderate-intensity exercise (k=2)[98,123] and an approximate 35-minute/week increase in moderate or total physical activity (k=2).[99,109] This increase in the amount of physical activity per week is similar to findings in our previous review in adults without cardiovascular risk factors.[55] It is clear that increased physical activity is associated with a decrease in CVD events and mortality.[162] Based on a meta-analysis by Stattelmair and colleagues of 33 observational studies to determine the dose-response between levels of physical activity and risk for CAD, it appears that persons who had 150 minutes per week of physical activity had a 14 percent lower CAD risk. Persons who were physically active at levels lower than recommended also had statistically significant lower risk.[163] This finding supports the 2008 Physical Activity Guidelines for Americans and the American College of Sports Medicine recommendations for 150 minutes per week of moderate-intensity exercise, with the caveat that adults who are unable or unwilling to meet this goal still benefit from engaging in amounts of exercise less than recommended.[162,164] Another review by Zheng and colleagues of 12 studies to quantify the dose-response between walking and CVD risk found that an increase of approximately 30 minutes per week was associated with a 19 percent lower CAD risk.[165] Based on extrapolation from observational studies, it is likely that even a modest increase in the percentage of persons meeting a recommended 150 minutes per week of moderate-intensity activity or a modest increase in total or moderate-intensity activity per week can lower incidence of CAD and CAD events.

Adverse Effects

We did not a priori hypothesize any serious harms for counseling intervention. Overall, a limited number of trials reported on adverse effects of interventions and only one trial in older adults found two events of serious harms resulting from physical activity.[98] Observational studies from our previous systematic review of lifestyle counseling interventions suggest an increased risk for serious cardiac events during vigorous physical activity, primarily in persons with low levels of habitual activity.[55] The absolute risk for serious cardiac events related to physical activity, however, appears to be extremely small. In these observational studies, minor musculoskeletal injuries were fairly common when participants increased their physical activity from their habitual levels. The type and total amount of activity and relative change in activity were all important factors in determining the risk for injury. Noncontact, low-impact activities had lower injury rates, including walking, bicycling, and swimming. Increasing physical activity in a series of small increments, each followed by an adaptation period, resulted in lower rates of injury.[166] Additional information regarding harms of physical activity are detailed in the DHHS 2008 report on physical activity.[166] Therefore, focusing on low-impact activities and increasing activity in small increments can mitigate serious harm or injury from counseling interventions in older adults or persons at high risk for injury.

Considerations for Applicability of Findings

Population Considerations

Our review's findings are widely applicable to a broad range of individuals with CVD risk factors, including dyslipidemia, hypertension, impaired fasting glucose, glucose intolerance, metabolic syndrome, obesity, and smoking. Our review did not include trials conducted exclusively in persons with diabetes or in populations selected exclusively for obesity. Nearly all trials included persons who were overweight or obese. Several trials also included some persons who were already diagnosed with diabetes. Included trials also involved persons who had not yet started antihypertension or lipid-lowering medications, as well as those already taking them. Although included trials provided little direct evidence of comparisons of findings between the two sexes and across different age or racial/ethnic groups, we have no reason to believe that the benefit of intensive counseling would not apply to both men and women, middle-aged and older adults, and nonwhite subpopulations (namely African and Latino Americans), given the fair representation of these groups across included trials. Serious harms from increased physical activity were reported in one trial in older adults. As such, older adults may be at increased risk for adverse events, but very sparse reporting of harms limits any definitive conclusions about harms, much less differential harms between subpopulations.

Trials varied in their recruitment strategies, the restrictiveness of the eligibility criteria, and recruitment and retention rates. Of the trials with adequate reporting about recruitment methods, 16 trials relied on volunteers as part (k=8) or all (k=8) of their recruitment strategy. Most trials had eligibility criteria excluding persons with acute medical conditions or any known serious medical conditions. The proportion of trial participants out of the entire eligible sample ranged from 15 to 100 percent (k=53). The majority of trials had very high recruitment rates, with only 10 trials having less than 50 percent of eligible participants randomized into the trial. Overall, retention rates in the trials were greater than 80 percent. Sixteen trials had retention rates less than 80 percent. Trials with volunteer participants, restrictive eligibility criteria, low recruitment rates, and/or high retention rates likely overestimate the true magnitude of benefit of these counseling interventions in real-world settings.

Intervention Considerations

Effective interventions were medium- to high-intensity combined lifestyle or diet-only counseling interventions. Medium-intensity interventions are defined as greater than 30 minutes up to 360 minutes of contact. Approximately two thirds of the medium-intensity interventions had 120 minutes of contact time or greater; the median number of contacts was five and median duration of the intervention was 9 months. Diet-only and physical activity–only counseling interventions were mostly medium-intensity. High-intensity interventions had greater than 360 minutes of contact; the median number of contacts was 16 and median duration of the intervention was 12 months. Specially trained individuals delivered these interventions, including dietitians or nutritionists, physiotherapists or exercise professionals, as well as health educators, nurses, or psychologists.

Counseling interventions generally focused on behavioral change and could include cointerventions. Ten trials explicitly reported medication adjustment or counseling on medication adherence as part of the intervention protocol. In one of these 10 trials, the intervention protocol for medication adjustment focused on withdrawal or tapering off of antihypertension medications.[117] Several trials explicitly stated provision of free or low-cost access to exercise classes (although supervised exercise was not mandatory). Only two trials reported provision of financial incentives for participation, and two other trials offered some provision of free food to intervention participants (but were not considered to be feeding trials). Adherence, and therefore effectiveness, in trials may be higher than in real-world practice, especially for higher-intensity interventions. Unfortunately, measures of adherence and fidelity were not consistently reported in included trials. Thirty-three of the 74 trials reported adherence.[72-74,76,77,80-82,84,86,87,89,90,92,94,98,99,105,107,114,116,118,122,127,129,130,132-134,137,146,167,168] Adherence in the 13 trials that reported the proportion of participants who attended all of the sessions ranged from 50 to 95 percent.[74,77,81,84,87,91,116,122,127,129,130,137,167] Adherence in the seven trials that reported the proportion of participants who received any intervention ranged from 46 to 99 percent.[72,82,86,99,105,133,134]

Based on included trials, we are not able to define the minimum necessary counseling components for an effective intervention. All included counseling interventions involved more than didactic education alone. Most of these trials included audit and feedback (including self-monitoring), problem solving skills, and individualized care plans. Using qualitative analyses and meta-regressions, we did not find that the intervention format (e.g., face-to-face, group, individual, phone), the person delivering the counseling, the number of sessions, or the duration of intervention significantly affected the direction or magnitude of benefit. Based on a meta-analysis by Michie and colleagues of combined lifestyle counseling interventions specifically using meta-regressions to examine a number of a priori–specified intervention components, it appears that interventions with "self-monitoring" and use of at least one "self-regulatory technique" derived from control theory (i.e., prompt intention formation, prompt specific goal setting, provide feedback on performance, prompt self-monitoring behavior, prompt review of behavioral goals) were significantly more effective than interventions not including these components.[169] This review found that the duration of the intervention, the person delivering the counseling, the intervention format (i.e., individual vs. group), the study setting, the number of included sessions, or the number of behavior change techniques employed did not distinguish between effective and ineffective interventions. Greaves and colleagues conducted a systematic review of existing reviews of diabetes prevention lifestyle counseling and found that interventions that targeted both diet and physical activity, mobilized social support, used well-established behavior change techniques, used self-regulatory techniques (i.e., goal setting, self-monitoring, feedback on performance, and goal review), and had greater contact time or frequency of contact had greater effectiveness.[170] The review by Greaves and colleagues did not identify a minimum threshold of time/intensity that was effective and did not find any clear associations between intervention effectiveness and the person delivering counseling, the study setting, or the intervention format.

Review Limitations

Eating a healthy diet and increasing physical activity clearly have health benefits beyond CVD prevention and CVD risk factor modification. To support the USPSTF recommendation process, however, our review focused narrowly on the primary prevention of CVD in persons with risk factors for CVD. Therefore, we excluded persons with known diabetes, coronary heart disease, cerebrovascular disease, peripheral artery disease, and chronic kidney disease. We previously conducted a similar review of behavioral counseling interventions for the primary prevention of

CVD focused on unselected populations and persons without known risk factors, as well as a review on the management of adult obesity, which included behavioral interventions.[55,57] Therefore, this systematic review represents only a subset of a much larger body of literature on diet and physical activity counseling interventions in other populations and similar interventions with different specific aims (i.e., to prevent other diseases [e.g., cancer] or conditions [e.g., falls/disability]). Our review also focused on interventions that were relevant to primary care (i.e., those that could be conducted in or referred from primary care). Therefore, our review excluded behavioral interventions delivered through worksites, schools, and community organizations (e.g., churches); for these, we refer the reader to the CDC's Community Preventive Services Task Force.[171] Additionally, we limited included studies of effectiveness to fair- to good-quality randomized, controlled trials or controlled clinical trials conducted in developed countries so as to identify the evidence with the least risk for bias and the highest applicability to current U.S. practice. We only included studies published after 1990. We also excluded trials without a true control arm (e.g., usual care, minimal intervention, attention control, wait list control). As a result, we did not address literature addressing the comparative effectiveness of different types of behavioral counseling and intervention elements.

We categorized and pooled clinically heterogeneous interventions and lengths of followup in order to synthesize the evidence. We categorized length of followup into short (<12 months), intermediate (12 to 24 months), and long (>24 months). We pooled outcomes according to these categorizations. Likewise, we categorized interventions by intensity (minutes of persons-contact) rather than total number of, or duration of contacts. While this categorization scheme is consistent with the definitions of intensity used in our previous work supporting the USPSTF healthy lifestyle counseling recommendation, it is somewhat arbitrary, and some "medium-intensity" interventions were still quite intensive (in terms of minutes, frequency, and duration of contacts). Furthermore, because of limitations in reporting of intervention characteristics in the published literature, we had to estimate the duration of contacts in several instances. Our assumptions in these instances, however, would not change the overall categorization of intensity (low, medium, high). Therefore, we use gross categorizations of "intensity" rather than report actual minutes of contact.

There were also limitations posed by the quantitative pooling of results. Of the 71 trials, only 14 trials could not be included in meta-analyses because of limitations in reporting at the primary study level (e.g., no measure of dispersion). Of the data included in the meta-analyses, some degree of calculation was necessary to include the trials in the meta-analyses, although only a small percentage required statistical judgment. These calculations included determining that an abnormally small value reported as a standard deviation was actually a standard error and estimating the correlation between baseline and followup values in order to calculate the standard deviation of the change score. In these instances, we erred on the side of avoiding a type I error or overestimation of effect size.

We purposefully pooled across a clinically heterogeneous body of counseling literature. For most outcomes, the statistical heterogeneity was moderate and, therefore, was still reasonable to allow for the interpretation of pooled estimates. Given the clinical heterogeneity and our use of random-effects analyses, confidence interval estimates should be primarily used to understand the magnitude of effects on the individual outcomes. There was considerable statistical heterogeneity for fasting blood glucose and weight outcomes. As a result, one should interpret pooled estimates with caution. Likewise, we believe the clinical significance of the overall reduction in weight across trials should be interpreted in the context of the accompanying reductions in lipids, blood pressure, and measures of glucose. Despite examining for a number of factors that may explain for the heterogeneity of findings across trials, we were unable to identify additional population, intervention, or study characteristics that explained the statistical heterogeneity in pooled analyses (other than at a gross level of population targeted and intervention type).

Other potential sources of risk for bias in our review includes limiting the search to English-only publications, only including published trials, potential selective reporting of outcomes, and including trials that used volunteer participants. Egger's statistical test for small-study effects was significant only for triglyceride outcomes, which we do not discuss at length.

Study Limitations and Future Research Needs

Behavioral counseling to prevent CVD is a very active field of research and numerous trials in persons at risk for CVD are currently underway (**Appendix B**). Despite a very large body of trial evidence, well-conducted trials (and funding for these trials) are still needed to understand the full impact of these behavioral interventions on important health outcomes. Additional studies should also determine if less-intensive interventions are as effective as higher-intensity counseling.

While medium- to high-intensity combined lifestyle and diet-only interventions are effective, many of the high-intensity interventions would require resources that are not currently available or paid for in the current health system (and real-world patient adherence to intensive counseling may be considerably lower than in included trials). Additional research on how best to disseminate and implement these types of intensive behavioral counseling interventions into current practice is needed. Details on the fidelity of and adherence to counseling interventions should be routinely reported to better understand the applicability of behavioral counseling trial findings. We found a wide range of intensity for effective interventions, from a couple hours to greater than 30 hours of contact time. Future research should also evaluate if lower-intensity counseling interventions (e.g., a couple hours) are as effective as higher-intensity counseling (e.g., DPP) or if there is a minimum intensity, frequency, or duration of contact that could still improve lipids, blood pressure, and diabetes incidence. Evaluating true low-intensity interventions may not be feasible given that the standard of care for persons with CVD risk factors is at least minimal counseling. Future research on different modalities that require minimal health care resources (i.e., technology-based counseling), and therefore "lower the intensity" of interventions, is advisable.

It is clear that healthy diet and physical activity behaviors both contribute to good cardiovascular and overall health. Additional research on the additive or differential benefit of different counseling messages (i.e., diet, physical activity, or both) in different populations would be helpful in determining whether clinical scenarios focusing on diet or physical activity alone is advisable (or preferable) to combined lifestyle counseling.

Only a limited number of trials (k=11) reported followup beyond 24 months.[69,89,91,93,107,115,117,118, 138,139,149] While it is clear that high-intensity counseling interventions can reduce diabetes incidence in the long term, additional trials are needed to determine if beneficial effects of reductions in other important intermediate health outcomes are reproducible in the longer term. Many of the trials that had longer-term followup were high-intensity interventions with ongoing maintenance sessions throughout the trial period. Therefore, relatively little is known about the maintenance of beneficial physiologic (or behavior) change after an active intervention ends. Trials evaluating lower-intensity interventions rarely report longer-term outcomes. If additional evidence supports the effectiveness of low- to medium-intensity interventions, longer-term followup for these interventions would also help us understand the benefits of these interventions.

Given the progress of medical care and other factors, CVD events are relatively low. Therefore, the sample sizes and length of followup for counseling trials are likely to be prohibitively large or long if powered to detect differences in CVD outcomes. For example, the Look AHEAD (Action for Health in Diabetes) trial (n=5,145) that evaluated a high-intensity lifestyle intervention in overweight or obese persons with diabetes found no reduction in the rate of CVD events at about 10 years despite reductions in intermediate health outcomes (i.e., weight, glucose) and improvements in physical activity levels.[172] Self-reported patient outcomes, namely health-related QOL measures, are in fact health outcomes (i.e., can be experienced by the patient) and are underutilized in this body of literature. Future research would benefit from measuring and consistently reporting QOL and related self-reported patient outcomes.

Given the mixed findings for physical activity–only counseling trials, future research replicating successful physical activity–only counseling interventions would help us determine if such types of counseling interventions work and the populations these interventions should target. Physical activity–only counseling trials were generally of lower intensity than other included trials. Future research on the effectiveness of higher-intensity counseling interventions, especially in persons with CVD risk factors, is advisable. We primarily found evidence of increases in self-reported measures of physical activity. Greater use of objective measures to assess physical activity (i.e., step counts using pedometers, VO_2max to measure cardiorespiratory fitness) would corroborate self-reported changes in physical activity level, which is especially important when the changes in magnitude are small.

Conclusions

In general, medium- to high-intensity diet and physical activity behavioral counseling in persons with CVD risk factors resulted in consistent improvements across a variety of important cardiovascular intermediate health outcomes, including total and LDL cholesterol, blood pressure, glucose, and weight outcomes up to 2 years. Overall, high-intensity combined lifestyle counseling can reduce diabetes incidence at 3 to 4 years. The applicability of intensive counseling interventions depends largely on their availability and real-world adherence to these interventions. Very limited evidence exists on health outcomes or harmful effects of these counseling interventions. Extrapolating from other bodies of literature, the improvements we observed in intermediate health outcomes could translate into long-term reduction in CVD events. It is unlikely that intensive counseling interventions have serious patient harms. Future research on behavioral counseling in this population should focus on the effectiveness of lower-intensity interventions and should consistently include self-reported measures of health-related QOL.

References

1. Caspersen CJ, Powell KE, Christenson GM. Physical activity, exercise, and physical fitness: definitions and distinctions for health-related research. *Public Health Rep.* 1985;100(2):126-31. PMID: 3290711.
2. Haskell WL, Lee IM, Pate RR, et al. Physical activity and public health: updated recommendation for adults from the American College of Sports Medicine and the American Heart Association. *Med Sci Sports Exerc.* 2007;39(8):1423-34. PMID: 17762377.
3. Nelson ME, Rejeski WJ, Blair SN, et al. Physical activity and public health in older adults: recommendation from the American College of Sports Medicine and the American Heart Association. *Med Sci Sports Exerc.* 2007;39(8):1435-45. PMID: 17762378.
4. U.S. Department of Health and Human Services. 2008 Physical Activity Guidelines for Americans. Washington, DC: U.S. Department of Health and Human Services; 2008.
5. D'Agostino RB Sr, Vasan RS, Pencina MJ, et al. General cardiovascular risk profile for use in primary care: the Framingham Heart Study. *Circulation.* 2008;117(6):743-53. PMID: 18212285.
6. Yusuf S, Hawken S, Ounpuu S, et al. Effect of potentially modifiable risk factors associated with myocardial infarction in 52 countries (the INTERHEART study): case-control study. *Lancet.* 2004;364(9438):937-52. PMID: 15364185.
7. Wilson PW, D'Agostino RB, Levy D, et al. Prediction of coronary heart disease using risk factor categories. *Circulation.* 1998;97(18):1837-47. PMID: 9603539.
8. Goldstein LB, Bushnell CD, Adams RJ, et al. Guidelines for the primary prevention of stroke: a guideline for healthcare professionals from the American Heart Association/American Stroke Association. *Stroke.* 2011;42(2):517-84. PMID: 21127304.
9. Norris SL, Kansagara D, Bougatsos C, et al. Screening for Type 2 Diabetes Mellitus: Update of 2003 Systematic Evidence Review for the U.S. Preventive Services Task Force. Evidence Synthesis No. 61. AHRQ Publication No. 08-05116-EF-1. Rockville, MD: Agency for Healthcare Research and Quality; 2008.
10. Mokdad AH, Marks JS, Stroup DF, et al. Actual causes of death in the United States, 2000. *JAMA.* 2004;291(10):1238-45. PMID: 15010446.
11. Murphy SL, Xu J, Kochanek KD. Deaths: final data for 2010. *Natl Vital Stat Rep.* 2013;61(4):1-117. PMID: 24979972.
12. Centers for Disease Control and Prevention. Vital signs: avoidable deaths from heart disease, stroke, and hypertensive disease - United States, 2001-2010. *MMWR Morb Mortal Wkly Rep.* 2013;62(35):721-7. PMID: 24005227.
13. Centers for Disease Control and Prevention. Million hearts: strategies to reduce the prevalence of leading cardiovascular disease risk factors--United States, 2011. *MMWR Morb Mortal Wkly Rep.* 2011;60(36):1248-51. PMID: 21918495.
14. Yoon SS, Burt V, Louis T, et al. Hypertension among adults in the United States, 2009-2010. *NCHS Data Brief.* 2012;(107):1-8. PMID: 23102115.
15. Carroll MD, Kit B, Lacher D. Total and high-density lipoprotein cholesterol in adults: National Health and Nutrition Examination Survey, 2009-2010. *NCHS Data Brief.* 2012;(92):1-8. PMID: 22617230.

16. Kuklina EV, Carroll MD, Shaw KM, et al. Trends in high LDL cholesterol, cholesterol-lowering medication use, and dietary saturated-fat intake: United States, 1976-2010. *NCHS Data Brief.* 2013;(117):1-8. PMID: 23759124.
17. Cowie CC, Rust KF, Ford ES, et al. Full accounting of diabetes and pre-diabetes in the U.S. population in 1988-1994 and 2005-2006. *Diabetes Care.* 2009;32(2):287-94. PMID: 19017771.
18. Ervin RB. Prevalence of Metabolic Syndrome Among Adults 20 Years of Age and Over, by Sex, Age, Race and Ethnicity, and Body Mass Index: United States, 2003–2006. Hyattsville, MD: National Center for Health Statistics; 2009. PMID: 19634296.
19. Schiller JS, Lucas JW, Peregoy JA. Summary health statistics for U.S. adults: National Health Interview Survey, 2010. *Vital Health Stat.* 2012;(252):1-207. PMID: 22834228.
20. Chobanian AV, Bakris GL, Black HR, et al. Seventh report of the Joint National Committee on Prevention, Detection, Evaluation, and Treatment of High Blood Pressure. *Hypertension.* 2003;42(6):1206-52. PMID: 14656957.
21. Centers for Disease Control and Prevention. Vital signs: prevalence, treatment, and control of high levels of low-density lipoprotein cholesterol---United States, 1999-2002 and 2005-2008. *MMWR Morb Mortal Wkly Rep.* 2011;60(4):109-14. PMID: 21293326.
22. Centers for Disease Control and Prevention. QuickStats: age-adjusted percentage of adults aged >20 years with hypertension, by poverty level---National Health and Nutrition Examination Survey, United States, 2003-2006. *MMWR Morb Mortal Wkly Rep.* 2008;57(20);557.
23. Ford ES, Bergmann MM, Boeing H, et al. Healthy lifestyle behaviors and all-cause mortality among adults in the United States. *Prev Med.* 2012;55(1):23-7. PMID: 22564893.
24. Nettleton JA, Polak JF, Tracy R, et al. Dietary patterns and incident cardiovascular disease in the Multi-Ethnic Study of Atherosclerosis. *Am J Clin Nutr.* 2009;90(3):647-54. PMID: 19625679.
25. Kant AK, Leitzmann MF, Park Y, et al. Patterns of recommended dietary behaviors predict subsequent risk of mortality in a large cohort of men and women in the United States. *J Nutr.* 2009;139(7):1374-80. PMID: 19474153.
26. Anderson AL, Harris TB, Tylavsky FA, et al. Dietary patterns and survival of older adults. *J Am Diet Assoc.* 2011;111(1):84-91. PMID: 21185969.
27. Lantz PM, Golberstein E, House JS, et al. Socioeconomic and behavioral risk factors for mortality in a national 19-year prospective study of U.S. adults. *Soc Sci Med.* 2010;70(10):1558-66. PMID: 20226579.
28. Mente A, de Koning L, Shannon HS, et al. A systematic review of the evidence supporting a causal link between dietary factors and coronary heart disease. *Arch Intern Med.* 2009;169(7):659-69. PMID: 19364995.
29. Crowe FL, Key TJ, Appleby PN, et al. Dietary fibre intake and ischaemic heart disease mortality: the European Prospective Investigation into Cancer and Nutrition-Heart study. *Eur J Clin Nutr.* 2012;66(8):950-6. PMID: 22617277.
30. Chowdhury R, Stevens S, Gorman D, et al. Association between fish consumption, long chain omega 3 fatty acids, and risk of cerebrovascular disease: systematic review and meta-analysis. *BMJ.* 2012;345:e6698. PMID: 23112118.

31. Eckel RH, Jakicic JM, Ard JD, et al. 2013 AHA/ACC guideline on lifestyle management to reduce cardiovascular risk: a report of the American College of Cardiology/American Heart Association Task Force on Practice Guidelines. *J Am Coll Cardiol.* 2014;63(25 Pt B):2960-84. PMID: 24239922.
32. U.S. Department of Health and Human Services. Healthy People 2020. Washington, DC: U.S. Department of Health and Human Services; 2014. Accessed at http://www.healthypeople.gov/2020/topicsobjectives2020/ on 22 July 2014.
33. U.S. Department of Health and Human Services. Nutrition and Your Health: Dietary Guidelines for Americans. 5th ed. Washington, DC: U.S. Department of Health and Human Services; 2000. Accessed at http://www.cnpp.usda.gov/Publications/DietaryGuidelines/2000/2000DGProfessionalBooklet.pdf on 22 July 2014.
34. Huffman MD, Capewell S, Ning H, et al. Cardiovascular health behavior and health factor changes (1988-2008) and projections to 2020: results from the National Health and Nutrition Examination Surveys. *Circulation.* 2012;125(21):2595-602. PMID: 22547667.
35. King DE, Mainous AG III, Carnemolla M, et al. Adherence to healthy lifestyle habits in US adults, 1988-2006. *Am J Med.* 2009;122(6):528-34. PMID: 19486715.
36. Mellen PB, Gao SK, Vitolins MZ, et al. Deteriorating dietary habits among adults with hypertension: DASH dietary accordance, NHANES 1988-1994 and 1999-2004. *Arch Intern Med.* 2008;168(3):308-14. PMID: 18268173.
37. Kirkpatrick SI, Dodd KW, Reedy J, et al. Income and race/ethnicity are associated with adherence to food-based dietary guidance among US adults and children. *J Acad Nutr Diet.* 2012;112(5):624-35. PMID: 22709767.
38. Oldroyd J, Burns C, Lucas P, et al. The effectiveness of nutrition interventions on dietary outcomes by relative social disadvantage: a systematic review. *J Epidemiol Community Health.* 2008;62(7):573-9. PMID: 18559438.
39. Trost SG, Owen N, Bauman AE, et al. Correlates of adults' participation in physical activity: review and update. *Med Sci Sports Exerc.* 2002;34(12):1996-2001. PMID: 12471307.
40. Zhou Q, Remsburg R, Caufield K, et al. Lifestyle behaviors, chronic diseases, and ratings of health between black and white adults with pre-diabetes. *Diabetes Educ.* 2012;(2):219-28. PMID: 22454406.
41. Beydoun MA, Gary TL, Caballero BH, et al. Ethnic differences in dairy and related nutrient consumption among US adults and their association with obesity, central obesity, and the metabolic syndrome. *Am J Clin Nutr.* 2008;87(6):1914-25. PMID: 18541585.
42. Dubowitz T, Heron M, Bird CE, et al. Neighborhood socioeconomic status and fruit and vegetable intake among whites, blacks, and Mexican Americans in the United States. *Am J Clin Nutr.* 2008;87(6):1883-91. PMID: 18541581.
43. Talbot LA, Morrell CH, Fleg JL, et al. Changes in leisure time physical activity and risk of all-cause mortality in men and women: the Baltimore Longitudinal Study of Aging. *Prev Med.* 2007;45(2-3):169-76. PMID: 17631385.
44. Allender S, Cowburn G, Foster C. Understanding participation in sport and physical activity among children and adults: a review of qualitative studies. *Health Educ Res.* 2006;21(6):826-35. PMID: 16857780.

45. American Academy of Family Physicians. Summary of Recommendations for Clinical Preventive Services. Leawood, KS: American Academy of Family Physicians; 2014. Accessed at http://www.aafp.org/dam/AAFP/documents/patient_care/clinical_recommendations/cps-recommendations.pdf on 22 July 2014.
46. American College of Physicians. ACP Clinical Practice Guidelines. Washington, DC: American College of Physicians; 2014. Accessed at http://www.acponline.org/clinical_information/guidelines/guidelines/ on 22 July 2014.
47. Artinian NT, Fletcher GF, Mozaffarian D, et al. Interventions to promote physical activity and dietary lifestyle changes for cardiovascular risk factor reduction in adults: a scientific statement from the American Heart Association. *Circulation.* 2010;122(4):406-41. PMID: 20625115.
48. Academy of Nutrition and Dietetics. Hypertension Evidence-Based Nutrition Practice Guideline. Chicago: Academy of Nutrition and Dietetics; 2008. Accessed at http://www.andeal.org/topic.cfm?cat=3259&auth=1 on 22 July 2014.
49. Academy of Nutrition and Dietetics. Disorders of Lipid Metabolism Update Evidence-Based Nutrition Practice Guideline. Chicago: Academy of Nutrition and Dietetics; 2011. Accessed at http://www.andeal.org/topic.cfm?cat=4528 on 22 July 2014.
50. Hiddink GJ, Hautvast JG, van Woerkum CM, et al. Consumers' expectations about nutrition guidance: the importance of primary care physicians. *Am J Clin Nutr.* 1997;65(6 Suppl):1974S-9. PMID: 9174506.
51. Ayala C, Neff LJ, Croft JB, et al. Prevalence of self-reported high blood pressure awareness, advice received from health professionals, and actions taken to reduce high blood pressure among US adults--Healthstyles 2002. *J Clin Hypertens (Greenwich).* 2005;7(9):513-9. PMID: 16227770.
52. Flocke SA, Clark A, Schlessman K, et al. Exercise, diet, and weight loss advice in the family medicine outpatient setting. *Fam Med.* 2005;37(6):415-21. PMID: 15933194.
53. Barnes PM, Schoenborn CA. Trends in adults receiving a recommendation for exercise or other physical activity from a physician or other health professional. *NCHS Data Brief.* 2012;(86):1-8. PMID: 22617014.
54. Hebert ET, Caughy MO, Shuval K. Primary care providers' perceptions of physical activity counselling in a clinical setting: a systematic review. *Br J Sports Med.* 2012;46(9):625-31. PMID: 22711796.
55. Lin JS, O'Connor E, Whitlock EP, et al. Behavioral counseling to promote physical activity and a healthful diet to prevent cardiovascular disease in adults: a systematic review for the U.S. Preventive Services Task Force. *Ann Intern Med.* 2010;153(11):736-50. PMID: 21135297.
56. Harris RP, Helfand M, Woolf SH, et al. Current methods of the US Preventive Services Task Force: a review of the process. *Am J Prev Med.* 2001;43(3 Suppl):21-35. PMID: 11306229.
57. LeBlanc E, O'Connor E, Whitlock EP, et al. Screening for and Management of Obesity and Overweight in Adults. Evidence Synthesis No. 89. AHRQ Publication No. 11-05159-EF-1. Rockville, MD: Agency for Healthcare Research and Quality; 2011. PMID: 22049569.

58. U.S. Preventive Services Task Force. Screening for and management of obesity in adults: U.S. Preventive Services Task Force recommendation statement. *Ann Intern Med.* 2012;157(5):373-8. PMID: 22733087.
59. U.S. Preventive Services Task Force. Behavioral counseling interventions to promote a healthful diet and physical activity for cardiovascular disease prevention in adults: U.S. Preventive Services Task Force recommendation statement. *Ann Intern Med.* 2012;157(5):367-71. PMID: 22733153.
60. U.S. Preventive Services Task Force. Procedure Manual. Rockville, MD: U.S. Preventive Services Task Force; 2011. Accessed at http://www.uspreventiveservicestaskforce.org/uspstf08/methods/procmanual.htm on 22 July 2014.
61. National Institute for Health and Clinical Excellence. The Guidelines Manual. London: National Institute for Health and Clinical Excellence; 2012. Accessed at http://publications.nice.org.uk/the-guidelines-manual-pmg6 on 22 July 2014.
62. DerSimonian R, Laird N. Meta-analysis in clinical trials. *Control Clin Trials.* 1986;7(3):177-88. PMID: 3802833.
63. Taylor BN, Thompson A (eds). The International System of Units. NIST Special Publication 330. Gaithersburg, MD: National Institute of Standards and Technology; 2008. Accessed at http://physics.nist.gov/Pubs/SP330/sp330.pdf on 22 July 2014.
64. Higgins JP, Thompson SG. Quantifying heterogeneity in a meta-analysis. *Stat Med.* 2002;21(11):1539-58. PMID: 12111919.
65. Egger M, Davey SG, Schneider M, et al. Bias in meta-analysis detected by a simple, graphical test. *BMJ.* 1997;315(7109):629-34. PMID: 9310563.
66. Terrin N, Schmid CH, Lau J. In an empirical evaluation of the funnel plot, researchers could not visually identify publication bias. *J Clin Epidemiol.* 2005;58(9):894-901. PMID: 16085192.
67. Voils CI, Coffman CJ, Yancy WS Jr, et al. A randomized controlled trial to evaluate the effectiveness of CouPLES: a spouse-assisted lifestyle change intervention to improve low-density lipoprotein cholesterol. *Prev Med.* 2013;56(1):46-52. PMID: 23146744.
68. Broekhuizen K, van Poppel MN, Koppes LL, et al. Can multiple lifestyle behaviours be improved in people with familial hypercholesterolemia? Results of a parallel randomised controlled trial. *PLoS One.* 2012;7(12):e50032. PMID: 23251355.
69. Ives DG, Kuller LH, Traven ND. Use and outcomes of a cholesterol-lowering intervention for rural elderly subjects. *Am J Prev Med.* 1993;9(5):274-81. PMID: 8257616.
70. Anderson JW, Garrity TF, Wood CL, et al. Prospective, randomized, controlled comparison of the effects of low-fat and low-fat plus high-fiber diets on serum lipid concentrations. *Am J Clin Nutr.* 1992;56(5):887-94. PMID: 1329482.
71. Stefanick ML, Mackey S, Sheehan M, et al. Effects of diet and exercise in men and postmenopausal women with low levels of HDL cholesterol and high levels of LDL cholesterol. *N Engl J Med.* 1998;339(1):12-20. PMID: 9647874.
72. Delahanty LM, Sonnenberg LM, Hayden D, et al. Clinical and cost outcomes of medical nutrition therapy for hypercholesterolemia: a controlled trial. *J Am Diet Assoc.* 2001;101(9):1012-23. PMID: 11573752.
73. Moy TF, Yanek LR, Raqueño JV, et al. Dietary counseling for high blood cholesterol in families at risk of coronary disease. *Prev Cardiol.* 2001;4(4):158-64. PMID: 11832672.

74. Ammerman AS, Keyserling TC, Atwood JR, et al. A randomized controlled trial of a public health nurse directed treatment program for rural patients with high blood cholesterol. *Prev Med.* 2003;36(3):340-51. PMID: 12634025.
75. Bloemberg BP, Kromhout D, Goddijn HE, et al. The impact of the guidelines for a healthy diet of the Netherlands Nutrition Council on total and high density lipoprotein cholesterol in hypercholesterolemic free-living men. *Am J Epidemiol.* 1991;134(1):39-48. PMID: 1853859.
76. Hyman DJ, Ho KS, Dunn JK, et al. Dietary intervention for cholesterol reduction in public clinic patients. *Am J Prev Med.* 1998;15(2):139-45. PMID: 9713670.
77. Johnston HJ, Jones M, Ridler-Dutton G, et al. Diet modification in lowering plasma cholesterol levels. A randomised trial of three types of intervention. *Med J Aust.* 1995;162(10):524-6. PMID: 7776913.
78. Neil HA, Roe L, Godlee RJ, et al. Randomised trial of lipid lowering dietary advice in general practice: the effects on serum lipids, lipoproteins, and antioxidants. *BMJ.* 1995;310(6979):569-73. PMID: 7888933.
79. van der Veen J, Bakx C, van den Hoogen H, et al. Stage-matched nutrition guidance for patients at elevated risk for cardiovascular disease: a randomized intervention study in family practice. *J Fam Pract.* 2002;51(9):751-8. PMID: 12366892.
80. Anderssen SA. Oslo Diet and Exercise Study: a one year randomized intervention trial. Effect on haemostatic variables and other coronary risk factors. *Nutr Metab Cardiovasc Dis.* 1995;5:189-200.
81. Keyserling TC, Ammerman AS, Davis CE, et al. A randomized controlled trial of a physician-directed treatment program for low-income patients with high blood cholesterol: the Southeast Cholesterol Project. *Arch Fam Med.* 1997;6(2):135-45. PMID: 9075448.
82. Stevens VJ, Glasgow RE, Toobert DJ, et al. One-year results from a brief, computer-assisted intervention to decrease consumption of fat and increase consumption of fruits and vegetables. *Prev Med.* 2003;36(5):594-600. PMID: 12689805.
83. Tomson Y, Johannesson M, Aberg H. The costs and effects of two different lipid intervention programmes in primary health care. *J Intern Med.* 1995;237(1):13-7. PMID: 7830025.
84. Bosworth HB, Olsen MK, Grubber JM, et al. Two self-management interventions to improve hypertension control: a randomized trial. *Ann Intern Med.* 2009;151(10):687-95. PMID: 19920269.
85. Janus ED, Best JD, Davis-Lameloise N, et al. Scaling-up from an implementation trial to state-wide coverage: results from the preliminary Melbourne Diabetes Prevention Study. *Trials.* 2012;13:152. PMID: 22929458.
86. Kanaya AM, Santoyo OJ, Gregorich S, et al. The Live Well, Be Well Study: a community-based, translational lifestyle program to lower diabetes risk factors in ethnic minority and lower-socioeconomic status adults. *Am J Pub Health.* 2012;102:1551-8. PMID: 22698027.
87. Ma J, Yank V, Xiao L, et al. Translating the Diabetes Prevention Program lifestyle intervention for weight loss into primary care: a randomized trial. *JAMA Intern Med.* 2013;173:113-21. PMID: 23229846.

88. Vermunt PW, Milder IE, Wielaard F, et al. Lifestyle counseling for type 2 diabetes risk reduction in Dutch primary care: results of the APHRODITE study after 0.5 and 1.5 years. *Diabetes Care*. 2011;34(9):1919-25. PMID: 21775759.
89. Knowler WC, Barrett CE, Fowler SE, et al. Reduction in the incidence of type 2 diabetes with lifestyle intervention or metformin. *New Engl J Med*. 2002;346:393-403. PMID: 11832527.
90. Oldroyd JC, Unwin NC, White M, et al. Randomised controlled trial evaluating the effectiveness of behavioural interventions to modify cardiovascular risk factors in men and women with impaired glucose tolerance: outcomes at 6 months. *Diabetes Res Clin Pract*. 2001;52(1):29-43. PMID: 11182214.
91. Penn L, White M, Oldroyd J, et al. Prevention of type 2 diabetes in adults with impaired glucose tolerance: the European Diabetes Prevention RCT in Newcastle upon Tyne, UK. *BMC Public Health*. 2009;9:342. PMID: 19758428.
92. Moore SM, Hardie EA, Hackworth NJ, et al. Can the onset of type 2 diabetes be delayed by a group-based lifestyle intervention? A randomised control trial. *Psychol Health*. 2011;26(4):485-99. PMID: 20945253.
93. Kosaka K, Noda M, Kuzuya T. Prevention of type 2 diabetes by lifestyle intervention: a Japanese trial in IGT males. *Diabetes Res Clin Pract*. 2005;67(2):152-62. PMID: 15649575.
94. Ockene IS, Tellez TL, Rosal MC, et al. Outcomes of a Latino community-based intervention for the prevention of diabetes: the Lawrence Latino Diabetes Prevention Project. *Am J Pub Health*. 2012;102(2):336-42. PMID: 22390448.
95. Kulzer B, Hermanns N, Gorges D, et al. Prevention of Diabetes Self-Management Program (PREDIAS): effects on weight, metabolic risk factors, and behavioral outcomes. *Diabetes Care*. 2009;32(7):1143-6. PMID: 19509014.
96. Mensink M, Corpeleijn E, Feskens EJ, et al. Study on Lifestyle-Intervention and impaired Glucose Tolerance Maastricht (SLIM): design and screening results. *Diabetes Res Clin Pract*. 2003;61:49-58. PMID: 12849923.
97. Watanabe M, Yamaoka K, Yokotsuka M, et al. Randomized controlled trial of a new dietary education program to prevent type 2 diabetes in a high-risk group of Japanese male workers. *Diabetes Care*. 2003;26(12):3209-14. PMID: 14633803.
98. Morey MC, Pieper CF, Edelman DE, et al. Enhanced fitness: a randomized controlled trial of the effects of home-based physical activity counseling on glycemic control in older adults with prediabetes mellitus. *J Am Geriatr Soc*. 2012;60(9):1655-62. PMID: 22985140.
99. Yates T, Davies M, Gorely T, et al. Effectiveness of a pragmatic education program designed to promote walking activity in individuals with impaired glucose tolerance: a randomized controlled trial. *Diabetes Care*. 2009;32(8):1404-10. PMID: 19602539.
100. Tiessen AH, Smit AJ, Broer J, et al. Randomized controlled trial on cardiovascular risk management by practice nurses supported by self-monitoring in primary care. *BMC Fam Pract*. 2012;13:90. PMID: 22947269.
101. Lakerveld J, Bot SD, Chinapaw MJ, et al. Primary prevention of diabetes mellitus type 2 and cardiovascular diseases using a cognitive behavior program aimed at lifestyle changes in people at risk: design of a randomized controlled trial. *BMC Endocr Disord*. 2008;8:6. PMID: 18573221.

102. Cochrane T, Davey R, Iqbal Z, et al. NHS health checks through general practice: randomised trial of population cardiovascular risk reduction. *BMC Public Health.* 2012;12:944. PMID: 23116213.
103. Harris MF, Fanaian M, Jayasinghe UW, et al. A cluster randomised controlled trial of vascular risk factor management in general practice. *Med J Aust.* 2012;197:387-93. PMID: 23025735.
104. Moreau KL, Degarmo R, Langley J, et al. Increasing daily walking lowers blood pressure in postmenopausal women. Med Sci Sports Exerc. 2001;33:1825-31. PMID: 11689731.
105. van Keulen HM, Mesters I, Ausems M, et al. Tailored print communication and telephone motivational interviewing are equally successful in improving multiple lifestyle behaviors in a randomized controlled trial. *Ann Behav Med.* 2011;41(1):104-18. PMID: 20878293.
106. Wood DA, Kotseva K, Connolly S, et al. Nurse-coordinated multidisciplinary, family-based cardiovascular disease prevention programme (EUROACTION) for patients with coronary heart disease and asymptomatic individuals at high risk of cardiovascular disease: a paired, cluster-randomised controlled trial. *Lancet.* 2008;371:1999-2012. PMID: 18555911.
107. Toft U, Kristoffersen L, Ladelund S, et al. The effect of adding group-based counselling to individual lifestyle counselling on changes in dietary intake. The Inter99 study--a randomized controlled trial. *Int J Behav Nutr Phys Act.* 2008;5:59. PMID: 19025583.
108. Hayashi T, Farrell MA, Chaput LA, et al. Lifestyle intervention, behavioral changes, and improvement in cardiovascular risk profiles in the California WISEWOMAN project. *J Womens Health (Larchmt).* 2010;19(6):1129-38. PMID: 20509780.
109. Murphy SM, Edwards RT, Williams N, et al. An evaluation of the effectiveness and cost effectiveness of the National Exercise Referral Scheme in Wales, UK: a randomised controlled trial of a public health policy initiative. *J Epidemiol Community Health.* 2012;66(8):745-53. PMID: 22577180.
110. Keyserling TC, Samuel Hodge CD, Jilcott SB, et al. Randomized trial of a clinic-based, community-supported, lifestyle intervention to improve physical activity and diet: the North Carolina enhanced WISEWOMAN project. *Prev Med.* 2008;46(6):499-510. PMID: 18394692.
111. Beckmann SL, Os I, Kjeldsen SE, et al. Effect of dietary counselling on blood pressure and arterial plasma catecholamines in primary hypertension. *Am J Hypertens.* 1995;8(7):704-11. PMID: 7546496.
112. Fagerberg B, Wikstrand J, Berglund G, et al. Mortality rates in treated hypertensive men with additional risk factors are high but can be reduced: a randomized intervention study. *Am J Hypertens.* 1998;11(1 Pt 1):14-22. PMID: 9504445.
113. Rodriguez MA. Is behavior change sustainable for diet, exercise, and medication adherence? *Diss Abstr Int B Sci Eng.* 2012;73(3B):1860.
114. Eakin E, Reeves M, Lawler S, et al. Telephone counseling for physical activity and diet in primary care patients. *Am J Prev Med.* 2009;36(2):142-9. PMID: 19062240.
115. Agewall S, Wikstrand J, Samuelsson O, et al. The efficacy of multiple risk factor intervention in treated hypertensive men during long-term follow up. *J Intern Med.* 1994;236(6):651-9. PMID: 7989900.

116. Appel LJ, Champagne CM, Harsha DW, et al. Effects of comprehensive lifestyle modification on blood pressure control: main results of the PREMIER clinical trial. *JAMA*. 2003;289:2083-93. PMID: 12709466.

117. Whelton PK, Appel LJ, Espeland MA, et al. Sodium reduction and weight loss in the treatment of hypertension in older persons: a randomized controlled trial of nonpharmacologic interventions in the elderly (TONE). *JAMA*. 1998;279(11):839-46. PMID: 9515998.

118. Tuomilehto J, Lindström J, Eriksson JG, et al. Prevention of type 2 diabetes mellitus by changes in lifestyle among subjects with impaired glucose tolerance. *New Engl J Med*. 2001;344:1343-50. PMID: 11333990.

119. Nilsson PM, Lindholm LH, Schersten BF. Life style changes improve insulin resistance in hyperinsulinaemic subjects: a one-year intervention study of hypertensives and normotensives in Dalby. *J Hypertens*. 1992;10(9):1071-8. PMID: 1328367.

120. Bruckert E, Giral P, Paillard F, et al. Effect of an educational program (PEGASE) on cardiovascular risk in hypercholesterolaemic patients. *Cardiovasc Drugs Ther*. 2008;22(6):495-505. PMID: 18830810.

121. Babazono A, Kame C, Ishihara R, et al. Patient-motivated prevention of lifestyle-related disease in Japan: a randomized, controlled clinical trial. *Dis Manage Health Outcomes*. 2007;15(2):119-26.

122. Fortier MS, Hogg W, O'Sullivan TL, et al. Impact of integrating a physical activity counsellor into the primary health care team: physical activity and health outcomes of the Physical Activity Counselling randomized controlled trial. *Appl Physiol Nutr Metab*. 2011;36(4):503-14. PMID: 21848444.

123. Elley CR, Kerse N, Arroll B, et al. Effectiveness of counselling patients on physical activity in general practice: cluster randomised controlled trial. *BMJ*. 2003;326:793. PMID: 12689976.

124. Uusitupa M, Peltonen M, Lindström J, et al. Ten-year mortality and cardiovascular morbidity in the Finnish Diabetes Prevention Study--secondary analysis of the randomized trial. *PLoS One*. 2009;4:e5656. PMID: 19479072.

125. Young DR, Coughlin J, Jerome GJ, et al. Effects of the PREMIER interventions on health-related quality of life. *Ann Behav Med*. 2010;40:302-12. PMID: 20799005.

126. Migneault JP, Dedier JJ, Wright JA, et al. A culturally adapted telecommunication system to improve physical activity, diet quality, and medication adherence among hypertensive African-Americans: a randomized controlled trial. *Ann Behav Med*. 2012;43(1):62-73. PMID: 22246660.

127. Applegate WB, Miller ST, Elam JT, et al. Nonpharmacologic intervention to reduce blood pressure in older patients with mild hypertension. *Arch Intern Med*. 1992;152(6):1162-6. PMID: 1599343.

128. Arroll B, Beaglehole R. Salt restriction and physical activity in treated hypertensives. *N Z Med J*. 1995;108(1003):266-8. PMID: 7637923.

129. Edelman D, Oddone EZ, Liebowitz RS, et al. A multidimensional integrative medicine intervention to improve cardiovascular risk. *J Gen Intern Med*. 2006;21(7):728-34. PMID: 16808774.

130. Van Roie E, Delecluse C, Opdenacker J, et al. Effectiveness of a lifestyle physical activity versus a structured exercise intervention in older adults. *J Aging Phys Act*. 2010;18(3):335-52. PMID: 20651418.

131. Sluijs EM, Poppel MN, Twisk JW, et al. Effect of a tailored physical activity intervention delivered in general practice settings: results of a randomized controlled trial. *Am J Public Health*. 2005;95:1825-31. PMID: 16186461.
132. Lakerveld J, Bot SD, Chinapaw MJ, et al. Motivational interviewing and problem solving treatment to reduce type 2 diabetes and cardiovascular disease risk in real life: a randomized controlled trial. *Int J Behav Nutr Phys Act*. 2013;10:47. PMID: 23597082.
133. Koelewijn-van Loon MS, van der Weijden T, van Steenkiste B, et al. Involving patients in cardiovascular risk management with nurse-led clinics: a cluster randomized controlled trial. *CMAJ*. 2009;181(12):E267-74. PMID: 19948811.
134. Muhlhauser I, Sawicki PT, Didjurgeit U, et al. Evaluation of a structured treatment and teaching programme on hypertension in general practice. *Clin Exp Hypertens*. 1993;15(1):125-42. PMID: 8467308.
135. Hyman DJ, Pavlik VN, Taylor WC, et al. Simultaneous vs sequential counseling for multiple behavior change. *Arch Intern Med*. 2007;167(11):1152-8. PMID: 17563023.
136. Svetkey LP, Pollak KI, Yancy WS Jr, et al. Hypertension Improvement Project: randomized trial of quality improvement for physicians and lifestyle modification for patients. *Hypertension*. 2009;54(6):1226-33. PMID: 19920081.
137. Kastarinen MJ, Puska PM, Korhonen MH, et al. Non-pharmacological treatment of hypertension in primary health care: a 2-year open randomized controlled trial of lifestyle intervention against hypertension in eastern Finland. *J Hypertens*. 2002;20(12):2505-12. PMID: 12473876.
138. Burke V, Beilin L, Cutt H, et al. A lifestyle program for treated hypertensives improves cardiovascular risk factors: a randomized controlled trial. *J Clin Epidemiol*. 2007;60(2):133-41. PMID: 17208119.
139. Ter Bogt NC, Bemelmans WJ, Beltman FW, et al. Preventing weight gain: one-year results of a randomized lifestyle intervention. *Am J Prev Med*. 2009;37(4):270-7. PMID: 19765497.
140. Wister A, Loewen N, Kennedy-Symonds H, et al. One-year follow-up of a therapeutic lifestyle intervention targeting cardiovascular disease risk. *CMAJ*. 2007;177(8):859-65. PMID: 17923653.
141. Kallings LV, Sierra JJ, Fisher RM, et al. Beneficial effects of individualized physical activity on prescription on body composition and cardiometabolic risk factors: results from a randomized controlled trial. *Eur J Cardiovasc Prev Rehabil*. 2009;16(1):80-4. PMID: 19237997.
142. Burke V, Beilin LJ, Cutt HE, et al. Effects of a lifestyle programme on ambulatory blood pressure and drug dosage in treated hypertensive patients: a randomized controlled trial. *J Hypertens*. 2005;23:1241-9. PMID: 15894901.
143. Svetkey LP, Erlinger TP, Vollmer WM, et al. Effect of lifestyle modifications on blood pressure by race, sex, hypertension status, and age. *J Human Hypertens*. 2005;19:21-31. PMID: 15385946.
144. Broekhuizen K, van Poppel MN, Koppes LL, et al. A tailored lifestyle intervention to reduce the cardiovascular disease risk of individuals with familial hypercholesterolemia (FH): design of the PRO-FIT randomised controlled trial. *BMC Public Health*. 2010;10:69. PMID: 20156339.

145. Burke V, Beilin LJ, Cutt HE, et al. Moderators and mediators of behaviour change in a lifestyle program for treated hypertensives: a randomized controlled trial (ADAPT). *Health Educ Res.* 2008;23:583-91. PMID: 17890759.

146. Bo S, Ciccone G, Baldi C, et al. Effectiveness of a lifestyle intervention on metabolic syndrome. A randomized controlled trial. *J Gen Intern Med.* 2007;22(12):1695-703. PMID: 17922167.

147. Lin PH, Yancy WS Jr, Pollak KI, et al. The influence of a physician and patient intervention program on dietary intake. *J Acad Nutr Diet.* 2013;113(11):1465-75. PMID: 23999279.

148. Anderssen S, Holme I, Urdal P, et al. Diet and exercise intervention have favourable effects on blood pressure in mild hypertensives: the Oslo Diet and Exercise Study (ODES). *Blood Press.* 1995;4(6):343-9. PMID: 8746601.

149. Roumen C, Feskens EJ, Corpeleijn E, et al. Predictors of lifestyle intervention outcome and dropout: the SLIM study. *Eur J Clin Nutr.* 2011;65(10):1141-7. PMID: 21587283.

150. Ammerman A, Pignone M, Fernandez L, et al. Counseling to Promote a Healthy Diet. Systematic Evidence Review No. 18. Rockville, MD: Agency for Healthcare Research and Quality; 2002. PMID: 20722113.

151. Eden KB, Orleans CT, Mulrow CD, et al. Clinician Counseling to Promote Physical Activity. Systematic Evidence Review No. 9. Rockville, MD: Agency for Healthcare Research and Quality; 2002. PMID: 20722178.

152. Baker MK, Simpson K, Lloyd B, et al. Behavioral strategies in diabetes prevention programs: a systematic review of randomized controlled trials. *Diabetes Res Clin Pract.* 2011;91(1):1-12. PMID: 20655610.

153. Gillett M, Royle P, Snaith A, et al. Non-pharmacological interventions to reduce the risk of diabetes in people with impaired glucose regulation: a systematic review and economic evaluation. *Health Technol Assess.* 2012;16(33):1-236. PMID: 22935084.

154. Hopper I, Billah B, Skiba M, et al. Prevention of diabetes and reduction in major cardiovascular events in studies of subjects with prediabetes: meta-analysis of randomised controlled clinical trials. *Eur J Cardiovasc Prev Rehabil.* 2011;18(6):813-23. PMID: 21878448.

155. Schellenberg ES, Dryden DM, Vandermeer B, et al. Lifestyle interventions for patients with and at risk for type 2 diabetes: a systematic review and meta-analysis. *Ann Intern Med.* 2013;159(8):543-51. PMID: 24126648.

156. Ebrahim S, Taylor F, Ward K, et al. Multiple risk factor interventions for primary prevention of coronary heart disease. *Cochrane Database Syst Rev.* 2011;(1):CD001561. PMID: 21249647.

157. Law MR, Wald NJ, Thompson SG. By how much and how quickly does reduction in serum cholesterol concentration lower risk of ischaemic heart disease? *BMJ.* 1994;308(6925):367-72. PMID: 8043072.

158. Cook NR, Cutler JA, Obarzanek E, et al. Long term effects of dietary sodium reduction on cardiovascular disease outcomes: observational follow-up of the Trials of Hypertension Prevention (TOHP). *BMJ.* 2007;334(7599):885-8. PMID: 17449506.

159. MacMahon S, Peto R, Cutler J, et al. Blood pressure, stroke, and coronary heart disease, 1: prolonged differences in blood pressure: prospective observational studies corrected for the regression dilution bias. *Lancet.* 1990;335(8692):765-74. PMID: 1969518.

160. Jensen MD, Ryan DH, Apovian CM, et al. 2013 AHA/ACC/TOS guideline for the management of overweight and obesity in adults: a report of the American College of Cardiology/American Heart Association Task Force on Practice Guidelines and the Obesity Society. *J Am Coll Cardiol.* 2014;63(25 Pt B):2985-3023. PMID: 24239920.
161. Danaei G, Ding EL, Mozaffarian D, et al. The preventable causes of death in the United States: comparative risk assessment of dietary, lifestyle, and metabolic risk factors. *PLoS Med.* 2009;6(4):e1000058. PMID: 19399161.
162. U.S. Department of Health and Human Services. 2008 Physical Activity Guidelines for Americans. Washington, DC: U.S. Department of Health and Human Services; 2008. Accessed at http://www.health.gov/paguidelines/pdf/paguide.pdf on 22 July 2014.
163. Sattelmair J, Pertman J, Ding EL, et al. Dose response between physical activity and risk of coronary heart disease: a meta-analysis. *Circulation.* 2011;124(7):789-95. PMID: 2180663.
164. Garber CE, Blissmer B, Deschenes MR, et al. American College of Sports Medicine position stand. Quantity and quality of exercise for developing and maintaining cardiorespiratory, musculoskeletal, and neuromotor fitness in apparently healthy adults: guidance for prescribing exercise. *Med Sci Sports Exerc.* 2011;43(7):1334-59. PMID: 21694556.
165. Zheng H, Orsini N, Amin J, et al. Quantifying the dose-response of walking in reducing coronary heart disease risk: meta-analysis. *Eur J Epidemiol.* 2009;24(4):181-92. PMID: 19306107.
166. U.S. Department of Health and Human Services. 2008 Physical Activity Guidelines for Americans Summary. Washington, DC: U.S. Department of Health and Human Services; 2014. Accessed at http://www.health.gov/paguidelines/guidelines/summary.aspx on 22 July 2014.
167. Murphy S, Raisanen L, Moore G, et al. A pragmatic randomised controlled trial of the Welsh National Exercise Referral Scheme: protocol for trial and integrated economic and process evaluation. *BMC Public Health.* 2010;10:352. PMID: 20565846.
168. Hardcastle S, Taylor A, Bailey M, et al. A randomised controlled trial on the effectiveness of a primary health care based counselling intervention on physical activity, diet and CHD risk factors. *Patient Educ Counsel.* 2008;70(1):31-9. PMID: 17997263.
169. Michie S, Abraham C, Whittington C, et al. Effective techniques in healthy eating and physical activity interventions: a meta-regression. *Health Psychol.* 2009;28(6):690-701.
170. Greaves CJ, Sheppard KE, Abraham C, et al. Systematic review of reviews of intervention components associated with increased effectiveness in dietary and physical activity interventions. *BMC Public Health.* 2011;11:119.
171. Zaza S, Lawrence RS, Mahan CS, et al. Scope and organization of the Guide to Community Preventive Services. *Am J Prev Med.* 2000;18(1 Suppl):27-34. PMID: 10806977.
172. Look AHEAD Research Group; Wing RR, Bolin P, et al. Cardiovascular effects of intensive lifestyle intervention in type 2 diabetes. *New Engl J Med.* 2013;369(2):145-54. PMID: 23796131.
173. Rodriguez Cristobal JJ, Alonso-Villaverde GC, Trave MP, et al. Randomised clinical trial of an intensive intervention in the primary care setting of patients with high plasma fibrinogen in the primary prevention of cardiovascular disease. *BMC Res Notes.* 2012;5:126. PMID: 22381072.

174. Keyserling TC, Ammerman AS, Atwood JR, et al. A cholesterol intervention program for public health nurses in the rural southeast: description of the intervention, study design, and baseline results. *Public Health Nurs.* 1999;16(3):156-67. PMID: 10388332.
175. Tomson Y, Aberg H. Risk factors for cardiovascular disease--a comparison between Swedes and immigrants. *Scand J Prim Health Care.* 1994;12(3):147-54. PMID: 7997691.
176. Kallings LV. Physical Activity on Prescription: Studies on Physical Activity Level, Adherence, and Cardiovascular Risk Factors [Dissertation]. Stockholm: Karolinska Institutet; 2008. Accessed at http://diss.kib.ki.se/2008/978-91-7409-111-3/thesis.pdf on 22 July 2014.

Figure 1. Analytic Framework: Behavioral Counseling to Promote a Healthy Lifestyle for Cardiovascular Disease Prevention in Persons With Cardiovascular Risk Factors

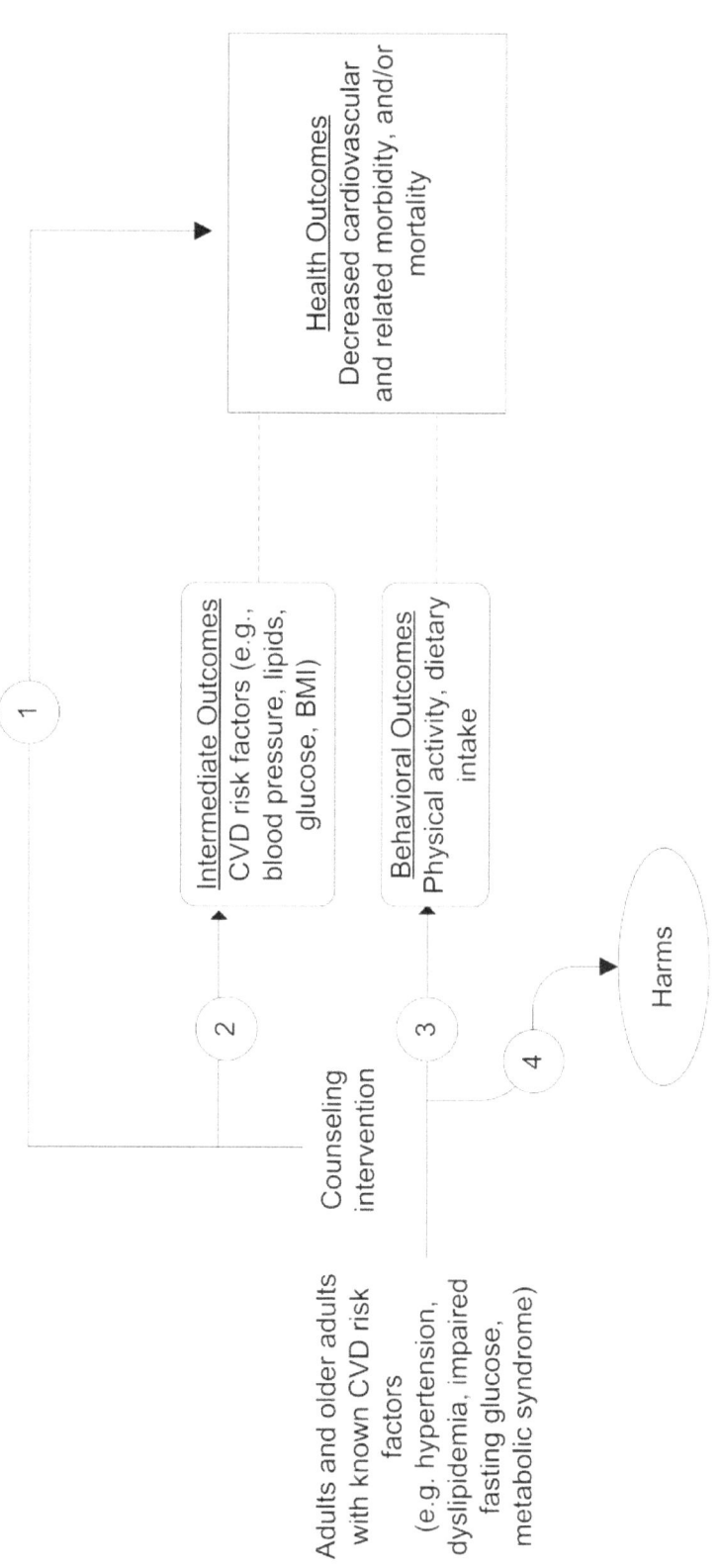

Abbreviations: CVD = cardiovascular disease; BMI = body mass index.

Figure 2. Pooled Analysis of Total Cholesterol in Persons With Dyslipidemia, Sorted by Length of Followup Time

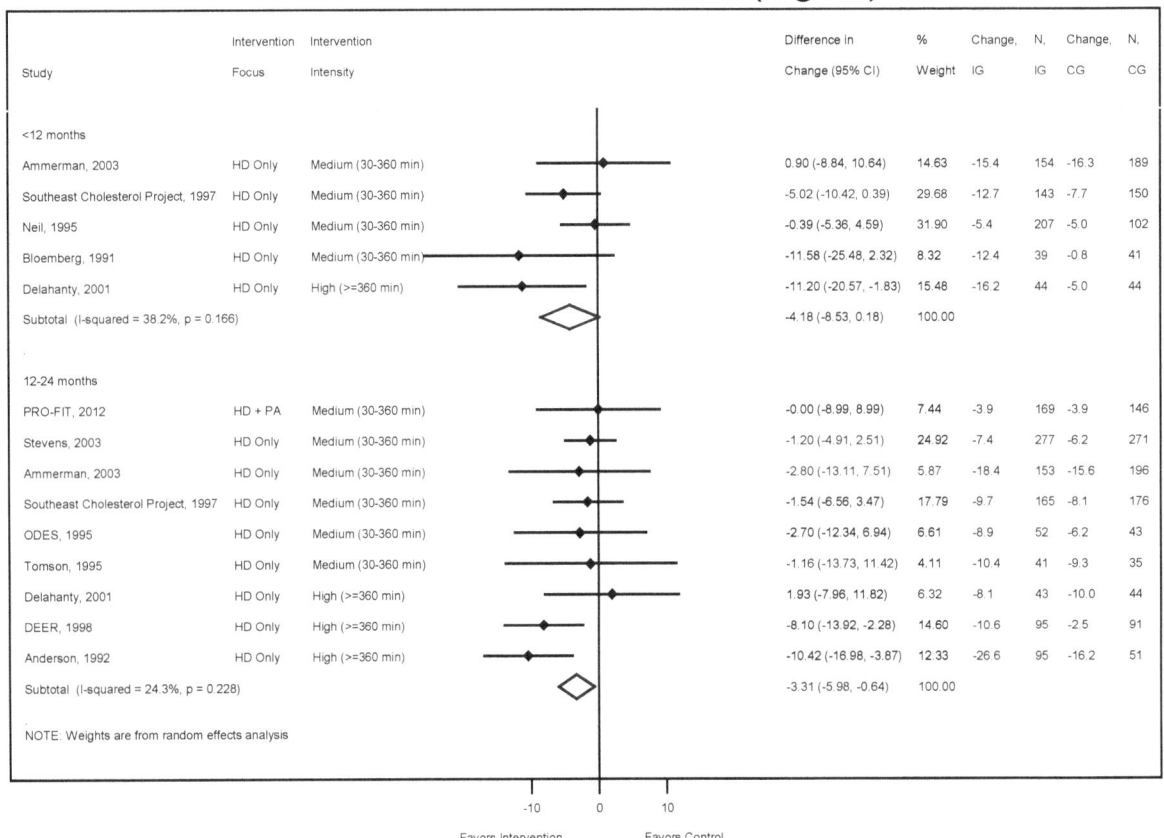

Figure 3. Pooled Analysis of Low-Density Lipoprotein Cholesterol in Persons With Dyslipidemia, Sorted by Length of Followup Time

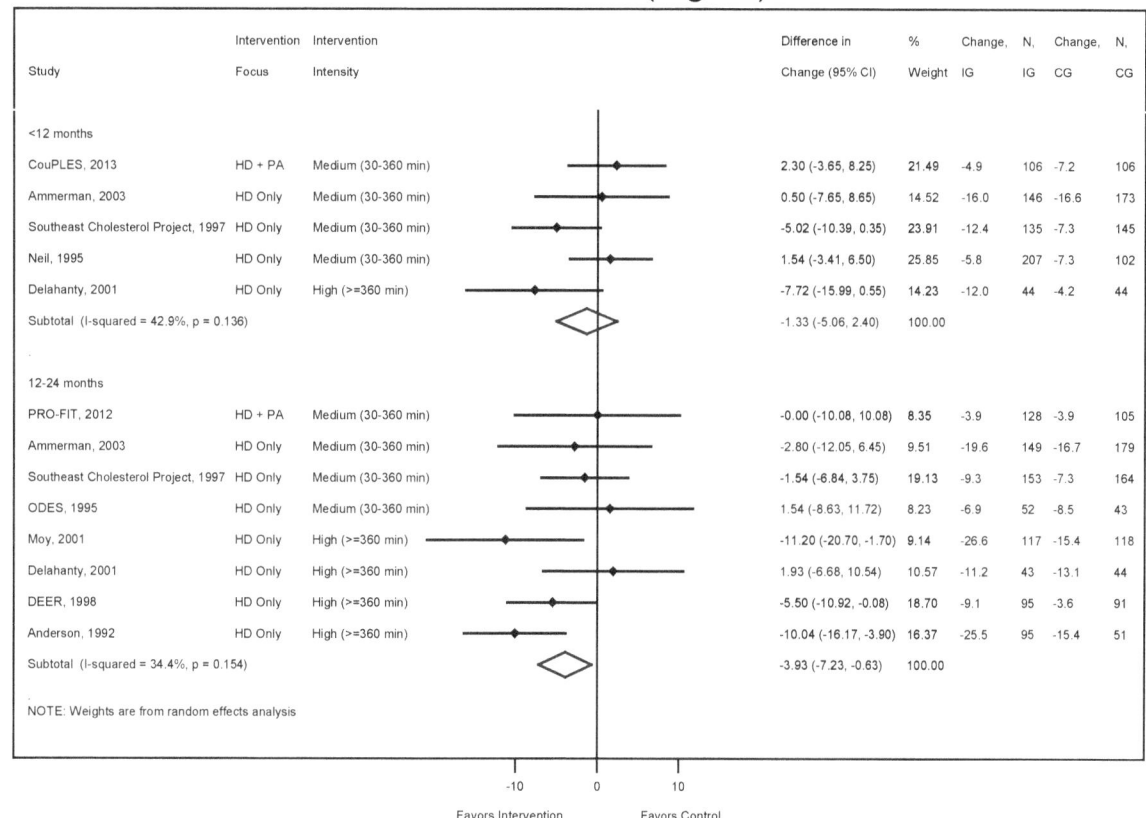

Figure 4. Pooled Analysis of Total Cholesterol in Persons With Dyslipidemia or Multiple Risk Factors, Sorted by Length of Followup Time

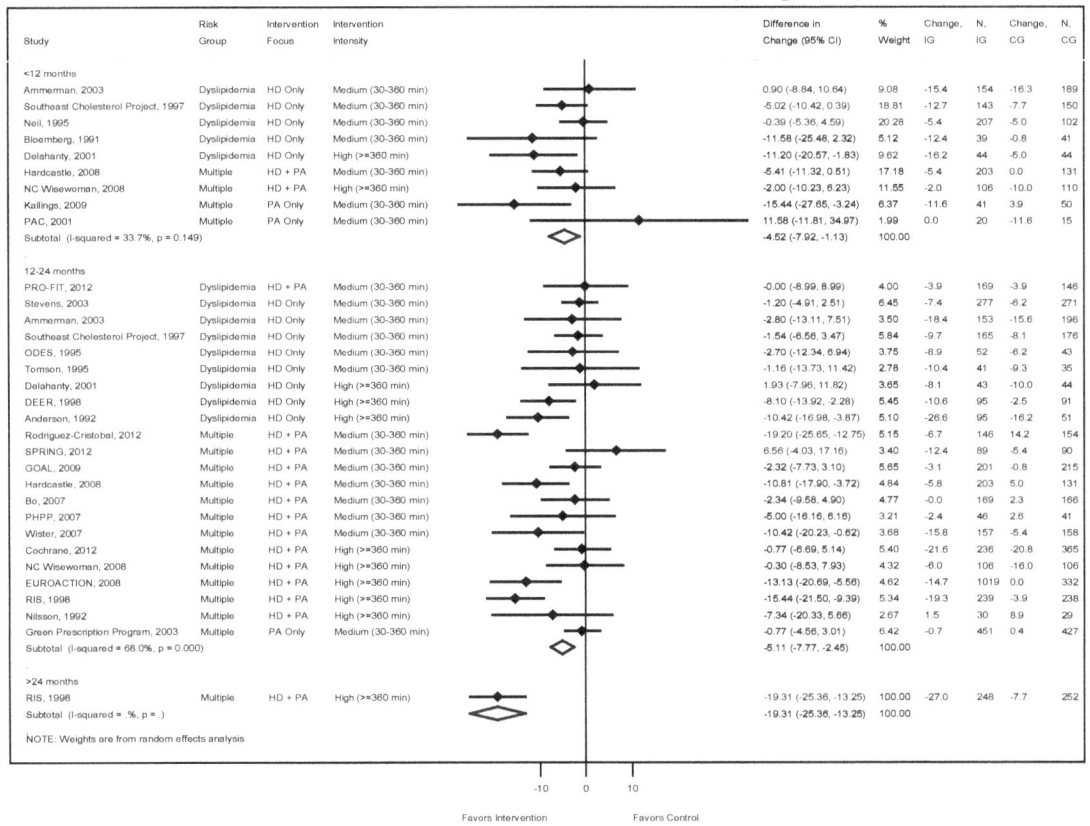

Figure 5. Pooled Analysis of Low-Density Lipoprotein Cholesterol in Persons With Dyslipidemia or Multiple Risk Factors, Sorted by Length of Followup Time

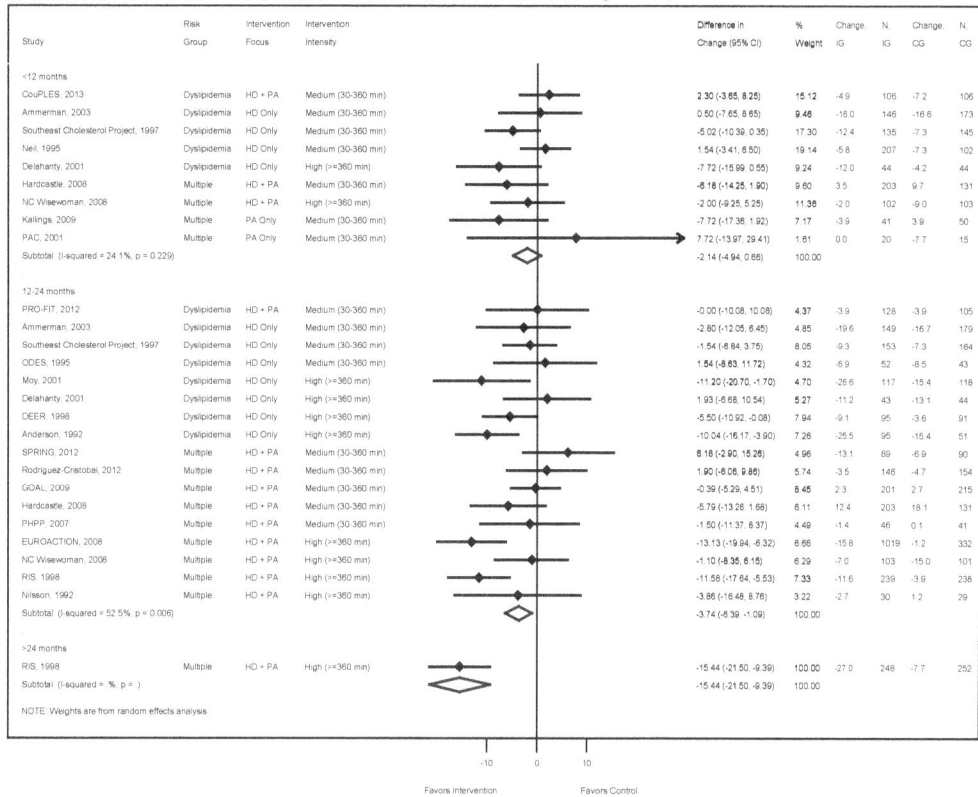

Figure 6. Pooled Analysis of Weight in Persons With Dyslipidemia or Multiple Risk Factors, Sorted by Length of Followup Time

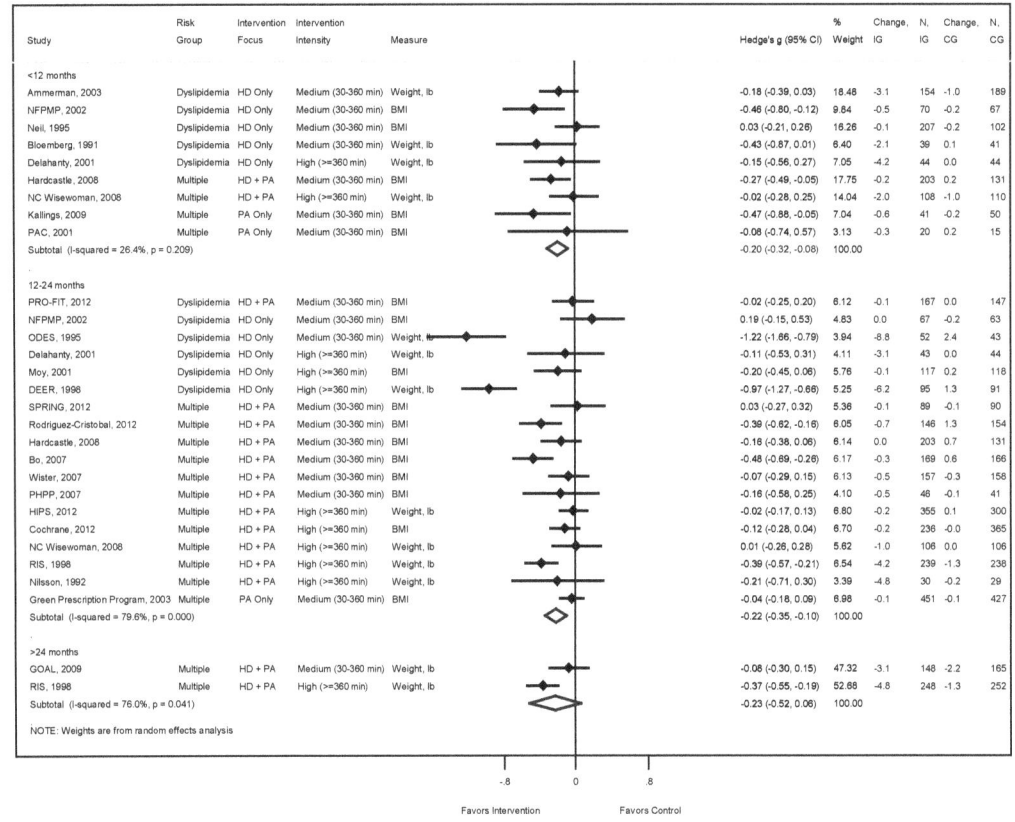

Figure 7. Pooled Analysis of Systolic Blood Pressure in Persons With Hypertension, Sorted by Length of Followup Time

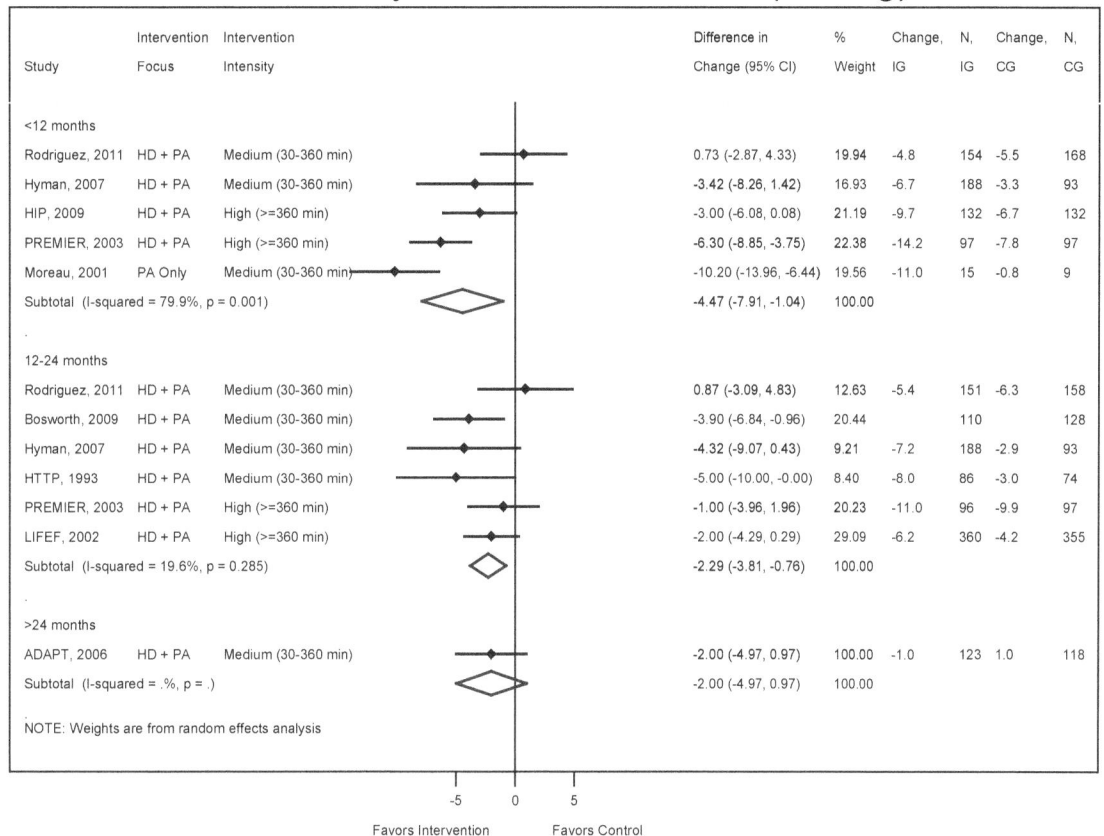

Figure 8. Pooled Analysis of Diastolic Blood Pressure in Persons With Hypertension, Sorted by Length of Followup Time

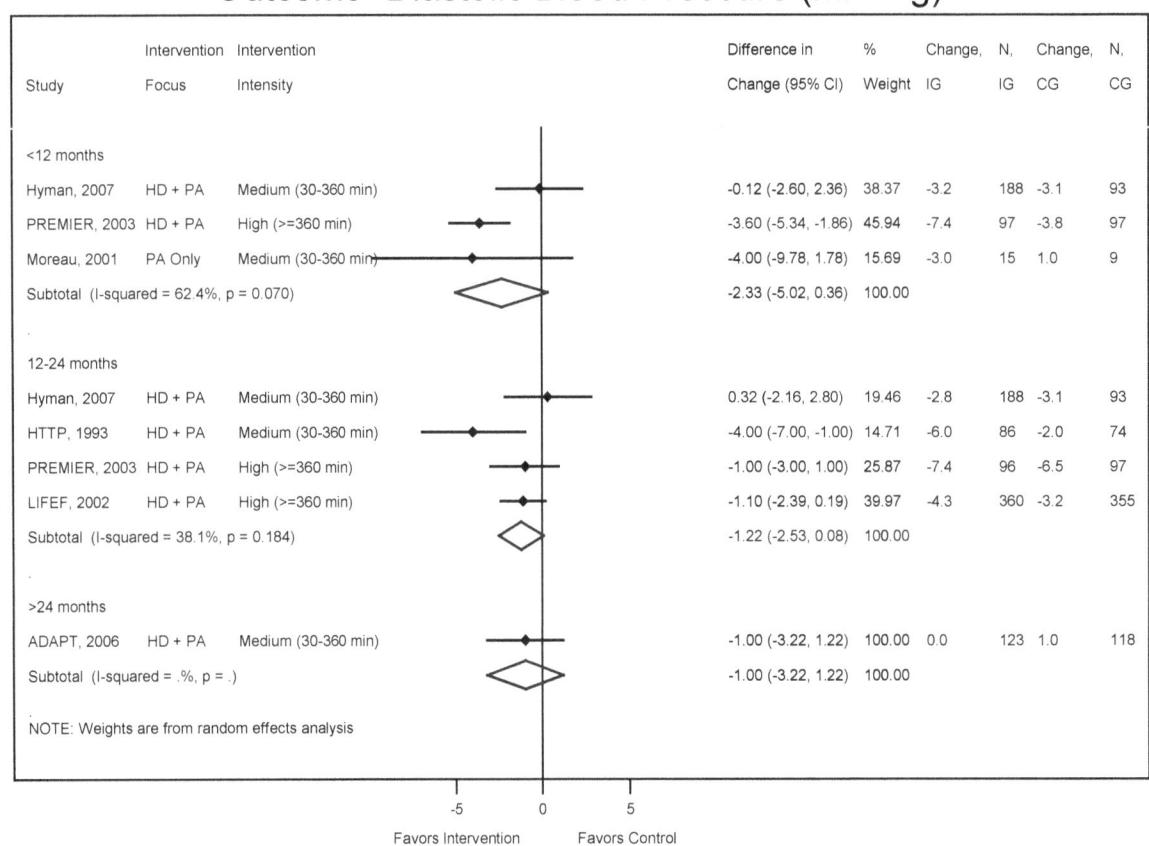

Figure 9. Pooled Analysis of Systolic Blood Pressure in Persons With Hypertension or Multiple Risk Factors, Sorted by Length of Followup Time

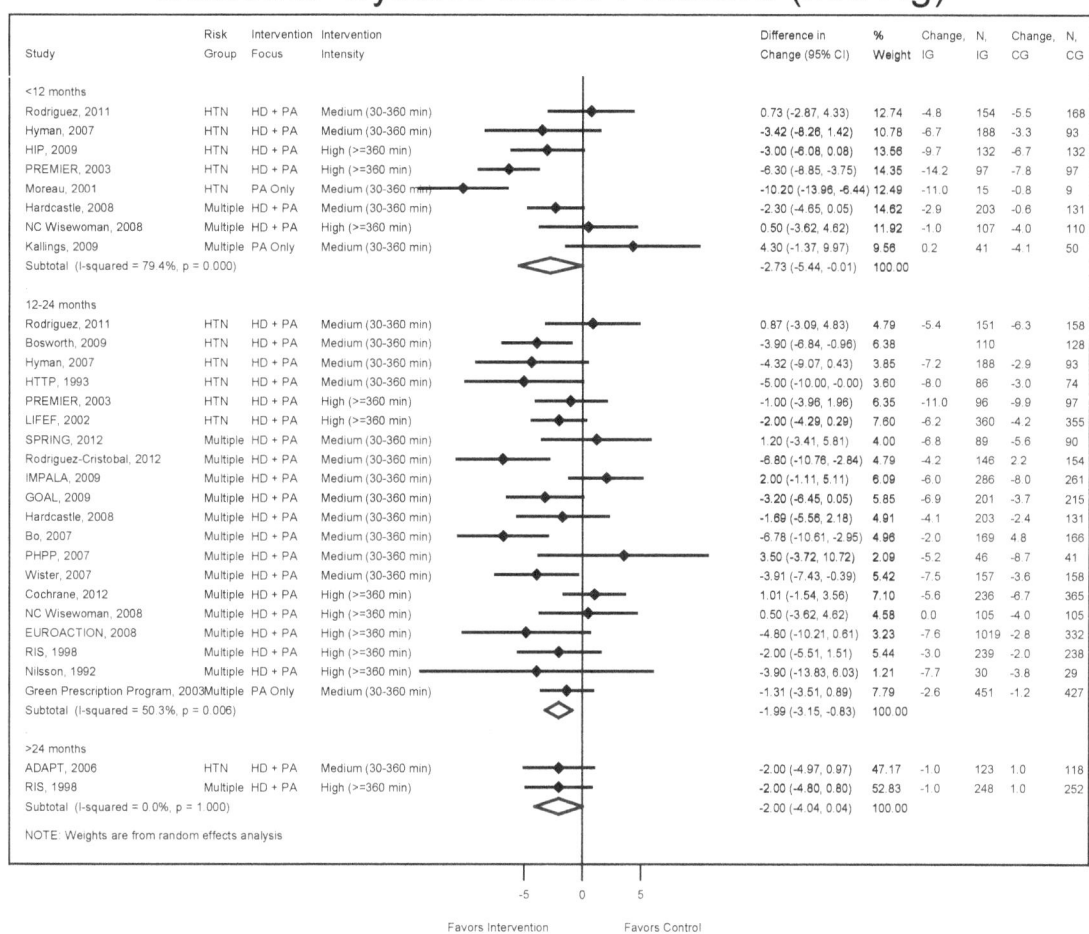

Figure 10. Pooled Analysis of Diastolic Blood Pressure in Persons With Hypertension or Multiple Risk Factors, Sorted by Length of Followup Time

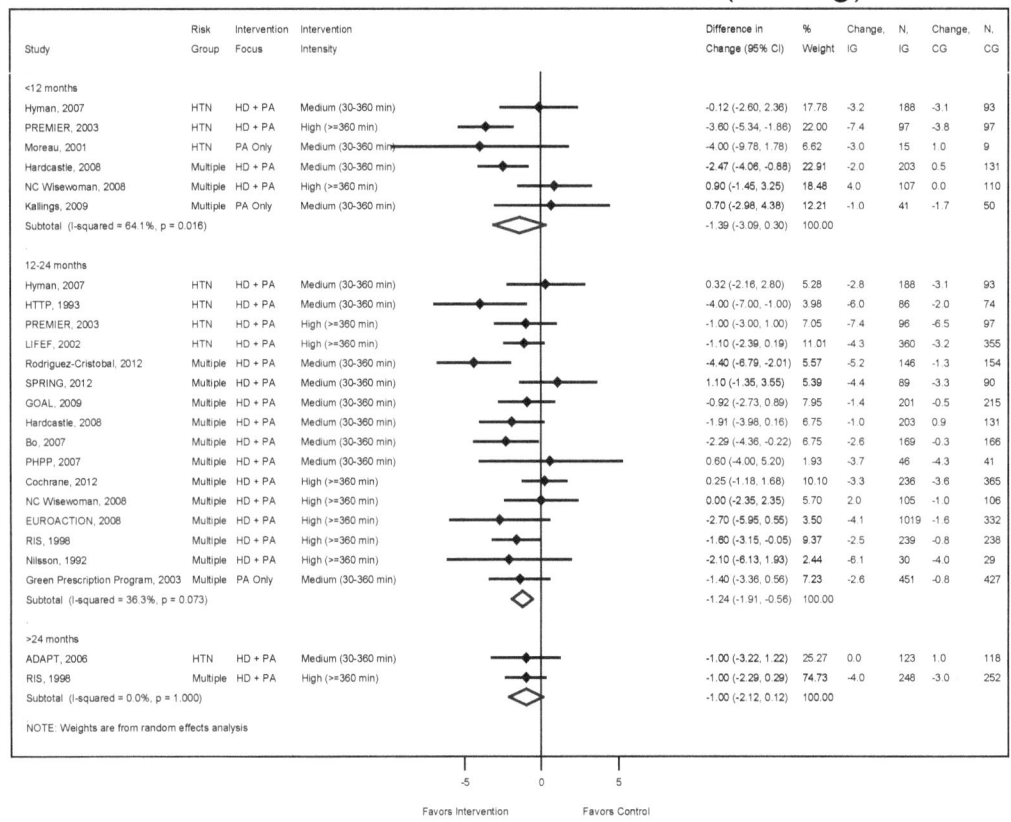

Figure 11. Pooled Analysis of Weight in Persons With Hypertension or Multiple Risk Factors, Sorted by Length of Followup Time

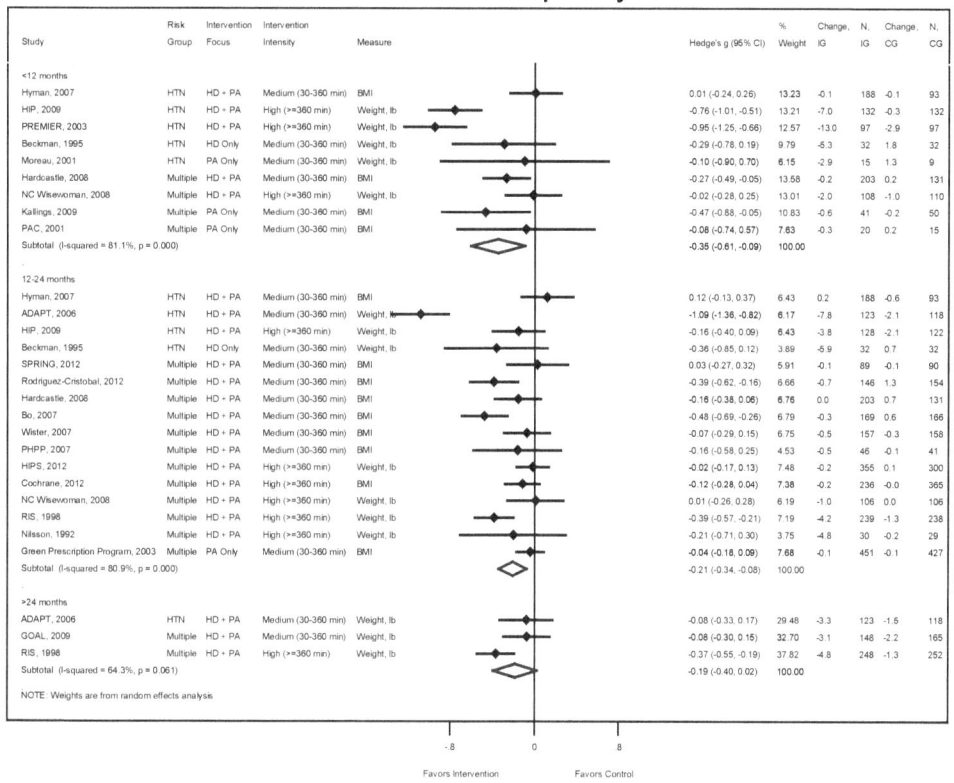

Figure 12. Pooled Analysis of Diabetes Incidence in Persons With Impaired Fasting Glucose or Impaired Glucose Tolerance, Sorted by Length of Followup Time

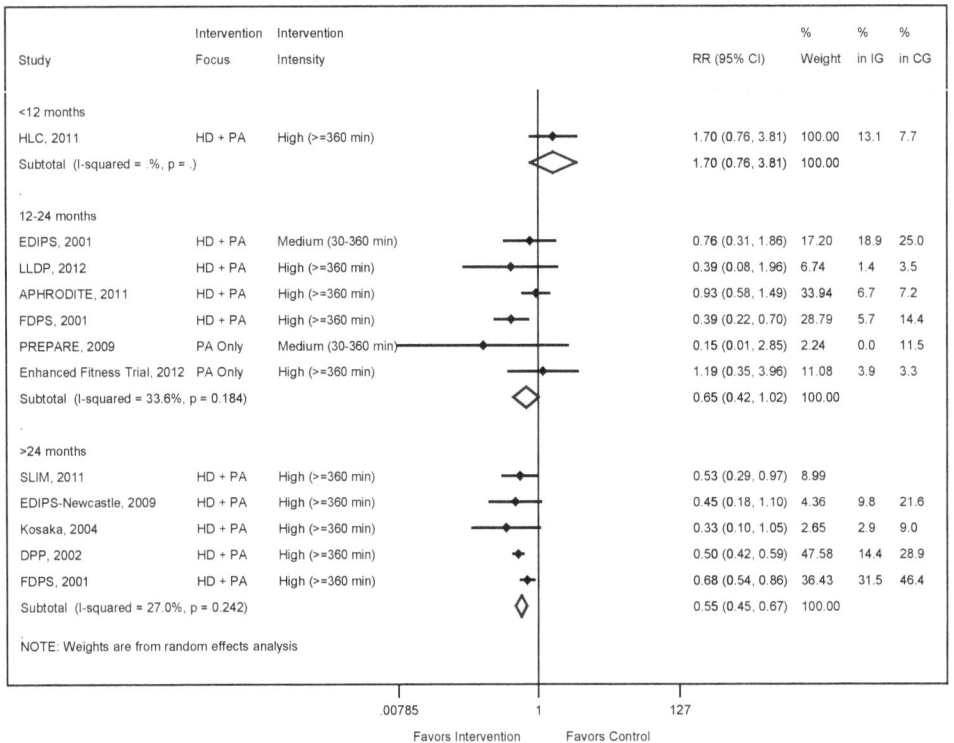

Figure 13. Pooled Analysis of Diabetes Incidence in Persons With Impaired Fasting Glucose, Impaired Glucose Tolerance, or Multiple Risk Factors, Sorted by Length of Followup Time

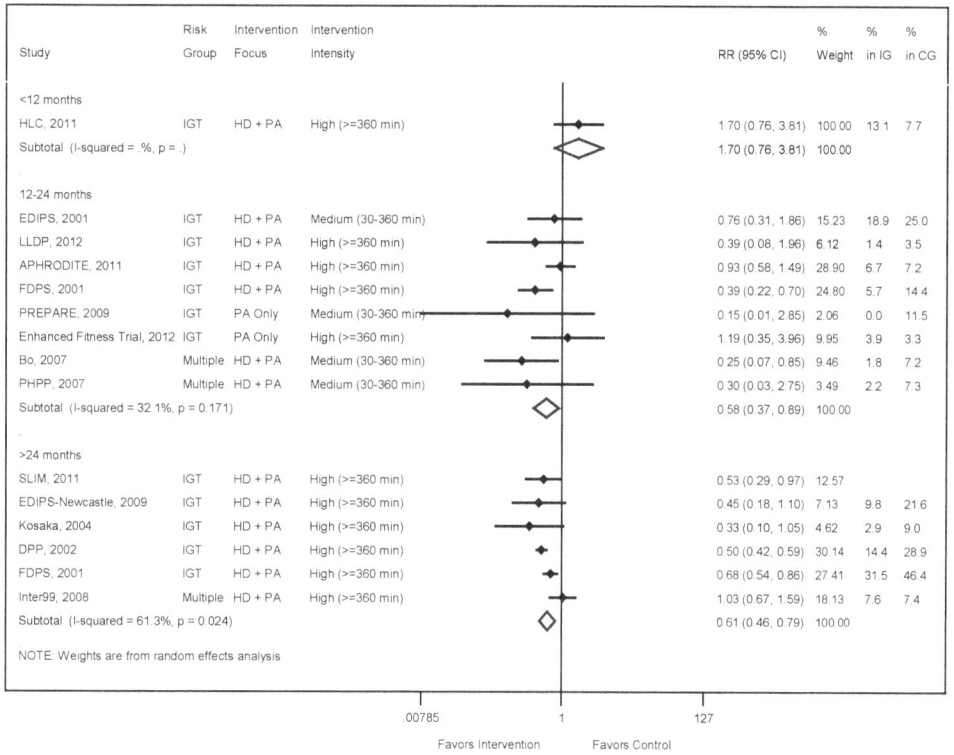

Figure 14. Pooled Analysis of Fasting Glucose in Persons With Impaired Fasting Glucose or Impaired Glucose Tolerance, Sorted by Length of Followup Time

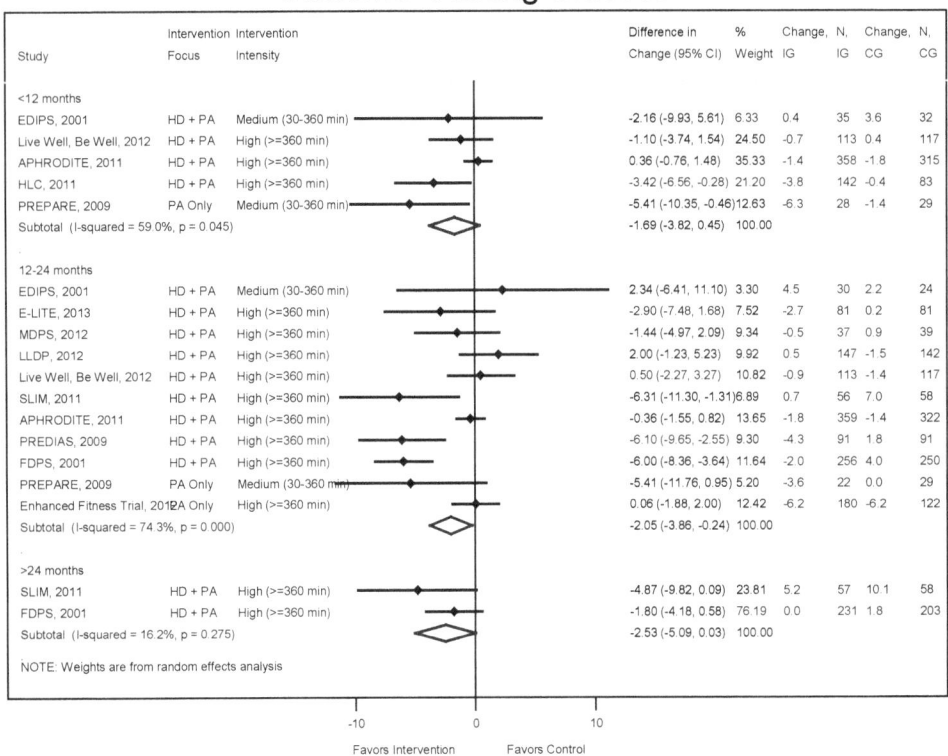

Figure 15. Pooled Analysis of Weight in Persons With Impaired Fasting Glucose, Impaired Glucose Tolerance, or Multiple Risk Factors, Sorted by Length of Followup Time

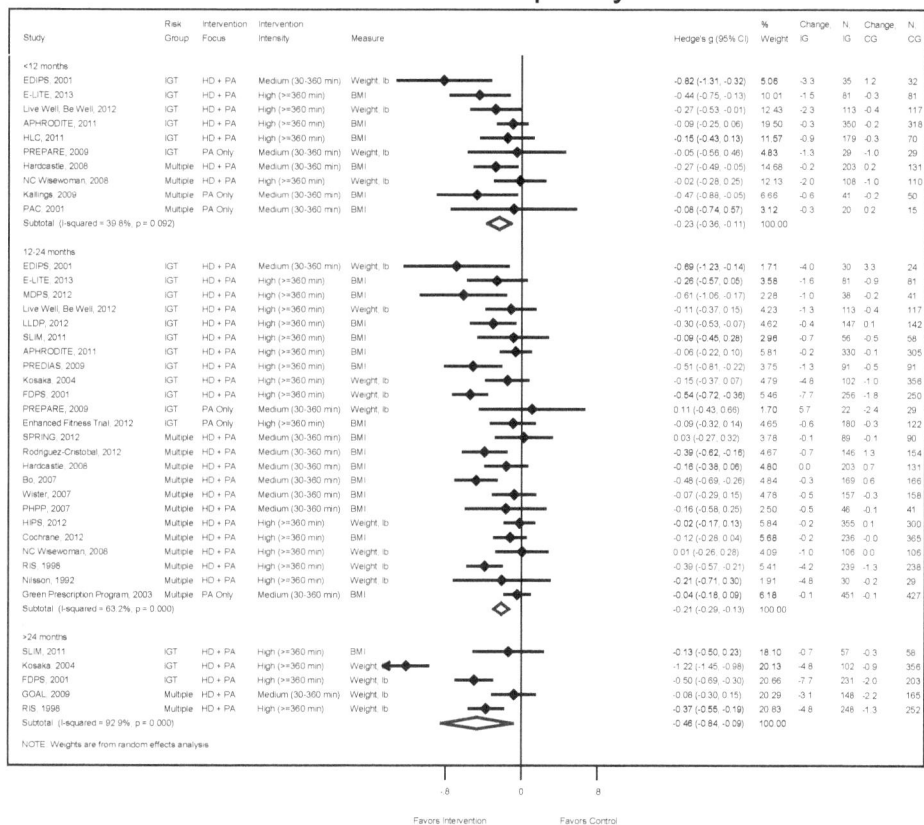

Figure 16. Pooled Analysis of Total Cholesterol for Combined Healthy Diet and Physical Activity Interventions in All Risk Groups, Sorted by Length of Followup Time

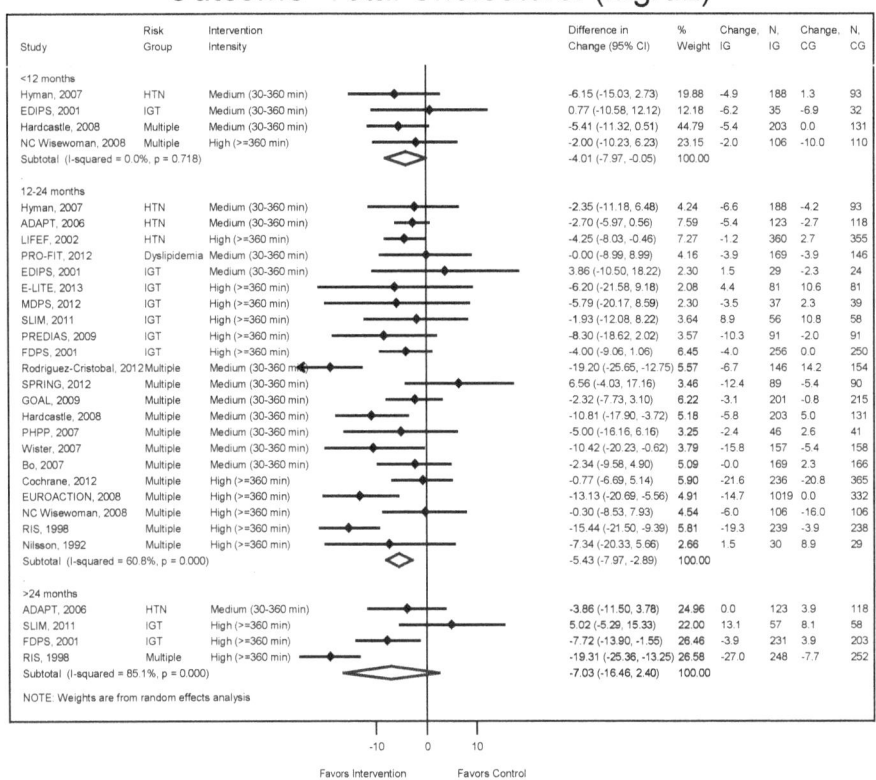

Figure 17. Pooled Analysis of Low-Density Lipoprotein Cholesterol for Combined Healthy Diet and Physical Activity Interventions in All Risk Groups, Sorted by Length of Followup Time

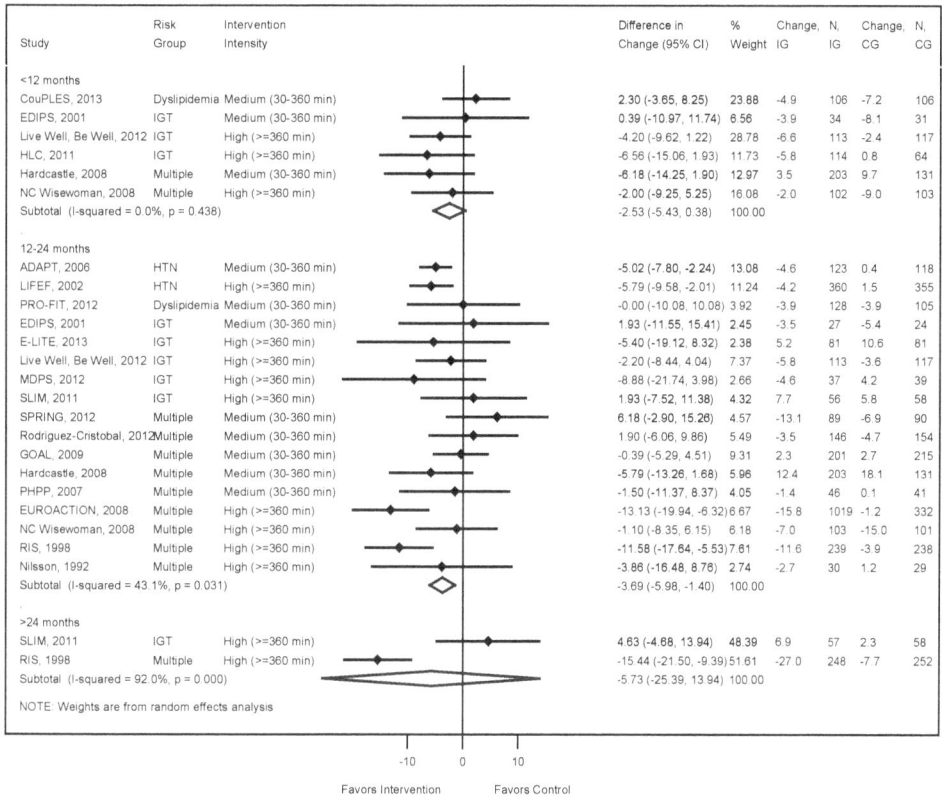

Figure 18. Pooled Analysis of Systolic Blood Pressure for Combined Healthy Diet and Physical Activity Interventions in All Risk Groups, Sorted by Length of Followup Time

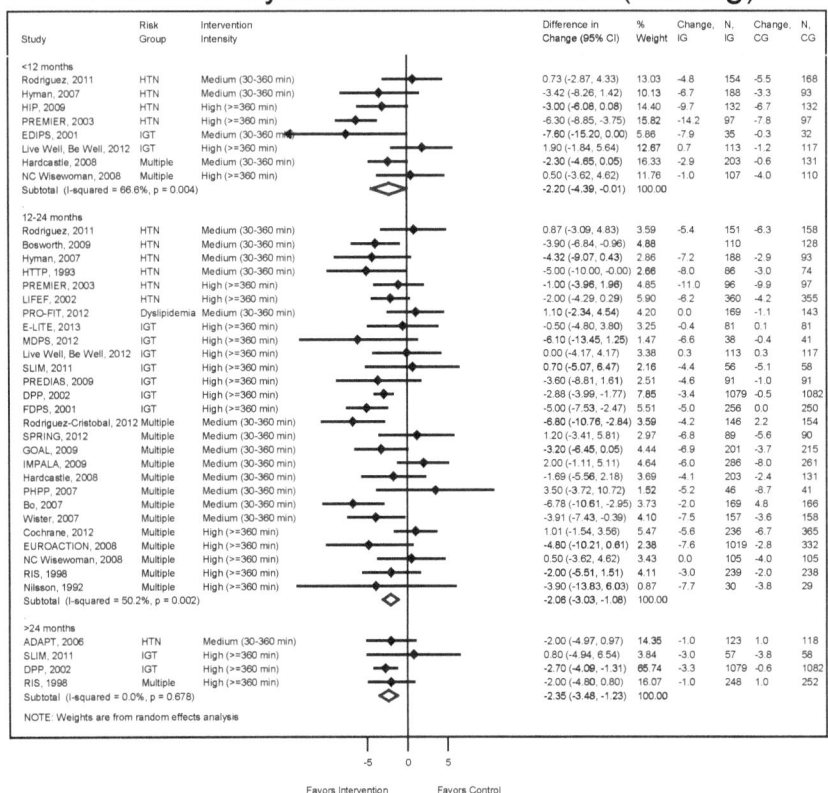

Figure 19. Pooled Analysis of Diastolic Blood Pressure for Combined Healthy Diet and Physical Activity Interventions in All Risk Groups, Sorted by Length of Followup Time

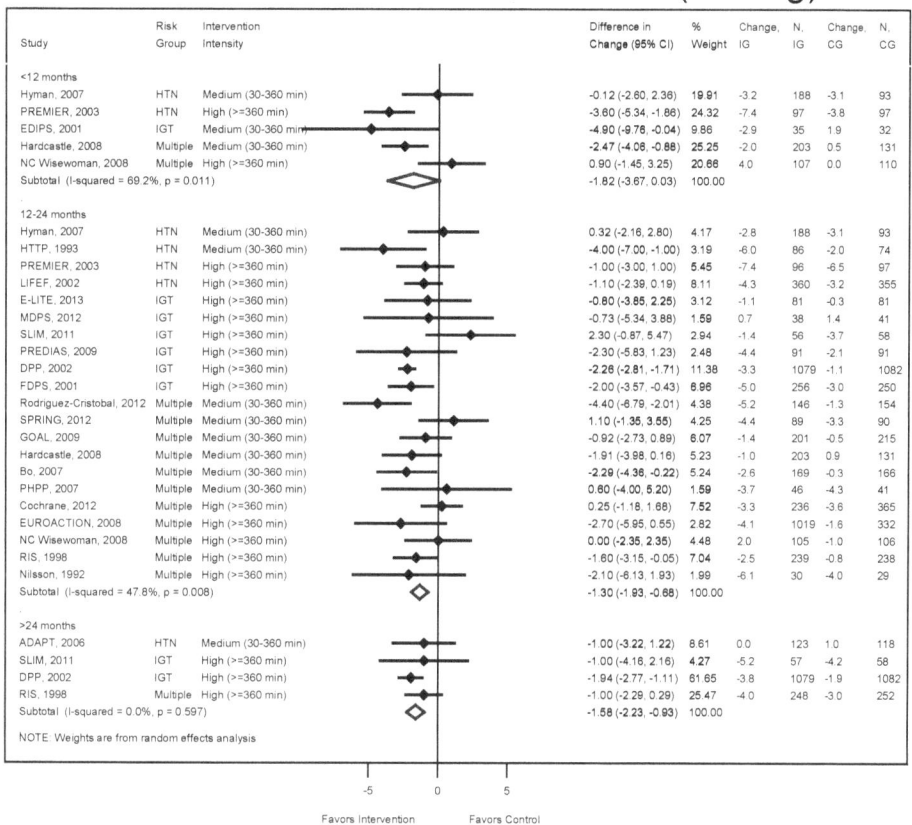

Figure 20. Pooled Analysis of Fasting Glucose for Combined Healthy Diet and Physical Activity Interventions in All Risk Groups, Sorted by Length of Followup Time

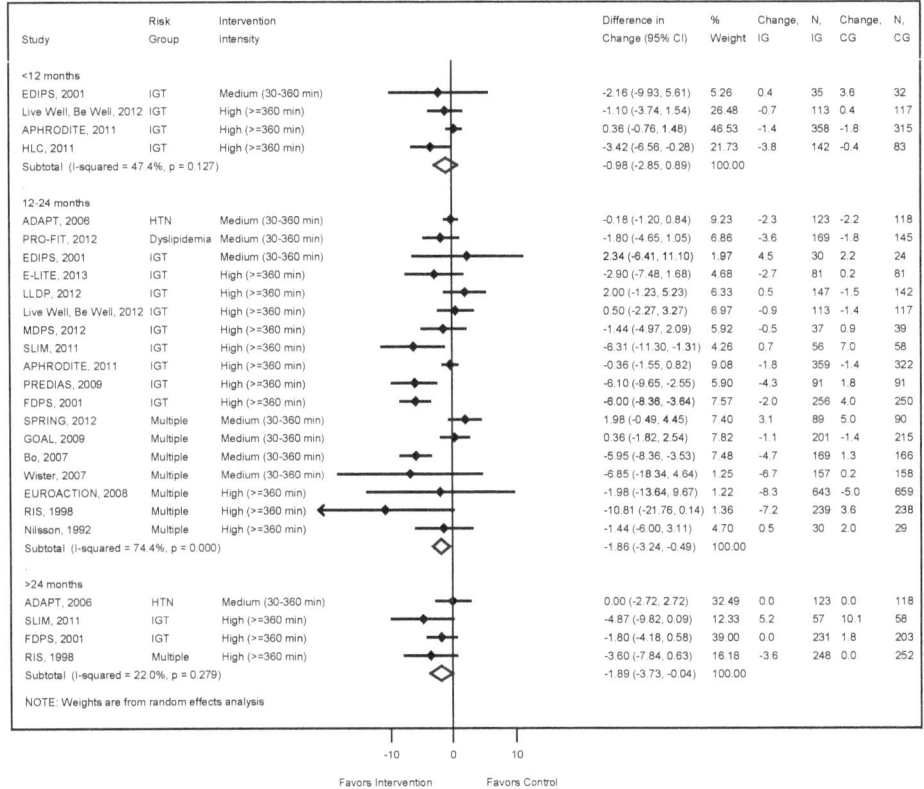

Figure 21. Pooled Analysis of Diabetes Incidence for Combined Healthy Diet and Physical Activity Interventions in All Risk Groups, Sorted by Length of Followup Time

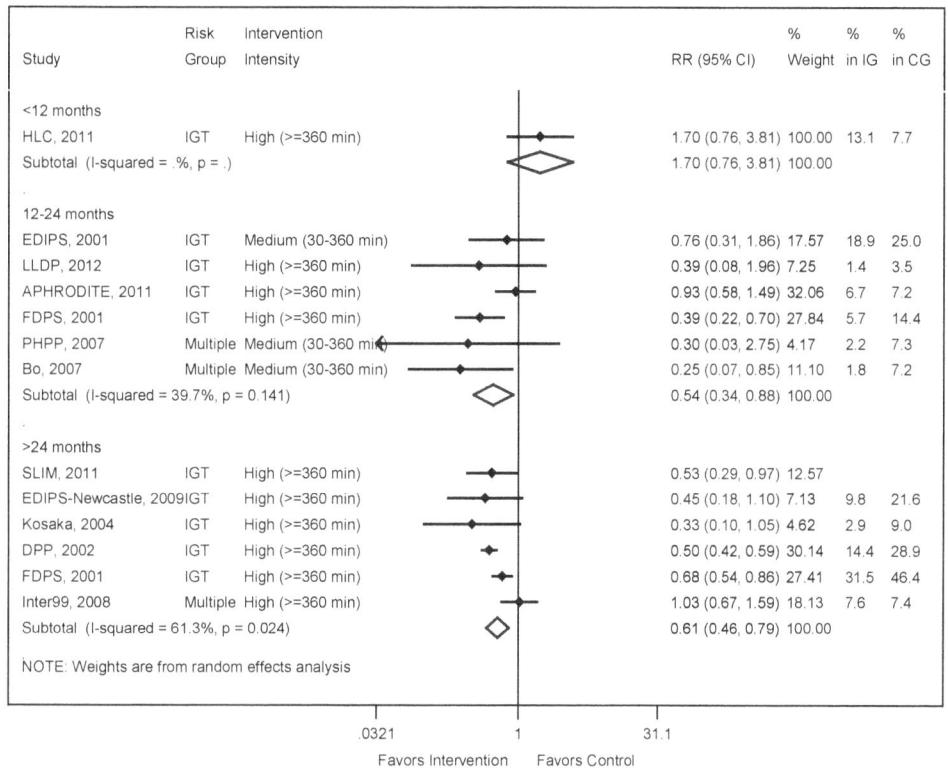

Table 1. Included Studies by Population and Key Question

Population	Study Reference	N	Intervention Focus	Intervention Intensity*	KQ1	KQ2	KQ3	KQ4
Dyslipidemia	CouPLES, 2013[67]	255	HD + PA	Medium		×	×	
Dyslipidemia	PRO-FIT, 2012[68]	340	HD + PA	Medium		×	×	
Dyslipidemia	RHPP Trial, 1993[69]	1,197	HD + PA	Medium (IG1+IG2)‡		×†		
Dyslipidemia	Anderson, 1992[70]	177	HD	High (IG1+IG2)‡		×	×	
Dyslipidemia	DEER, 2010[71]	189	HD	High		×	×	
Dyslipidemia	Delahanty, 2001[72]	90	HD	High		×	×	
Dyslipidemia	Moy, 2001[73]	235	HD	High		×	×	
Dyslipidemia	Ammerman, 2003[74]	468	HD	Medium		×		
Dyslipidemia	Bloemberg, 1991[75]	80	HD	Medium		×		
Dyslipidemia	Hyman, 1998[76]	123	HD	Medium		×†	×	
Dyslipidemia	Johnston, 1995[77]	179	HD	Medium (IG1+IG2)‡		×†		
Dyslipidemia	Neil, 1995[78]	309	HD	Medium (IG1+IG2)‡		×		
Dyslipidemia	NFPMP, 2004[79]	143	HD	Medium		×	×	
Dyslipidemia	ODES, 1997[80]	98	HD	Medium		×	×	
Dyslipidemia	Southeast Cholesterol Project, 1997[81]	372	HD	Medium		×	×	
Dyslipidemia	Stevens, 2003[82]	616	HD	Medium		×		
Dyslipidemia	Tomson, 1995[83]	92	HD	Medium		×		
HTN	Applegate, 1992[127]	56	HD + PA	High		×†	×	
HTN	LIHEF, 2003[137]	715	HD + PA	High		×	×	
HTN	Migneault, 2012[126]	337	HD + PA	High		×†	×	
HTN	PREMIER, 2009[116]	304	HD + PA	High (IG1+IG2)§	×	×	×	×
HTN	TONE, 1998[117]	975	HD + PA	High (IG2+IG3)§	×	×†	×	×
HTN	HIP[136]	574	HD + PA	High (Pt, MD+pt) Medium (MD only)		×	×	
HTN	Arroll, 1995[128]	208	HD + PA	Medium		×†	×	
HTN	ADAPT, 2008[138]	241	HD + PA	Medium		×	×	×
HTN	Bosworth, 2009[84§]	477	HD + PA	Medium (IG1+IG2)		×		
HTN	Hyman, 2007[135]	281	HD + PA	Medium (IG1+IG2)‡		×	×	
HTN	HTTP, 1993[134]	200	HD + PA	Medium		×		
HTN	Rodriguez, 2012[113]	533	HD + PA	Medium		×	×	×
HTN	Vitalum, 2008-2011[105]	1,629	HD + PA	Medium (IG2+IG3)§ Low (IG1)			×	
HTN	TONE, 1998[117]	975	HD	High (IG1)	×	×†	×	×
HTN	Arroll, 1995[128]	208	HD	Medium		×†	×	
HTN	Beckman, 1995[111]	64	HD	Medium		×	×	
HTN	Arroll, 1995[128]	208	PA	Medium		×†	×	
HTN	Moreau, 2001[104]	24	PA	Medium		×	×	
Glucose	APHRODITE, 2011[88]	925	HD + PA	High		×	×	
Glucose	DPP, 2002[89]	2,161	HD + PA	High	×	×	×	×
Glucose	EDIPS-Newcastle, 2009[91]	102	HD + PA	High		×	×	
Glucose	E-LITE, 2013[87]	162	HD + PA	High		×		
Glucose	FDPS, 2001[118]	522	HD + PA	High	×	×	×	
Glucose	HLC, 2012[92]	307	HD + PA	High	×	×	×	
Glucose	Kosaka, 2004[93]	482	HD + PA	High		×		
Glucose	Live Well, Be Well, 2012[86]	238	HD + PA	High	×	×	×	
Glucose	Melbourne DPS, 2012[85]	92	HD + PA	High	×	×	×	
Glucose	LLDP, 2012[94]	312	HD + PA	High	×	×	×	×
Glucose	PREDIAS, 2009[95]	182	HD + PA	High	×	×	×	
Glucose	SLIM, 2011[149]	147	HD + PA	High		×	×	
Glucose	EDIPS, 2006[90]	78	HD + PA	Medium		×	×	
Glucose	Watanabe, 2003[97]	173	HD	Low		×†	×	
Glucose	Enhanced Fitness Trial, 2012[98]	302	PA	High (IG1+IG2)	×	×	×	×
Glucose	Prepare Trial, 2009[99]	98	PA	Medium (IG1+IG2)§		×	×	
Mixed	Cochrane, 2012[102]	601	HD + PA	High		×	×	
Mixed	Edelman, 2006[129]	154	HD + PA	High		×†	×	
Mixed	EURO-ACTION, 2008[106]	2,385	HD + PA	High		×	×	
Mixed	HIPS, 2012[103]	814	HD + PA	High		×	×	
Mixed	Inter99, 2011[107]	4,503	HD + PA	High		×	×	

Table 1. Included Studies by Population and Key Question

Population	Study Reference	N	Intervention Focus	Intervention Intensity*	KQ1	KQ2	KQ3	KQ4
Mixed	Nilsson, 1992[119]	63	HD + PA	High	×	×	×	
Mixed	RIS, 1994[115]	508	HD + PA	High	×	×		
Mixed	WISEWOMAN North Carolina, 2008[110]	236	HD + PA	High	×	×	×	
Mixed	Bo, 2007[146]	375	HD + PA	Medium		×	×	×
Mixed	GOAL, 2011[139]	457	HD + PA	Medium		×	×	
Mixed	Hardcastle, 2008[168]	334	HD + PA	Medium		×	×	
Mixed	Hoorn, 2013[132]	622	HD + PA	Medium		×	×	
Mixed	Logan Healthy Living, 2010[114]	434	HD + PA	Medium			×	×
Mixed	PEGASE, 2008[120]	640	HD + PA	Medium	×	×†	×	
Mixed	PHPP, 2007[121]	99	HD + PA	Medium	×	×	×	
Mixed	SPRING, 2012[100]	201	HD + PA	Medium		×	×	
Mixed	WISEWOMAN California, 2012[108]	1,093	HD + PA	Medium		×†	×	
Mixed	Wister, 2007[140]	315	HD + PA	Medium		×	×	
Mixed	IMPALA, 2009[133]	615	HD + PA	Medium		×	×	
Mixed	Rodriguez-Cristobal, 2012[173]	436	HD + PA	Medium		×		
Mixed	LIFE, 2010[130]	186	PA	High		×†	×	×
Mixed	Green Prescription Programme, 2003[123]	878	PA	Medium		×	×	×
Mixed	NERS, 2012[109]	2,160	PA	Medium			×	
Mixed	PAC, 2001[122]	120	PA	Medium	×	×	×	
Mixed	PACE, 2005[131]	771	PA	Medium		×†	×	
Mixed	Kallings, 2009[141]	101	PA	Medium			×	

* Low: ≤30 min; medium: 30–360 min; high: ≥360 min.
† Not included in meta-analyses because of limitations in reporting of outcomes.
‡ Meta-analysis combines the two intervention groups.
§ Meta-analysis included higher-intensity intervention.

Abbreviations: ADAPT = Activity Diet and Blood Pressure Trial; APHRODITE = Active Prevention in High-Risk Individuals of Diabetes Type 2 in and Around Eindhoven; CouPLES = Couples Partnering for Lipid Enhancing Strategies; DPP = Diabetes Prevention Program; DPS = Diabetes Prevention Study; EDIPS = European Diabetes Prevention Study; E-Lite = Evaluation of Lifestyle Interventions to Treat Elevated Cardiometabolic Risk in Primary Care; FDPS = Finnish Diabetes Prevention Study; GOAL = Groningen Overweigh and Lifestyle Study; HD = healthy diet; HIP = Hypertension Improvement Project; HIPS = Health Improvement and Prevention Study; HLC = Healthy Living Course; HTN = hypertension; HTTP = Hypertension Teaching and Treatment Program; IG = intervention group; IMPALA = Improving Patient Adherence to Lifestyle Advice ; KQ = key question; LIFE = Lifestyle Interventions and Independence for Elder; LIHEF = Lifestyle Intervention against Hypertension in Eastern Finland; LLDP = Lawrence Latino Diabetes Prevention Project; MD = physician; N = study population; NERS = National Exercise Referral Scheme; PA = physical activity; PAC = Physical Activity Counseling; PACE = Physician-based Assessment and Counseling for Exercise; PEGASE = Pan European Grid Advanced Simulation and State Estimation; PHPP = Patient-motivated Health Promotion Program; PREDIAS = Prevention of Diabetes Self-Management Program; pt = patient; RIS = Risk Factor Intervention Study; SLIM = Study on Lifestyle Interventions and IGT Maastricht; SPRING = Self-monitoring and Prevention of Risk Factors; TONE = Trial of Non-Pharmacological Interventions in the Elderly.

Table 2. Included Studies by Intervention Focus and Key Question

Intervention Focus	Study Reference	N	Intervention Intensity*	Population	KQ1	KQ2	KQ3	KQ4
HD + PA	Applegate, 1992[127]	56	High	HTN		×†	×	
HD + PA	HIP[136]	574	High	HTN		×	×	
HD + PA	LIHEF, 2003[137]	715	High	HTN		×	×	
HD + PA	Migneault, 2012[126]	337	High	HTN		×†	×	
HD + PA	PREMIER, 2009[116]	304	High	HTN	×	×	×	×
HD + PA	TONE, 1998[117]	975	High	HTN	×	×†	×	×
HD + PA	APHRODITE, 2011[88]	925	High	IFG		×	×	
HD + PA	EDIPS-Newcastle, 2009[91]	102	High	IFG		×	×	
HD + PA	E-LITE, 2013[87]	162	High	IFG		×		
HD + PA	DPP, 2002[89]	2,161	High	IFG	×	×	×	×
HD + PA	FDPS, 2001[118]	522	High	IFG	×	×	×	
HD + PA	HLC, 2012[92]	307	High	IFG	×	×	×	
HD + PA	Kosaka, 2005[93]	482	High	IFG		×		
HD + PA	Live Well, Be Well, 2012[86]	230	High	IFG	×	×	×	
HD + PA	LLDP, 2012[94]	312	High	IFG	×	×	×	×
HD + PA	Melbourne DPS, 2012[85]	92	High	IFG	×	×	×	
HD + PA	PREDIAS, 2009[95]	182	High	IFG	×	×	×	
HD + PA	SLIM, 2011[149]	147	High	IFG		×	×	
HD + PA	Cochrane, 2012[102]	601	High	Mixed		×	×	
HD + PA	Edelman, 2006[129]	154	High	Mixed		×†	×	
HD + PA	EURO-ACTION, 2008[106]	2,385	High	Mixed		×	×	
HD + PA	HIPS, 2012[103]	814	High	Mixed		×	×	
HD + PA	Inter99, 2008[107]	4,503	High	Mixed		×	×	
HD + PA	Nilsson, 1992[119]	63	High	Mixed	×	×	×	
HD + PA	PEGASE, 2008[120]	640	High	Mixed	×	×†	×	
HD + PA	RIS, 1994[115]	508	High	Mixed	×	×		
HD + PA	WISEWOMAN North Carolina, 2008[110]	236	High	Mixed	×	×	×	
HD + PA	PRO-FIT, 2012[68]	340	Medium	Dyslipidemia		×	×	
HD + PA	RHPP Trial, 1993[69]	1,197	Medium	Dyslipidemia		×†		
HD + PA	CouPLES, 2013[67]	255	Medium	Dyslipidemia		×	×	
HD + PA	ADAPT, 2008[138]	241	Medium	HTN		×	×	×
HD + PA	Arroll, 1995[128]	208	Medium	HTN		×†		
HD + PA	Bosworth, 2009[84]‡	477	Medium	HTN		×		
HD + PA	HTTP, 1993[134]	200	Medium	HTN		×		
HD + PA	Hyman, 2007[135]	281	Medium	HTN		×	×	
HD + PA	Rodriguez, 2012[113]	533	Medium	HTN		×	×	×
HD + PA	Vitalum, 2011[105]	1,629	Medium	HTN			×	
HD + PA	EDIPS, 2006[90]	78	Medium	IFG		×	×	
HD + PA	Hoorn, 2013[132]	622	Medium	Mixed		×	×	
HD + PA	Logan Healthy Living, 2010[114]	434	Medium	Mixed			×	×
HD + PA	Rodriguez-Cristobal, 2012[173]	436	Medium	Mixed		×		
HD + PA	SPRING, 2012[100]	201	Medium	Mixed		×	×	
HD + PA	Bo, 2007[146]	375	Medium	Mixed		×	×	×
HD + PA	PHPP, 2007[121]	99	Medium	Mixed	×	×	×	
HD + PA	Hardcastle, 2008[168]	334	Medium	Mixed		×	×	
HD + PA	GOAL, 2011[139]	457	Medium	Mixed		×	×	
HD + PA	WISEWOMAN California, 2012[108]	1,093	Medium	Mixed		×†	×	
HD + PA	Wister, 2007[140]	315	Medium	Mixed		×	×	
HD + PA	IMPALA, 2009[133]	615	Medium	Mixed		×	×	
HD	Anderson, 1992[70]	177	High	Dyslipidemia		×	×	
HD	DEER, 2010[71]	189	High	Dyslipidemia		×	×	
HD	Delahanty, 2001[72]	90	High	Dyslipidemia		×	×	
HD	Moy, 2001[73]	235	High	Dyslipidemia		×	×	
HD	TONE, 1998[117]	975	High	HTN	×	×†	×	×
HD	Ammerman, 2003[74]	468	Medium	Dyslipidemia		×		

Table 2. Included Studies by Intervention Focus and Key Question

Intervention Focus	Study Reference	N	Intervention Intensity*	Population	KQ1	KQ2	KQ3	KQ4
HD	Bloemberg, 1991[75]	80	Medium	Dyslipidemia		×		
HD	Hyman, 1998[76]	123	Medium	Dyslipidemia		×†	×	
HD	Johnston, 1995[77]	179	Medium	Dyslipidemia		×†		
HD	Neil, 1995[78]	309	Medium	Dyslipidemia		×		
HD	NFPMP, 2002[79]	143	Medium	Dyslipidemia		×	×	
HD	ODES, 1997[80]	98	Medium	Dyslipidemia		×	×	
HD	Southeast Cholesterol Project, 1997[81]	372	Medium	Dyslipidemia		×	×	
HD	Stevens, 2003[82]	616	Medium	Dyslipidemia		×		
HD	Tomson, 1994[83]	92	Medium	Dyslipidemia		×		
HD	Arroll, 1995[128]	208	Medium	HTN		×†	×	
HD	Beckman, 1995[111]	64	Medium	HTN		×	×	
HD	Watanabe, 2003[97]	173	Low	IFG		×†	×	
PA	Enhanced Fitness Trial, 2012[98]	302	High	IFG	×	×	×	×
PA	PAC, 2001[122]	120	Medium	Mixed	×	×	×	
PA	Arroll, 1995[128]	208	Medium	HTN		×†	×	
PA	Moreau, 2001[104]	24	Medium	HTN		×	×	
PA	Prepare Trial, 2009[99]	98	Medium	IFG		×	×	
PA	LIFE, 2010[130]	186	High	Mixed		×†	×	×
PA	Green Prescription Programme, 2003[123]	878	Medium	Mixed		×	×	×
PA	Kallings, 2009[141]	101	Medium	Mixed		×	×	
PA	NERS, 2012[109]	2,160	Medium	Mixed			×	
PA	PACE, 2005[131]	771	Medium	Mixed		×†	×	

* Low: ≤30 min; medium: 30–360 min; high ≥360 min.
† Not included in meta-analyses because of limitations in reporting of outcomes.
‡ Meta-analysis included higher-intensity intervention.

Abbreviations: ADAPT = Activity Diet and Blood Pressure Trial; APHRODITE = Active Prevention in High-Risk Individuals of Diabetes Type 2 in and Around Eindhoven; CouPLES = Couples Partnering for Lipid Enhancing Strategies; DEER = Diet and Exercise for Elevated Risk; DPP = Diabetes Prevention Program; DPS = Diabetes Prevention Study; EDIPS = European Diabetes Prevention Study; E-Lite = Evaluation of Lifestyle Interventions to Treat Elevated Cardiometabolic Risk in Primary Care; FDPS = Finnish Diabetes Prevention Study; GOAL = Groningen Overweigh and Lifestyle Study; HD = healthy diet; HIP = Hypertension Improvement Project; HIPS = Health Improvement and Prevention Study; HLC = Healthy Living Course; HTN = hypertension; HTTP = Hypertension Teaching and Treatment Program; IFG = impaired fasting glucose; IMPALA = Improving Patient Adherence to Lifestyle Advice; KQ = key question; LIFE = Lifestyle Interventions and Independence for Elder; LIHEF = Lifestyle Intervention against Hypertension in Eastern Finland; LLDP: Lawrence Latino Diabetes Prevention Project; N = study population; NERS = National Exercise Referral Scheme; NFPMP = Nijmegen Family Practices Monitoring Project; ODES = Oslo Diet and Exercise Study; PA = physical activity; PAC = Physical Activity Counseling; PACE = Physician-based Assessment and Counseling for Exercise; PEGASE = Pan European Grid Advanced Simulation and State Estimation; PHPP = Patient-motivated Health Promotion Program; PREDIAS = Prevention of Diabetes Self-Management Program; RIS = Risk Factor Intervention Study; SLIM = Study on Lifestyle Interventions and IGT Maastricht; SPRING = Self-monitoring and Prevention of Risk Factors; TONE = Trial of Non-Pharmacological Interventions in the Elderly.

Table 3. Behavioral Counseling Trials in Persons With Dyslipidemia or Elevated Cholesterol: Study and Population Characteristics

Study, Year	Quality	Country	N	Mean Age, y	% Men	Mean TC and LDL, mg/dL	% On Lipid-Lowering Medications	Mean BMI, kg/m²	% DM
Healthy diet and physical activity interventions									
CouPLES, 2009, 2013[67]	Fair	US	255	61	94.9	TC: NR LDL: 126.3	46.3	NR	NR
PRO-FIT, 2012[68]	Fair	The Netherlands	340	45	44.0†	TC: 204.6† LDL: 142.8†	69.0†	26.5†	NR
RHPP Trial, 1993[69]	Fair	US	1,197	71	43.2†	TC: 266.9† LDL: NR	NR	% with BMI >30: 30.8†	16.3†
Healthy diet-only interventions									
Anderson, 1992[70]	Fair	US	177	41†	56.6†	TC: 233.2 LDL: 158.3†	0	NR	0
Ammerman, 2003[74] Keyserling, 1999[174]	Fair	US	468	55	29.0	TC: 257† LDL: 180†	0	28.8†	3.6†
Bloemberg, 1991[75]	Fair	The Netherlands	80	47†	100.0	TC: 268.3† LDL: NR	NR	26.2†	0
DEER, 1998[71]	Fair	US	189	52†	51.8†	TC: 232.5† LDL: 158.2†	0	26.7†	0
Delahanty, 2001[72]	Good	US	90	49	66.7†	TC: 238.6† LDL: 164.9†	0	NR	0
Hyman, 1998[76]	Fair	US	123	57†	25.2†	TC: 272.8† LDL: NR	0	31.2†	NR
Johnston, 1995[77]	Fair	Australia	179	57†	31.0†	TC: 245.2† LDL: 156.4†	NR	25.1†	0
Moy, 2001[73]	Fair	US	235	46*	51.9*	TC: NR LDL: 173.7*	NR	29.0*	NR
Neil, 1995[78]	Fair	UK	309	55*	52.8†	TC: 273.4* LDL: 199.6	0	26.4	NR
NFPMP, 2002[79]	Fair	The Netherlands	143	58	37.0	TC: NR LDL: NR	NR	28.7	8.0
ODES, 1995[80]	Fair	Norway	98	45†	85.3†	TC: 249.8† LDL: 170.3†	0‡	29.0†	0
Southeast Cholesterol Project, 1997[81]	Fair	US	372	56	38.0†	TC: 253.3† LDL: 180.3†	0	% with BMI >30: 23	0
Stevens, 2003[82]	Fair	US	616	54†	0	NR	0	30.3†	NR
Tomson, 1995[83] Tomson, 1994[175]	Fair	Sweden	92	43†	56.6†	TC: 281.5† LDL: NR	NR	25.0†	0

* Median.
† Calculated.
‡ Assumed.

Abbreviations: BMI = body mass index; CouPLES = Couples Partnering for Lipid Enhancing Strategies; DEER = Diet and Exercise for Elevated Risk; DM = diabetes mellitus; LDL = low-density lipoprotein; N = study population; NFPMP = Nijmegen Family Practice Monitoring Project; NR = not reported; ODES = Oslo Diet and Exercise Study; RHPP = Rural Health Promotion Project; UK = United Kingdom; US = United States; TC = total cholesterol.

Table 4. Behavioral Counseling Trials in Persons With Hypertension: Study and Population Characteristics

Study, Year	Quality	Country	N	Mean Age, y	% Men	Mean SBP and DBP, mm HG	% on HTN Medications	Mean BMI, kg/m²	% DM
Healthy diet and physical activity interventions									
ADAPT, 2006[138]	Fair	Australia	241	56*	44.4*	SBP: 126.5* DBP: 76.5*	100	30.1*	0
Applegate, 1992[127]	Fair	US	56	65*	44.7*	SBP: 144.0* DBP: 87.0*	0	NR	0
Arroll, 1995[128] *(Also arms in HD- & PA-only sections)*	Fair	New Zealand	208	55	52.0*	SBP: 144.6 DBP: 89.4	100	NR	NR
Bosworth, 2009[84]	Fair	US	478	61*	36.0*	SBP: 125* DBP: 71*	100	32.3*	36.0*
HIP, 2009[136]	Fair	US	574	61	39.0	SBP: 133.1 DBP: 74.1	97	32.5	30.0
HTTP, 1993[134]	Fair	Germany	200	51*	43.1*	SBP: 161.5* DBP: 96.5*	81.5*	NR	NR
Hyman, 2007[135]	Fair	US	281	53*	32.7*	SBP: 138.9 DBP: 85.3	NR	32.4	18.5
LIHEF, 2002[137]	Fair	Finland	715	54*	47.0*	SBP: 148.5* DBP: 91.0*	52.5*	28.7*	NR
Migneault, 2012[126]	Fair	US	337	57*	29.7	SBP: 131.2* DBP: 80.6*	100	34.4*	38.3*
PREMIER, 2003[116]	Good	US	304	52	36.5	SBP: 143.9 DBP: 87.5	0	% with BMI >30: women, 63%*; men, 66%*	0
Rodriguez, 2012[113]	Fair (poor for diet)	US	533	67	98.7	SBP: NR DBP: NR	NR	30.4*	NR
TONE, 1998[117] *(Also arm in HD-only section)*	Good	US	975	67	52.0	SBP: 127.5 DBP: 71.3	100	28.9*	0
Vitalum, 2011[105]	Fair	The Netherlands	1,629	57	55.0	SBP: NR DBP: NR	NR	27.5*	10.0*
Healthy diet–only interventions									
Arroll, 1995[128] *(Also arms in HD+PA & PA-only sections)*	Fair	New Zealand	208	55	52.0*	SBP: 144.6 DBP: 89.4	100	NR	NR
Beckman, 1995[111]	Fair	Norway	64	NR	100.0	SBP: NR DBP: NR	NR	27.3*	NR
TONE, 1998[117] *(Also arm in HD+PA section)*	Good	US	975	67	52.0	SBP: 127.5 DBP: 71.3	100	28.9*	0
Physical activity–only interventions									
Arroll, 1995[128] *(Also arms in HD+PA & HD-only sections)*	Fair	New Zealand	208	55	52.0*	SBP: 144.6 DBP: 89.4	100	NR	NR
Moreau, 2001[104]	Fair	US	24	54*	0	SBP: NR DBP: NR	42.0	NR	NR

* Calculated.

Abbreviations: ADAPT = Activity Diet and Blood Pressure Trial; BMI = body mass index; DBP = diastolic blood pressure; DM = diabetes mellitus; HIP = Hypertension Improvement Project; HTN = hypertension; HTTP = Hypertension Teaching and Treatment Programme; LIHEF = Lifestyle Intervention against Hypertension in Eastern Finland; N = study population; NR = not reported; SBP = systolic blood pressure; TONE = Trial of Non-Pharmacological Interventions in the Elderly; US = United States.

Table 5. Behavioral Counseling Trials in Persons With Impaired Fasting Glucose or Impaired Glucose Tolerance: Study and Population Characteristics

Study, Year	Quality	Country	N	Mean Age, y	% Men	Mean Glucose (FBG/GTT/HbA1c)	Mean BMI, kg/m^2	% HTN	% Dyslipidemia
Healthy diet and physical activity interventions									
APHRODITE, 2011[88]	Fair	The Netherlands	925	58	38.3	FBG: 100.9*	28.8	NR	NR
DPP, 2002[89]	Good	US	2,161	51	32.3	FBG: 106.5	34.0	26.9	34.6
EDIPS, 2001[90]	Fair	UK	78	58	56.7	FBG: 109.9*	30.2	NR	NR
EDIPS-Newcastle, 2009[91]	Fair	UK	102	57	40.2	FBG: 104.5*	33.8	NR	NR
E-LITE, 2013[87]	Good	US	162	52.0*	54*	FBG: 99.7	32.0	NR	NR
FDPS, 2001[118]	Good	Finland	522	55	33.0	FBG: 109.5*	31.2	30.5†	5.5†
HLC, 2011[92]	Fair	Australia	307	63	41.0*	FBG: 105.9*	29.7*	NR	NR
Kosaka, 2005[93]	Fair	Japan	NR (reports participants still present at 1-year observation [482])	50s	100	NR	23.9	NR	NR
Live Well, Be Well, 2012[86]	Good	US	238	56*	26.0*	FBG: 93.7*	30.0*	47.0*	NR
LLDP, 2012[94]	Good	US	312	52	25.6	FBG: 105	33.9	NR	NR
Melbourne DPS, 2012[85]	Fair	Australia	92	65*	27.0*	FBG: 93.2	30.8*	NR	NR
PREDIAS, 2009[95]	Fair	Germany	182	56	57.0	FBG: 105.7*	31.5	NR	NR
SLIM, 2011[149]	Fair	The Netherlands	147	57	51.0	FBG: 108.1*	29.8	26.5†	7.5†
Healthy diet–only interventions									
Watanabe, 2003[97]	Fair	Japan	173	55	100	FBG: 104.5*	24.4	NR	NR
Physical activity–only interventions									
Enhanced Fitness Trial, 2012[98]	Fair	US	302	67	97.0	FBG: 110.6	31.2	72	NR
Prepare Trial, 2009[99]	Fair	UK	98	65	66.0	FBG: 100.9*	29.2	54†	55†

* Calculated.
† Percent on medication.

Abbreviations: APHRODITE = Active Prevention in High-Risk Individuals of Diabetes Type 2 in and Around Eindhoven; BMI = body mass index; DPP = Diabetes Prevention Program; DPS = Diabetes Prevention Study; EDIPS = European Diabetes Prevention Study; E-Lite = Evaluation of Lifestyle Interventions to Treat Elevated Cardiometabolic Risk in Primary Care; FBG = fasting blood glucose; FDPS = Finnish Diabetes Prevention Study; GTT = glucose tolerance test; HbA1c = glycated hemoglobin; HLC = Healthy Living Course; HTN = hypertension; LLDP = Lawrence Latino Diabetes Prevention Project; N = study population; NR = not reported; PREDIAS = Prevention of Diabetes Self-Management Program; SLIM = Study on Lifestyle Intervention and IGT Maastricht; UK = United Kingdom; US = United States.

Table 6. Behavioral Counseling Trials in Persons With Mixed Cardiovascular Risk Factors: Study and Population Characteristics

Study, Year Quality	Country	N	Mean Age, y	% Men	% HTN	Mean BP, mm HG	% Dyslipidemia	Mean TC & LDL, mg/dL	% IFG or IGT	% DM	Mean FBG, mg/dL	Mean BMI, kg/m²
Healthy diet and physical activity interventions												
Bo, 2007[145] Fair	Italy	375	56*	41.7*	93.8*	SBP: 142.0* DBP: 88*	16.7†	TC: 227.8* LDL: NR	38*	0	104.5*	29.7*
Cochrane, 2012[102] Fair	UK	601	64*	88.2*	NR	SBP: 145.4* DBP: 85.1*	NR	TC: 185.3* LDL: NR	NR	NR	99.1*	28.1*
Edelman, 2006[129] Fair	US	154	53*	19.5*	37.7*	NR	NR	LDL: 134.7*	NR	15.6*	NR	33.7*
EURO-ACTION, 2008[106] Fair	France, Italy, Poland, Spain, Sweden, Denmark, The Netherlands, UK	2,385	62*	53.6*	63.0*	NR	75.2	NR	NR	28.7*	NR	NR
GOAL, 2009[139] Good	The Netherlands	457	56*	48.1*	61.7*	SBP: 145.5 DBP: 86.5*	39.2*	TC: 216.6* LDL: 133.9*	NR	0	93.7*	29.6*
Hardcastle, 2008[168] Fair	UK	334	50*	33	35	SBP: 133.7* DBP: 83.0*	57	TC: 210.4* LDL: 115.0*	NR	NR	NR	34.0*
HIPS, 2012[103] Fair	Australia	814	40-64 (range)	42.6*	8.7*	NR	88.0	NR	NR	0	NR	NR
Hoorn, 2013[132] Fair	The Netherlands	622	44.0*	41.6*	NR	SBP: 129.0* DBP: 73.4*	NR	NR	NR	0	NR	NR
IMPALA, 2009[133] Fair	The Netherlands	615	57	45	65.2*	SBP: 146.9 DBP: NR	43.3*	TC: NR LDL: 144.8*	NR	14.1*	106.3*	29
Inter99, 2008[107] Fair	Denmark	4,053	47	50.1*	NR	SBP: 140.5* DBP: NR	NR	TC: 223.9* LDL: NR	NR	9.9	NR	29.8*
Logan Healthy Living, 2009[114] Fair	Australia	434	58	38.9	85.5	NR	NR	NR	NR	45.4	NR	31.1
Nilsson, 1992[119] Fair	Sweden	63	56*	78.0*	78.0	SBP: 149.6* DBP: 85.9*	NR	TC: 220.1* LDL: 154.4*	NR	NR	FBG: 92.8*	28.4*
PEGASE, 2008[120] Fair	France	640	57*	60.0*	34.0*	NR	81.0*	TC: NR LDL: 148.5*	NR	8.7*	NR	% with BMI >30: 19.9*
PHPP, 2007[121] Fair	Japan	99	64*	42.4*	30.3*	SBP: 129.8* DBP: 78.8*	NR	TC: 205.7* LDL: 122.4*	NR	17.2*	NR	NR
RIS, 1994[115] Good (KQ1), Fair (KQ2)	Sweden	508	66	100.0	100.0	SBP: 155 DBP: 91	74	TC: 258.7* LDL: 177.6	3.0	22	104.5	27.1
Rodriguez-Cristobal, 2012[173] Fair	Spain	436	58*	37*	42*	SBP: 134.3* DBP: 81.2*	NR	TC: 210.6* LDL: 134.5*	NR	13.5*	NR	30.4*
SPRING, 2012[100] Fair	The Netherlands	201	65*	62.0*	76.0*	SBP: 158.0* DBP: 92.0*	78.0*	TC: 216.2* LDL: 139.0*	NR	0	97.3*	28.0*
WISEWOMAN California, 2010[108] Fair	US	1093	52*	0	17.3	SBP: 125.1* DBP: 76.7*	13.0	TC: 198.1* LDL: NR	NR	22.0	NR	31.9*

Table 6. Behavioral Counseling Trials in Persons With Mixed Cardiovascular Risk Factors: Study and Population Characteristics

Study, Year Quality	Country	N	Mean Age, y	% Men	% HTN	Mean BP, mm HG	% Dyslipidemia	Mean TC & LDL, mg/dL	% IFG or IGT	% DM	Mean FBG, mg/dL	Mean BMI, kg/m²
WISEWOMAN NC, 2006, 2008[110] Fair	US	236	53*	0	47.9*	SBP: 127* DBP: 78*	33.7*	TC: 210.5* LDL: 126.5*	NR	11.5*	FBG: 111.8*	31
Wister, 2007[140] Good	Canada	315	55*	41.6*	NR	SBP: 137.5* DBP: NR	NR	TC: 220.1* LDL: NR	NR	NR	Glucose: 147.8*	32.5
Physical activity–only interventions												
Green Prescription Programme (Walk to Heart, Health & Activity study), 2003[123] Fair	New Zealand	878	58	34	52*	SBP: 135.2* DBP: 82.1*	NR	TC: 220.1* LDL: NR	NR	11	NR	30
NERS, 2012[109] Fair	UK	2,160	52	34	NR	NR	NR	NR	NR	NR	NR	NR
PAC, 2001, 2007[122] Fair	Canada	120	47*	32*	34.2*	NR	NR	TC: 191.1* LDL: 112.0*	NR	10.8*	FBG: 104.5*	30.7*
PACE, 2005[131] Fair	The Netherlands	771	56	51	NR	NR	NR	NR	NR	NR	NR	28.9
Kallings, 2009[141] Good	Sweden	101	68*	43	NR	SBP: 140.1 DBP: 80.8	NR	TC: 212.3 LDL: 127.4	NR	NR	97.3*	30.1
LIFE, 2010[130] Fair	Belgium	126	67*	52.4*	NR	SBP: 145.6* DBP: 86.2*	NR	TC: 239.2* LDL: 148.5*	NR	0	94.5*	26.7*

* Calculated.
† Patients with low HDL cholesterol.

Abbreviations: BP = blood pressure; DBP = diastolic blood pressure; DM = diabetes mellitus; FBG = fasting blood glucose; GOAL = Groningen Overweight and Lifestyle Study; HIPS = Health Improvement and Prevention Study; HTN = hypertension; IFG = impaired fasting glucose; IGT = impaired glucose tolerance; IMPALA = Improving Patient Adherence to Lifestyle Advice; LDL = low-density lipoprotein; LIFE = Lifestyle Intervention and Independence for elder; N = study population; NERS = National Exercise Referral Scheme; NR = not reported; PAC = Physical Activity Counseling; PACE = Physician-based Assessment and Counseling for Exercise; PEGASE = Pan European Grid Advanced Stimulation and State Examination; PHPP = Patient-motivated Health Promotion Program; RIS = Risk Factor Intervention Study; SBP = systolic blood pressure; SPRING = Self-monitoring and Prevention of Risk Factors; TC = total cholesterol; US = United States; UK = United Kingdom.

Table 7. Behavioral Counseling Trials in Persons With Dyslipidemia or Elevated Cholesterol: Intervention Characteristics

Study, Year	Quality	N	Intervention Intensity	# of Contacts Interactive (I), Other (O)	Duration of Intervention	Type of Control
Healthy diet and physical activity interventions						
CouPLES, 2013[67]	Fair	255	Medium: phone only; included medication adherence, included spouse	I: 16 O: 0	10 months	MI
PRO-FIT, 2012[68]	Fair	340	Medium	I: 6 O: 0	12 months	UC
RHPP Trial, 1993[69]	Fair	1,197	IG1: Medium† *(hospital-based)*	I: range, 1 to 5 (mean, 4.2) O: 0	12 months	UC
			IG2: Medium† *(clinic-based)*	I: range, 1 to 5 (mean, 3.4) O: 0		
Healthy diet–only interventions						
Anderson, 1992[70]	Fair	177	IG1: High *(AHA diet)*	I: 29 O: 0	12 months	UC
			IG2: High *(AHA high fiber)*	I: 29 O: 0		
Ammerman, 2003[74] Keyserling, 1999[174]	Fair	468	Medium	I: 7 O: 2	12 months	UC
Bloemberg, 1991[75]	Fair	80	Medium	I: 3 O: 5	6 months*	No advice
DEER, 1998[71]	Fair	189	High	I: 17 O: 0	11 months	No advice
Delahanty, 2001[72]	Good	90	High	I: 6 O: 0	6 months	UC
Hyman, 1998[76]	Fair	123	Medium	I: 16 O: 12	6 months	UC
Johnston, 1995[77]	Fair	179	IG1: Medium *(group)*	I: 3 O: 0	6 months*	UC
			IG2: Medium *(individual)*	I: 3 O: 0		
Moy, 2001[73]	Fair	235	High	I: 13 O: 0	2 years*	UC
Neil, 1995[78]	Fair	309	IG1: Medium (40 min) *(nurse)*	I: 2 O: 0	8 weeks	UC
			IG2: Medium (40 min) *(dietician)*	I: 2 O: 0		
NFPMP, 2002[79]	Fair	143	Medium	I: 6 O: 0	14 weeks	UC
ODES, 1995[80]	Fair	98	Medium	I: 3 O: 0	9 months	Waitlist control
Southeast Cholesterol Project, 1997[81]	Fair	372	Medium	I: 6 O: 4	12 months	UC
Stevens, 2003[82]	Fair	616	Medium	I: 4 O: 0	9 weeks	AC

Table 7. Behavioral Counseling Trials in Persons With Dyslipidemia or Elevated Cholesterol: Intervention Characteristics

Study, Year	Quality	N	Intervention Intensity	# of Contacts Interactive (I), Other (O)	Duration of Intervention	Type of Control
Tomson, 1995[83] Tomson, 1994[175]	Fair	92	Medium	I: 6 O: 0	12 months	UC

* Assumed.
† Based on means.

Abbreviations: AC = attention control; AHA = American Health Association; CouPLES = Couples Partnering for Lipid Enhancing Strategies; DEER = Diet and Exercise for Elevated Risk; IG = intervention group; MI = minimal intervention; N = study population; NFPMP = Nijmegen Family Practices Monitoring Project; ODES = Oslo Diet and Exercise Study; UC = usual care.

Table 8. Behavioral Counseling Trials in Persons With Hypertension: Intervention Characteristics

Study, Year Intervention Focus	Quality	N	Intervention Intensity	# of Contacts Interactive (I), Other (O)	Duration of Intervention	Type of Control
Healthy diet and physical activity interventions						
ADAPT, 2006[138]	Fair	241	Medium	I: 6 O: 4	12 months	UC with partial AC
Applegate, 1992[127]	Fair	56	High	I: 14 O: 0	6 months	No advice
Arroll, 1995[128] *(Also has arms in HD- and PA-only sections)*	Fair	208	IG1: Medium *(PA + Salt)*	I: 1 O: 0	Unknown	UC
Bosworth, 2009[84]	Fair	478	IG1: Medium *(self-management + incentives)*	I: 12 O: 0	24 months	UC
			IG2: Medium *(combined + incentives)*	I: 12 O: 0		
HIP, 2009[136]	Fair	574	IG1: High *(pt only)*	I: 32 O: 0	18 months	UC
			IG2: High *(MD + pt)*	I: 32 O: 4		
			CG2: Medium *(MD only)*	I: 2 O: 4		
HTTP, 1993[134]	Fair	200	Medium (6 hr)	I: 4 O: 0	1 month	MI
Hyman, 2007[135]	Fair	281	IG1: Medium (6 hr) *(addressed 3 target areas at each clinic session)*	I: 24 O: 3	18 months	MI
			IG2: Medium (6 hr) *(addressed 1 at each session [in random order])*	I: 24 O: 3		
LIHEF, 2002[137]	Fair	715	High	I: 9 O: 0	18 months	UC
Migneault, 2012[125]	Fair	337	High	I: 33 O: 0	8 months	MI (manual + pedometer + scale)
PREMIER, 2003[116]	Good	304	IG1: High	I: 33 O: 0	18 months	UC
			IG2: High *(DASH diet)*	I: 33 O: 0	18 months	
Rodriguez, 2012[113]	Fair (poor for diet)	533	Medium *(phone only)*	I: 6 O: 0	6 months	CG1: MI CG2: UC
TONE, 1998[117] *(Also has arm in HD-only section)*	Good	975	IG2: High *(weight loss)*	I: 32 O: 0	15–36 months; median, 29 months	UC with partial AC
			IG3: High *(decreased sodium + weight loss)*	I: 32 O: 0		
Vitalum, 2011[105]	Fair	1,629	IG1: Low *(mail only)*	I: 0 O: 4	3.6 months	UC
			IG2: Medium *(phone)*	I: 4 O: 0		
			IG3: Medium *(mail + phone)*	I: 2 O: 2		

Table 8. Behavioral Counseling Trials in Persons With Hypertension: Intervention Characteristics

Study, Year Intervention Focus	Quality	N	Intervention Intensity	# of Contacts Interactive (I), Other (O)	Duration of Intervention	Type of Control
Healthy diet–only interventions						
Arroll, 1995[128] *(Also has arms in HD+PA and PA-only sections)*	Fair	208	IG3: Medium *(salt only)*	I: 1 O: 0	Unknown	UC
Beckman, 1995[111]	Fair	64	Medium	I: 5 O: 0	12 months	Waitlist control
TONE, 1998[117] *(Also has arms in HD+PA section)*	Good	975	IG1: High *(decreased sodium only)*	I: 32 O: 0	15–36 months; median, 29 months	UC with partial AC
Physical activity–only interventions						
Arroll, 1995[128] *(Also has arms in HD+PA and PA-only sections)*	Fair	208	IG2: Medium *(PA only)*	I: 1 O: 0	Unknown	UC
Moreau, 2001[104]	Fair	24	Medium (assumed)	I: assumed ≥1 O: 0	Unknown	No advice

Abbreviations: AC = attention control; ADAPT = Activity Diet and Blood Pressure Trial; CG = control group; HIP = Hypertension Improvement Project; HTTP = Hypertension Teaching and Treatment Programme; IG = intervention group; LIHEF = Lifestyle Intervention against Hypertension in Eastern Finland; MD = physician; MI = minimal intervention; N = study population; pt = patient; TONE = Trial of Non-Pharmacological Interventions in the Elderly; UC = usual care.

Table 9. Behavioral Counseling Trials in Persons With Impaired Fasting Glucose or Impaired Glucose Tolerance: Intervention Characteristics

Study, Year	Quality	N	Intervention Intensity	# of Contacts Interactive (I), Other (O)	Duration of Intervention	Type of Control
Healthy diet and physical activity interventions						
APHRODITE, 2011[88]	Fair	925	High	I: 18 O: 0	18 months	UC
DPP, 2002[89]	Good	2,161	High	I: ≥32* O: 0	6 months core curriculum + 1.8–4.6 years maintenance (mean, 2.8 years)	MI†
EDIPS, 2001[90]	Fair	78	Medium	I: 12 O: 0	24 months	No advice
EDIPS-Newcastle, 2009[91]	Fair	102	High	I: 24 O: 20	5 years	UC
E-LITE, 2013[87]	Good	162	High	I: 2 O: 42	15 months	UC
FDPS, 2001[118]	Good	522	High	I: 16‡ O: 0	Mean, 38.4 months	UC
HLC, 2011[92]	Fair	307	High	I: 7 O: 0	6 months	Waitlist control
Kosaka, 2005[93]	Fair	NR§	High	I: 16 O: 0	48 months	MI
Live Well, Be Well, 2012[86]	Good	238	High	I: 20 O: 12	12 months	Waitlist control
LLDP, 2012[94]	Good	312	High	I: 16 O: 0	12 months	UC
Melbourne DPS, 2012[85]	Fair	92	High	I: 7 O: 0	8 months	Waitlist control
PREDIAS, 2009[95]	Fair	182	High	I: 12 O: 0	12 months	MI
SLIM, 2011[149]	Fair	147	High	I: 15 (+ option to join exercise program for 1 hr/wk) O: 0	3 years‖	UC (single session)
Healthy diet–only interventions						
Watanabe, 2003[97]	Fair	173	Low (30 min)	I: 1 O: 1	6 months	UC
Physical activity–only interventions						
Enhanced Fitness Trial, 2012[98]	Fair	302	IG1: High (same content) IG2: High (same content)	I: 23 O: 5 I: 26 O: 5	12 months	MI (referral to program)
Prepare Trial, 2009[99]	Fair	98	IG1: Medium (counseling) IG2: Medium (counseling + pedometer)	I: 3 O: 0 I: 3 O: 0	6 months	UC (mailed info)

* Based on the 1.8-years maintenance phase.

Table 9. Behavioral Counseling Trials in Persons With Impaired Fasting Glucose or Impaired Glucose Tolerance: Intervention Characteristics

† Recommendations reviewed annually.
‡ Based on a mean followup of 38.4 months +optional supervised exercise twice per week.
§ Only participants still present at 1-year observation (n=482) are reported.
‖ Mean followup of 4.1 years (49.2 months).

Abbreviations: APHRODITE = Active Prevention in High-Risk Individuals of Diabetes Type 2 in and Around Eindhoven; DPP = Diabetes Prevention Program; DPS = Diabetes Prevention Study; EDIPS = European Diabetes Prevention Study; E-LITE = Evaluation of Lifestyle Interventions to Treat Elevated Cardiometabolic Risk in Primary Care; FDPS = Finnish Diabetes Prevention Study; HLC = Healthy Living Course; IG = intervention group; LLDP = Lawrence Latino Diabetes Prevention Project; MI = minimal intervention; N = study population; NR = not reported; PREDIAS = Prevention of Diabetes Self-Management Program; SLIM = Study on Lifestyle Intervention and IGT Maastricht; UC = usual care.

Table 10. Behavioral Counseling Trials in Persons With Mixed Cardiovascular Risk Factors: Intervention Characteristics

Study, Year	Quality	N	Intervention Intensity	# of Contacts Interactive (I), Other (O)	Duration of Intervention	Type of Control
Healthy diet and physical activity interventions						
Bo, 2007[145]	Fair	375	Medium	I: 5 O: 0	12 months	UC
Cochrane, 2012[102]	Fair	601	High	I: 7 O: 0	12 months	MI
Edelman, 2006[129]	Fair	154	High	I: 52 O: 0	10 months	UC
EURO-ACTION, 2008[106]	Fair	2,384	High	I: 8 O: 0	16 weeks*	UC
GOAL, 2009[139]	Good	457	Medium	I: 5 O: 0	8 months	UC
Hardcastle, 2008[168]	Fair	334	Medium	I: 5 O: 0	6 months	UC
HIPS, 2012[103]	Fair	814	High	I: 6 O: 0	12 months	Waitlist control
Hoorn, 2013[132]	Fair	622	Medium	I: 9 O: 0	16 months	UC
IMPALA, 2009[133]	Fair	615	Medium (50 min)	I: 3 O: 0	12 weeks	UC
Inter99, 2008[107]	Fair	4,053	High	I: 10 O: 0	5 years	MI (annual session)
Logan Healthy Living, 2009[114]	Fair	434	Medium (6 hr; phone only)	I: 18 O: 1	12 months	MI (3 sessions with brief, tailored feedback)
Nilsson, 1992[119]	Fair	63	High	I: 15 O: 0	12 months	UC
PEGASE, 2008[120]	Fair	640	High	I: 6 O: 0	6 months	UC
PHPP, 2007[121]	Fair	99	Medium	I: 6 O: 0	12 months	UC
RIS, 1994[115]	Good (KQ1) Fair (KQ2)	508	High	I: 7 (+5 for smokers [29%]) O: 0	4 months	UC
Rodriguez-Cristobal, 2012[173]	Fair	436	Medium†	I: 12 O: 0	2 years	UC
SPRING, 2012[100]	Fair	201	Medium	I: 5§ O: 0	12 months	MI
WISEWOMAN California, 2010[108]	Fair	1,093	Medium	I: 3 (+ telephone sessions‡ + incentives) O: 0	6 months	UC
WISEWOMAN NC, 2008[110]	Fair	236	High	I: 16 O: 4	12 months	UC
Wister, 2007[140]	Good	315	Medium	I: 2 (+4 more for quitting smokers [<15%]) O: 1	1 year	UC

Table 10. Behavioral Counseling Trials in Persons With Mixed Cardiovascular Risk Factors: Intervention Characteristics

Study, Year	Quality	N	Intervention Intensity	# of Contacts Interactive (I), Other (O)	Duration of Intervention	Type of Control
Physical activity-only interventions						
Green Prescription Programme (Walk to Heart, Health & Activity study), 2003[123]	Fair	878	Medium	I: ≥4 O: 4	12 months	Waitlist control
NERS, 2012[109]	Fair	2,160	Medium	I: 5 (+ option for exercise sessions) O: 0	8 months	Waitlist control
PAC, 2011[122]	Fair	120	Medium	I: 7 O: 0	13 weeks	MI (tailored PA prescription)
PACE, 2005[131]	Fair	771	Medium	I: 4 O: 0	8 weeks	UC
Kallings, 2009[141] Kallings, 2008[176]	Good	101	Medium	I: 4 O: 1	6 months	UC
LIFE, 2010[130]	Fair	126	High	I: 23 O: 0	11 months	UC

* Assumed.
† Possibly high, but intervention NR.
‡ Number NR.
§ Median of 4.9 sessions.

Abbreviations: GOAL = Groningen Overweight and Lifestyle Study; IMPALA = Improving Patient Adherence to Lifestyle Advice; KQ = key question; LIFE = Lifestyle Interventions and Independence for elder; MI = minimal intervention; N = study population; NERS = National Exercise Referral Scheme; PA = physical activity; PAC = Physical Activity Counseling; PACE = Physician-based Assessment and Counseling for Exercise; PEGASE = Pan European Grid Advanced Simulation and State Examination; PHPP = Patient-motivated Health Promotion Program; RIS = Risk Factor Intervention Study; SPRING = Self-monitoring and Prevention of Risk Factors; UC = usual care.

Table 11. Behavioral Counseling Trials: Key Question 1 Outcomes

Study, year Quality	N	Risk Population	Mean Age, y % Men	Intervention Type Intensity	Followup Time, mo	CVD Outcomes	Self-Reported QOL
PREMIER, 2003[116] Good	304	HTN	52 36.5	HD+PA High	Short: 6	Stroke↔† TIA↔† MI↔†	NR##
					Intermediate: 18	NR	NR
					Long: NR	--	--
TONE, 1998[117] Good	975	HTN	67 52.0	HD+PA High	Short: 9	NR	NR
					Intermediate: 18¶¶	NR	NR
					Long: 30 or 36¶¶	Stroke↔ TIA↔ MI↔ Angina↔ CHF↔ Other CV↔ Total CV↔	NR
DPP, 2002[89] Good	2,161	IFG	51 32.3	HD+PA High	Short: NR	--	--
					Intermediate: 12 + 24	NR	NR
					Long: 36	CVD-related deaths↔ Nonfatal CVD events↔	NR
FDPS, 2001[118] Good	522	IFG	55 33.0	HD+PA High	Short: 12	NR	NR
					Intermediate: 24	NR	NR
					Long: 120	Mortality↔ CVD events↔	NR
HLC, 2011[92] Fair	307	IFG	62 41.0*	HD+PA High	Short: 6	NR	Depression score‡↔
					Intermediate: NR	--	--
					Long: NR	--	--
Live Well, Be Well, 2012[86] Good	238	IFG	56 26.0*	HD+PA High	Short: 6	--	Health Status***↑ QOL↑↑↑↑
					Intermediate: 12	NR	Health Status***↔ QOL↑↑↑↑
					Long: NR	--	--
LLDP, 2012[94] Good	312	IFG	52 25.6	HD+PA High	Short: NR	--	--
					Intermediate: 12	NR	Depression score§↔
					Long: NR	--	--
Melbourne DPS, 2012[85] Fair	92	IFG	65 27.0	HD+PA High	Short: NR	--	--
					Intermediate: 12	NR	Depression score‡‡‡↔
					Long: NR	--	--
PREDIAS, 2009[95] Fair	182	IFG	56 57.0	HD+PA High	Short: NR	--	--
					Intermediate: 12	NR	% Depression§↔ QOL‖↔
					Long: NR	--	--
Enhanced Fitness Trial, 2012[98] Fair+	302	IFG	67 97.0	PA only High	Short: NR	--	--
					Intermediate: 12	NR	QOL¶↔
					Long: NR	--	--

Table 11. Behavioral Counseling Trials: Key Question 1 Outcomes

Study, year Quality	N	Risk Population	Mean Age, y % Men	Intervention Type Intensity	Followup Time, mo	CVD Outcomes	Self-Reported QOL
Nilsson, 1992[119] Fair	63	Mixed	56* 78.0*	HD+PA High	Short: NR Intermediate: 12 Long: NR	-- NR --	-- Health status§§↑ --
PEGASE, 2008[120] Fair	640	Mixed	57* 60.0*	HD+PA High	Short: 6 Intermediate: NR Long: NR	NR -- --	QOL (PCS)††↔ QOL (MCS)††↔ --
RIS, 1998[112] Good	508	Mixed	66 100.0	HD+PA High	Short: NR Intermediate:12 Long: 36‡‡	-- Total mortality↔ Total mortality↔ CVD mortality↔ MI↔ Stroke↔ First CV event↔ CVD events↔	-- NR NR
WISEWOMAN NC, 2008[110] Fair	236	Mixed	53 0	HD+PA High	Short: 6 Intermediate: 12 Long: NR	NR NR --	QOL**↔ QOL**↔ --
PHPP, 2007[121] Fair	99	Mixed	64* 42.4*	HD+PA Medium	Short: NR Intermediate: 12 Long: NR	-- NR --	-- QOL#↔ --
PAC, 2011[122] Fair	120	Mixed	47* 32*	PA only Medium	Short: 6 Intermediate: NR Long: NR	NR -- --	QOL‖‖↔ -- --

* Calculated.
† Health outcomes for entire study population, not stratified by HTN status.
‡ Based on DASS-21.
§ Based on CES-D.
‖ Psychological well-being using WHO-5.
¶ SF-36, general health and physical function.
# Using GHQ-30.
** Based on SF-8, PCS and MCS both↔.
†† SF-36.
‡‡ Health outcomes not reported at 72-month followup.
§§ Visual analogue scale.
‖‖ Based on SF-12, PCS and MCS.
¶¶ Results for combined salt reduction and weight loss arm; results similar for sodium reduction arm alone.
QOL outcomes were not reported separately for persons with HTN.
*** Self-rated health using Likert Scale.
††† Psychological Well-being II Scale.
‡‡‡ Hospital Anxiety and Depression Scale.

Abbreviations: CES-D = Center for Epidemiologic Studies Depression Scale; CHF = congestive heart failure; CV = cardiovascular; CVD = cardiovascular disease; DASS = Depression Anxiety & Stress Scale; DPP = Diabetes Prevention Program; DPS = Diabetes Prevention Study; FDPS = Finnish Diabetes Prevention Study; HD = healthy diet; HLC = Healthy Living Course; HTN = hypertension; IFG = impaired fasting glucose; LLDP = Lawrence Latino Diabetes Prevention Project; MCS = Mental Component Summary; MI = myocardial infarction; N = study population; NR = not reported; PA = physical activity; PAC = Physical Activity Counseling; PCS = Physical Component Summary; PEGASE = Pan European Grid Advanced Simulation and State Estimation; PHPP = Patient-motivated Health Promotion Program; PREDIAS = Prevention of Diabetes Self-Management Program; QOL = quality of life; SF = Short-form Health Survey; TIA = transient ischemic attack; TONE = Trial of Non-Pharmacological Interventions in the Elderly.

Table 12. Behavioral Counseling Trials in Persons With Dyslipidemia or Elevated Cholesterol: Key Question 2 Outcomes

Study, Year Quality	N	Followup Time, mo	TC	LDL	TG	Weight/BMI	Other Intermediate Outcomes
Healthy diet and physical activity interventions							
CouPLES, 2013[57] Fair	255	Short: 11	NR	↔	NR	NR	Changes in meds (%): no difference
		Intermediate: NA	--	--	--	--	--
		Long: NA	--	--	--	--	--
PRO-FIT, 2012[68] Fair	340	Short: NA	--	--	--	--	--
		Intermediate: 12	↔	NR	NR	BMI↔	HDL↔ SBP↔ FBG↔
		Long: NA	--	--	--	--	--
RHPP Trial, 1993[69] Fair	1,197	Short: NA	--	--	--	--	--
		Intermediate: NA	--	--	--	--	--
		Long: 30§	↔	NR	NR	NR	NR
Healthy diet–only interventions							
Anderson, 1992[70] Fair	177	Short: NA	--	--	--	--	--
		Intermediate: 12	↓	↓*	↔	Weight↔**	HDL↔ Started meds (%): no difference
		Long: NA	--	--	--	--	--
Ammerman, 2003[74] Keyserling, 1999[174] Fair	468	Short: 6	↔	↔	↔	Weight↑	HDL↔ Started meds (%): increase#
		Intermediate: 12	↔	↔	↔	Weight↔	HDL↔ Started meds (%): no difference
		Long: NA	--	--	--	--	--
Bloemberg, 1991[75] Fair	80	Short: 6	↓	NR	NR	Weight↑	HDL↔
		Intermediate: NA	--	--	--	--	--
		Long: NA	--	--	--	--	--
DEER, 1998[71]	189	Short: NA	--	--	--	--	--
		Intermediate: 12†	↓	↓	↔	Weight↑	HDL↔ SBP↔ DBP↔ FBG↑ 2-GTT↑# METS incidence, n (%)↑
		Long: NA	--	--	--	--	--
Delahanty, 2001[72] Good	90	Short: 6	↓	↔	↔	Weight↑**	HDL↔
		Intermediate: 12	↔	↔	↔	Weight↔	HDL↔
		Long: NA	--	--	--	--	--
Hyman, 1998[76] Fair	123	Short: 6	↔	NR	NR	Weight↔	Started meds (%): no difference
		Intermediate: NA	--	--	--	--	--
		Long: NA	--	--	--	--	--
Johnston, 1995[77] Fair	179	Short: 6§	↔	↔	NR	BMI↔ Weight↔	HDL↔
		Intermediate: NA	--	--	--	--	--
		Long: NA	--	--	--	--	--

Table 12. Behavioral Counseling Trials in Persons With Dyslipidemia or Elevated Cholesterol: Key Question 2 Outcomes

Study, Year Quality	N	Followup Time, mo	TC	LDL	TG	Weight/BMI	Other Intermediate Outcomes
Moy, 2001[73] Fair	235	Short: NA	--	--	--	--	--
		Intermediate: 24	NR	↑	↔	BMI↔	HDL↔
		Long: NA	--	--	--	--	--
Neil, 1995[78] Fair	309	Short: 6§	↔	↔	↔	BMI↔	HDL↔
		Intermediate: NA	--	--	--	--	--
		Long: NA	--	--	--	--	--
NFPMP, 2002[79]	143	Short: 6	NR	NR	NR	BMI↑ Weight↑	NR
		Intermediate: 12	↔	↔	↔	BMI↑ Weight↑	HDL↔ Started meds (%): no difference
		Long: NA	--	--	--	--	--
ODES, 1995[80] Fair	98	Short: NA	--	--	--	--	--
		Intermediate: 12	↔	↔	↔	BMI↑ Weight↑	HDL↑ SBP↑ DBP↔ FBG↑ 1-GTT↓ METS (%)↑
		Long: NA	--	--	--	--	--
Southeast Cholesterol Project, 1997[81] Fair	372	Short: 7	↔∥	↔∥	NR	NR	On meds (%): decrease
		Intermediate: 12	↔∥	↔∥	NR	NR	On meds (%): no difference
		Long: NA	--	--	--	--	--
Stevens, 2003[82] Fair	616	Short: NA	--	--	--	--	--
		Intermediate: 12	↔	NR	NR	NR	NR
		Long: NA	--	--	--	--	--
Tomson, 1995[83] Tomson, 1994[175] Fair	92	Short: NA	--	--	--	--	--
		Intermediate: 12	↔	NR	↔	NR	HDL↓¶
		Long: NA	--	--	--	--	--

* IG2 only.
† Outcome by men and women separately; no difference between sexes.
§ Results for IG1 and IG2 combined; no difference between groups.
∥ ↑ in persons not taking lipid-lowering medications.
¶ HDL cholesterol was statistically significantly higher in control group. Authors state that more women were in the control group and that HDL is generally higher in women. Outcome not adjusted for sex.
# p-value NR.
** Because of the adjustment of some reported data, values may be different than the unadjusted values reported in meta-analysis.

Abbreviations: BMI = body mass index; CouPLES = Couples Partnering for Lipid Enhancing Strategies; DBP = diastolic blood pressure; DEER = Diet and Exercise for Elevated Risk; FBG = fasting blood glucose; GTT = glucose tolerance test; HDL = high-density lipoprotein; LDL = low-density lipoprotein; meds = medications; METS = metabolic syndrome; N = study population; n = sample population; NA = not available; NFPMP = Nijmegen Family Practices Monitoring Project; NR = not reported; ODES = Oslo Diet and Exercise Study; RHPP = Rural Health Promotion Project; TC = total cholesterol; TG = triglycerides.

Table 13. Behavioral Counseling Trials in Persons With Hypertension: Key Question 2 Outcomes

Study, Year Quality	N	Followup Time, mo	SBP	DBP	Weight/ BMI	Other Intermediate Outcomes
Healthy diet and physical activity interventions						
ADAPT, 2006[138] Fair	241	Short: NA	--	--	--	--
		Intermediate: 12	NR	NR	Weight↑	TC (mg/dL)↔ HDL (mg/dL)↔ LDL (mg/dL)↑ TG (mg/dL)↔ FBG (mg/dL)↔
		Long: 36	↔	↔	Weight↔	Composite CVD risk*↔ Change in need for antiHTN meds (%): no difference Started statins (%)↔ Statin dose decreased (%)↔ TC (mg/dL)↑## HDL (mg/dL)↔ LDL (mg/dL) NR TG (mg/dL)↔ FBG (mg/dL)↔
Applegate, 1992[127] Fair	56	Short: 6	↑	↑	Weight↑	NR
		Intermediate: NA	--	--	--	--
		Long: NA	--	--	--	--
Arroll, 1995[128] Fair *(Also arms in HD- & PA-only sections)*	208	Short: 6	↔	↔	NR	HDL↑
		Intermediate: NA	--	--	--	--
		Long: NA	--	--	--	--
Bosworth, 2009[84] Fair	477	Short: NA	--	--	--	--
		Intermediate: 12	↑***	↑***	NR	NR
		Long: 24	↑***	↑***	NR	NR
HIP, 2009[136] Fair	574	Short: 6	MD↔ Pt↑	MD↔ Pt↑	Weight: MD↔ Pt↔	NR
		Intermediate: 18	MD↔ Pt↔	MD↔ Pt↔	Weight: MD↔ Pt↔	NR
		Long: NA	--	--	--	--
HTTP, 1993[134] Fair	200	Short: NA	--	--	--	--
		Intermediate: 18	↔	↑	NR	Number of meds per person: decrease
		Long: NA	--	--	--	--
Hyman, 2007[135] Fair	281	Short: 6	↔	↔	BMI↔	TC (mg/dL)↔
		Intermediate: 18[†]	↔	↔	BMI↔	TC (mg/dL)↔
		Long: NA	--	--	--	--
LIHEF, 2002[137] Fair	715	Short: NA	--	--	--	--
		Intermediate: 12 and 24[‡]	↔	↔§	Weight↑	TC (mg/dL)↑§ HDL (mg/dL)↔ LDL (mg/dL)↑¶¶ TG (mg/dL)↔
		Long: NA	--	--	--	--

Table 13. Behavioral Counseling Trials in Persons With Hypertension: Key Question 2 Outcomes

Study, Year Quality	N	Followup Time, mo	SBP	DBP	Weight/ BMI	Other Intermediate Outcomes
Migneault, 2012[126] Fair	337	Short: 8	↔	↔	NR	% with BP control (<140/90 mm Hg)↔
		Intermediate: 12 ‖	↔	↔	NR	NR
		Long: NA	--	--	--	--
PREMIER, 2003[116] Good	304	Short: 6	↑	↑	Weight↔	% optimal BP control (<120/80 mm Hg)↑ Use of meds (%): decrease % HTN↑¶ TC (mg/dL)#↑ LDL (mg/dL)#↔ HDL (mg/dL)#↔ TG (mg/dL)#↑ Glucose (mg/dL)#↑ Composite CVD risk*↔
		Intermediate: 18††	↔	↔	NR	Use of meds (%): decrease % HTN↑ Change in HTN status↔‡‡
		Long: NA	--	--	--	--
Rodriguez, 2012[113] Fair (poor for diet)	533	Short: 6	↔	NR	NR	NR
		Intermediate: 12	↔	NR	NR	NR
		Long: NA	--	--	--	--
TONE, 1998[117] Good (Also arm in HD-only section)	975	Short: 9	NR	NR	Weight↑	NR
		Intermediate: 18	NR	NR	Weight↑	% Free of CVD events, HTN↑ % Free of meds: increase
		Long: 30 or 36§§	NR	NR	Weight↑	% at BP goal (<140/90 mm Hg)↔ % Free of CVD events, HTN↑ % Free of meds: increase
Vitalum[105] Fair	1,629	Short: 6	NR	NR	NR	NR
		Intermediate: 18	NR	NR	NR	NR
		Long: NA	--	--	--	--
Healthy diet–only interventions						
Arroll, 1995[128] Fair (Also arms in HD+PA & PA-only sections)	208	Short: 6	↔	↔	NR	NR
		Intermediate: NA	--	--	--	--
		Long: NA	--	--	--	--
Beckman, 1995[111] Fair	64	Short: 6	NR	NR	NR	NR
		Intermediate: 12	↑‖	↑‖	Weight↔ BMI↔	TC (mg/dL)↔ HDL (mg/dL)↔ TG (mg/dL)↔
		Long: NA	--	--	--	--
TONE, 1998[117] Good (Also listed in HD+PA section)	975	Short: 9	NR	NR	NR	NR
		Intermediate: 18	NR	NR	NR	% Free of CVD events, HTN↑ % Free of meds: increase
		Long: 30 or 36§§	NR	NR	Weight↑	% Free of CVD events, HTN↑ % Free of meds: increase

Table 13. Behavioral Counseling Trials in Persons With Hypertension: Key Question 2 Outcomes

Study, Year Quality	N	Followup Time, mo	SBP	DBP	Weight/ BMI	Other Intermediate Outcomes
Physical activity–only interventions						
Arroll, 1995[128] Fair *(Also arms in HD+PA & HD-only sections)*	208	Short: 6	↔	↔	NR	HDL↑
		Intermediate: NA	--	--	--	--
		Long: NA				
Moreau, 2001[104] Fair	24	Short: 6	↑	↔	Weight↔ % body fat↔	FBG (mg/dL)↔
		Intermediate: NA	--	--	--	--
		Long: NA	--	--	--	--

* Using 10-year FRS.
† Results are for IG1 and IG2 combined.
‡ Outcomes for 12 and 24 months unless otherwise noted.
§ Significant at 12 months, not at 24 months.
‖ Outcomes derived from figure only.
¶ Among participants with HTN, those with HTN at followup.
# Patients with metabolic syndrome only.
** Health outcomes for entire study population, not stratified by HTN status.
†† IG1 and IG2 combined; outcomes for subgroup with HTN unless otherwise noted.
‡‡ Among participants with HTN, percent with normal BP and no medications at 18 months.
§§ Outcomes for IG2 (weight loss) and IG3 (sodium + weight loss) unless otherwise noted.
‖‖ Reports mean arterial pressure only.
¶¶ Significant at 24 months, not significant at 12 months.
Because of the adjustment of some reported data, values may be different than the unadjusted values reported in the meta-analysis.
*** Significant for IG2 only (BP reduction not significant for IG1 at 24 months).

Abbreviations: ADAPT = Activity Diet and Blood Pressure Trial; BMI = body mass index; CVD = cardiovascular disease; DBP = diastolic blood pressure; FBG = fasting blood glucose; HD = healthy diet; HDL = high-density lipoprotein; HIP = Health Improvement Project; HTN = hypertension; HTTP = Hypertension Teaching and Treatment Programme; LDL = low-density lipoprotein; LIHEF = Lifestyle Intervention against Hypertension in Eastern Finland; MD = physician; meds = medications; N = study population; NA = not available; NR = not reported; PA = physical activity; pt = patient; SBP = systolic blood pressure; TC = total cholesterol; TG = triglycerides; TONE = Trial of Non-Pharmacological Interventions in the Elderly.

Table 14. Behavioral Counseling Trials in Persons With Impaired Fasting Glucose or Impaired Glucose Tolerance: Key Question 2 Outcomes

Study, Year Quality	N	Followup Time, mo	DM Incidence	Glucose (FBG/GTT/HbA1c)	BP, mm Hg	Lipids, mg/dL	Weight (lb, BMI)	Other Intermediate Outcomes
Healthy diet and physical activity interventions								
APHRODITE, 2011[88] Fair	925	Short: 6	NR	FBG↔ 2h-GTT↔	NR	NR	BMI↔	NR
		Intermediate: 18	↔	FBG↔ 2h-GTT↔	NR	NR	BMI↔	NR
		Long: NA	--	--	--	--	--	--
DPP, 2002[89] Good	2,161	Short: N/A	--	--	--	--	--	--
		Intermediate: 12 + 24	NR	FBG↑	SBP↑ DBP↑	TG↑ HDL↑↑↑↑	Weight↑	NR
		Long: 36	↑	FBG↑	SBP↑ DBP↑	TC↔ LDL↔ TG↑ HDL↑↑↑↑	Weight↑	METs incidence↑
EDIPS, 2001[90] Fair	78	Short: 6	NR	FBG↔ 2h-GTT↔ A1c↔	SBP: NR DBP↔	TC↔ LDL↔ HDL↔ TG↔	Weight↑ BMI↑	NR
		Intermediate: 24	↔	FBG↔ 2h-GTT↔	NR	TC↔ LDL↔	Weight↑	NR
		Long: NR	--	--	--	--	--	--
EDIPS-Newcastle, 2009[91] Fair	102	Short: NA	NR	--	--	--	--	NR
		Intermediate: 12	↔	--	--	--	Weight↑	NR
		Long: 36 (mean followup)	↔	NR	NR	NR	Weight↔	NR
E-LITE, 2013[87] Good	162	Short: 6	NR	NR	NR	NR	Weight↑ BMI↑	NR
		Intermediate: 15	↔	FBG↑	SBP↔ DBP↔	TC↑ LDL↔ HDL↔ TG↔	Weight↑ BMI↑	NR
		Long: NA	--	--	--	--	--	--
FDPS, 2001[118] Good	522	Short: 12	↑	FBG↑ GTT↑ A1c↑	SBP↑ DBP↑	TC↔ HDL↔ TG↑	Weight↑ BMI↑	Cholesterol-lowering drugs (%): no difference AntiHTN drugs (%): no difference
		Intermediate: 24	↑	FBG↑ GTT↑	SBP↑ DBP↑	TC↔ TG↑ HDL↔	Weight↑	NR
		Long: 36	↑#	FBG↔ GTT↔ A1c↑	NR	TC↔ HDL↔ TG↑↑↑↑	BMI↑	NR

Table 14. Behavioral Counseling Trials in Persons With Impaired Fasting Glucose or Impaired Glucose Tolerance: Key Question 2 Outcomes

Study, Year Quality	N	Followup Time, mo	DM Incidence	Glucose (FBG/GTT/HbA1c)	BP, mm Hg	Lipids, mg/dL	Weight (lb, BMI)	Other Intermediate Outcomes
HLC, 2011[92] Fair	307	Short: 6	(%)↔	FBG↑ 2h-GTT↔	NR↑	LDL↔ HDL↔ TG↔	Weight↑ BMI↑↑↑↑	NR
		Intermediate: NA	--	--	--	--	--	--
		Long: NA	--	--	--	--	--	--
Kosaka, 2005[93] Fair	NR**	Short: 12	NR	NR	NR	NR	NR	NR
		Intermediate: 24	NR	NR	NR	NR	NR	NR
		Long: 48	↑	GTT↑‡	NR	NR	Weight↑	NR
Live Well, Be Well, 2012[86] Good	238	Short: 6	NR	FBG↔	SBP↔	LDL↔ HDL↔ TG↑	Weight↑	NR
		Intermediate: 12	NR	FBG↔	SBP↔	LDL↔ HDL↔ TG↔	Weight↔	NR
		Long: NA	--	--	--	--	--	--
LLDP[94] Good	312	Short: NA	--	--	--	--	--	--
		Intermediate: 12	↔	FBG↔ HbA1c↑	NR	NR	Weight↑ BMI↑	NR
		Long: NA	--	--	--	--	--	--
Melbourne DPS, 2012[85] Fair	92	Short: NA	--	--	--	--	--	--
		Intermediate: 12	NR	FBG↔ 2h-GTT↔ A1c↔	SBP↔ DBP↔	TC↔ LDL↔ HDL↔ TG↔	Weight↑ BMI↑	5% weight loss goal (%)↑
		Long: NA	--	--	--	--	--	--
PREDIAS, 2009[95] Fair	182	Short: NA	--	--	--	--	--	--
		Intermediate: 12	NR	FBG↑ 2h-GTT↔ A1c↔	SBP↔ DBP↔	TC↔	Weight↑ BMI↑	NR
		Long: NA	--	--	--	--	--	--
SLIM[149] Fair	147	Short: NA	--	--	--	--	--	--
		Intermediate: 12 + 24	NR	FBG↔-↑↑↑ 2h-GTT↑ A1c↔	SBP↔ DBP↔	TC↔ LDL↔ HDL↔ TG↑††	Weight↑ BMI↑	NR
		Long: 36–72‡‡	↑	FBG↔ 2h-GTT↑ A1c↔	SBP↔ DBP↔	TC↔ LDL↔ HDL↔ TG↔	Weight↑ BMI↑	% meds§§: no difference

Table 14. Behavioral Counseling Trials in Persons With Impaired Fasting Glucose or Impaired Glucose Tolerance: Key Question 2 Outcomes

Study, Year Quality	N	Followup Time, mo	DM Incidence	Glucose (FBG/GTT/HbA1c)	BP, mm Hg	Lipids, mg/dL	Weight (lb, BMI)	Other Intermediate Outcomes
Healthy diet–only interventions								
Watanabe, 2003[97] Fair	173	Short: NA	--	--	--	--	--	--
		Intermediate: 12	NR	FBG↔ 1h-GTT↔ 2h-GTT↑	NR	NR	NR	NR
		Long: NA	--	--	--	--	--	--
Physical activity–only interventions								
Enhanced Fitness Trial, 2012[98] Fair	302	Short: NA	--	--	--	--	--	--
		Intermediate: 12	↔	FBG↔ A1c↔	NR	TC↔ LDL↔ HDL↔ TG↔	Weight↔ BMI↔	NR
		Long: NA	--	--	--	--	--	--
Prepare Trial, 2009[99] Fair	98	Short: 6[∥]	NR	FBG↑ A1c↔	SBP↔*** DBP: NR	TC↔ HDL↔ TG↔	Weight↔	NR
		Intermediate: 12 + 24[¶¶]	↔	FBG↔/## A1c↔	SBP↔*** DBP: NR	TC↔ HDL↔*** TG↔***	Weight↔	NR
		Long: NA	--	--	--	--	--	--

‡ Percent conversion from IGT to nonIGT.
§ Based on CES-D.
∥ Psychological well-being using WHO-5.
¶ SF-36, general health and physical function.
# Up to 48 months.
** Trial only reports participants still present at 1-year observation (n=482).
†† ↔ at 12 months.
‡‡ Mean followup of 4.1 years.
§§ On BP-, lipid-, or glucose-lowering medications.
∥∥ Results for IG1 and IG2 unless otherwise noted.
¶¶ Results for 12 and 24 months unless otherwise noted.
↑ at 12 months.
*** 12-month outcome only.
††† Because of the adjustment of some reported data, values may be different than the unadjusted values reported in the meta-analysis.

Abbreviations: APHRODITE = Active Prevention in High-Risk Individuals of Diabetes Type 2 in and Around Eindhoven; BMI = body mass index; BP = blood pressure; CES-D = Center for Epidemiologic Studies Depression Scale; DASS = Depression Anxiety & Stress Scale; DBP = diastolic blood pressure; DM = diabetes mellitus; DPP = Diabetes Prevention Program; DPS = Diabetes Prevention Study; EDIPS = European Diabetes Prevention Study; E-LITE = Evaluation of Lifestyle Interventions to Treat Elevated Cardiometabolic Risk in Primary Care; FBG = fasting blood glucose; FDPS = Finnish Diabetes Prevention Study; GTT = glucose tolerance test; HbA1c = glycated hemoglobin; HDL = high-density lipoprotein; HLC = Healthy Living Course; HTN = hypertension; LDL = low-density lipoprotein; LLDP = Lawrence Latino Diabetes Prevention Project; METS = metabolic syndrome; meds = medications; N = study population; NA = not available; NR = not reported; PREDIAS = Prevention of Diabetes Self-Management Program; SBP = systolic blood pressure; SF = Short-form Health Survey; SLIM = Study on Lifestyle Intervention and IGT Maastricht; TC = total cholesterol; TG = triglycerides.

Table 15. Behavioral Counseling Trials in Persons With Mixed Cardiovascular Risk Factors: Key Question 2 Outcomes

Study, Year Quality	N	Followup Time, Mo	BP, mm Hg	Lipids, mg/dL	Glucose (FBG/GTT/HbA1c)	Weight (lb/BMI)	Other Intermediate Outcomes
Healthy diet and physical activity interventions							
Bo, 2007[145] Fair	375	Short: NA	--	--	--	--	--
		Intermediate: 12	SBP↑ DBP↑	TC↔ HDL↓ TG↑	FBG↑	Weight↑ BMI↑	DM incidence (%)↑ HTN incidence (%)↔
		Long: NA	--	--	--	--	--
Cochrane, 2012[102] Fair	601	Short: NA	--	--	--	--	--
		Intermediate: 12	SBP↔ DBP↔	TC↔	NR	Weight↔ BMI↔	Composite CVD risk#↔
		Long: NA	--	--	--	--	--
Edelman, 2006[129] Fair	154	Short: 10	NR	LDL↔	NR	BMI↔	Good BP control (%)↑
		Intermediate: NA	--	--	--	--	--
		Long: NA	--	--	--	--	--
EURO-ACTION, 2008[106] Fair	2,384	Short: NA	--	--	--	--	--
		Intermediate: 12	SBP↔ DBP↔	TC↔ LDL↑	FBG↔ HbA1c↔	BMI↑	BP <140/90 (%)↑ DM incidence (%)↔ Started meds (%)↑↑↑
		Long: NA	--	--	--	--	--
GOAL, 2009[139] Good	457	Short: NA	--	--	--	--	--
		Intermediate: 12	SBP↔ DBP↔	TC↔ LDL↔ HDL↔	FBG↔	Weight↑§§§	Composite CVD risk*↔
		Long: 36	NR	NR	NR	Weight↔§§§	--
Hardcastle, 2008[168] Fair	334	Short: 6	SBP↔ DBP↑	TC↔ LDL↔ HDL↔ TG↔	NR	Weight↑ BMI↑	NR
		Intermediate: 18	SBP↔ DBP↑	TC↑ LDL↔ HDL↔ TG↔	NR	BMI↑	NR
		Long: NA	--	--	--	--	--
HIPS, 2012[103] Fair	814	Short: NA	--	--	--	--	--
		Intermediate: 12	SBP↔	LDL↔ HDL↔ TG↔	NR	Weight↔ BMI↔	Composite CVD risk↔ Started meds (%)↔
		Long: NA	--	--	--	--	--
Hoorn, 2013[132] Fair	622	Short: 6	NR	NR	NR	NR	Composite CVD risk*↔
		Intermediate: 12	NR	NR	NR	NR	Composite CVD risk*↔
		Long: NA	--	--	--	--	--

Table 15. Behavioral Counseling Trials in Persons With Mixed Cardiovascular Risk Factors: Key Question 2 Outcomes

Study, Year Quality	N	Followup Time, Mo	BP, mm Hg	Lipids, mg/dL	Glucose (FBG/GTT/HbA1c)	Weight (lb/BMI)	Other Intermediate Outcomes
IMPALA, 2009[133] Fair	615	Short term: NA	--	--	--	--	--
		Intermediate: 12	SBP↑ DBP: NR	Cholesterol ratio ↔	NR	NR	Composite CVD risk *↑
		Long: NA	--	--	--	--	--
Inter99, 2008[107] Fair	4,053	Short: NA	--	--	--	--	--
		Intermediate: NA	--	--	--	--	--
		Long: 60	NR	NR	FBG↑ GTT↔	BMI↔	DM incidence (%)↔
Logan Healthy Living, 2009[114] Fair	434	Short: 12	NR	NR	NR	NR	NR
		Intermediate: 18	NR	NR	NR	NR	NR
		Long: NA	--	--	--	--	--
Nilsson, 1992[119] Fair	63	Short: NA	--	--	--	--	--
		Intermediate: 12	SBP↔ DBP↔	TC↔ LDL↔ HDL↔ TG↔	FBG↔ 1h-GTT↔ 2h-GTT↑	Weight↔	NR
		Long: NA	--	--	--	--	--
PEGASE, 2008[120] Fair	640	Short: 6	SBP↔ DBP: NR	TC↔ LDL↑ HDL↔	NR	NR	Composite CVD risk#↔
		Intermediate: NA	--	--	--	--	--
		Long: NA	--	--	--	--	--
PHPP, 2007[121] Fair	99	Short: NA	--	--	--	--	--
		Intermediate: 12	SBP↔ DBP↔	TC↔ LDL↔ HDL↔ TG↔	HbA1c↔	Weight↔ BMI↔	DM incidence (%)↔
		Long: NA	--	--	--	--	--
RIS[112] Good (KQ1), Fair (KQ2)	508	Short: NA	--	--	--	--	--
		Intermediate: 12	SBP↔ DBP↑	TC↑ LDL↑ HDL↔ TG↔	FBG↔	Weight↑ BMI↑	NR
		Long: 79	SBP↔**** DBP↔****	TC↑ LDL↑ HDL↔**** TG↑	FBG↔‖‖	Weight↑‖‖ BMI↔‖‖	Started lipid meds (%): increase
Rodriguez-Cristobal, 2012[173] Fair	436	Short: NA	--	--	--	--	--
		Intermediate: 24	SBP↑ DBP↑	TC↑ LDL↔ HDL↔ TG↔	NR‡‡	BMI↑	NR
		Long: NA	--	--	--	--	--

Table 15. Behavioral Counseling Trials in Persons With Mixed Cardiovascular Risk Factors: Key Question 2 Outcomes

Study, Year Quality	N	Followup Time, Mo	BP, mm Hg	Lipids, mg/dL	Glucose (FBG/GTT/HbA1c)	Weight (lb/BMI)	Other Intermediate Outcomes
SPRING, 2012[100] Fair	201	Short: NA	--	--	--	--	--
		Intermediate: 12	SBP↔ DBP↔	TC↔ LDL↔ HDL↔ TG↔	FBG↔	BMI↔	Composite CVD risk *↔ Started HTN meds (%): increase Started lipid meds (%): no change
		Long: NA	--	--	--	--	--
WISEWOMAN California, 2010[108] Fair	1,093	Short: NA	--	--	--	--	--
		Intermediate: 12	SBP↑ DBP↔	TC↔ HDL↔	NR	BMI↔	Composite CVD risk# ¶¶¶↔ Dyslipidemia (%)↔ Started lipid meds (%)###
		Long: NA	--	--	--	--	--
WISEWOMAN North Carolina, 2008[110] Fair	236	Short: 6	SBP↔ DBP↔	TC↔ LDL↔ HDL↔	NR	Weight↔	NR
		Intermediate: 12	SBP↔ DBP↔	TC↔ LDL↔ HDL↔	NR	Weight↔	NR
		Long: NA	--	--	--	--	--
Wister, 2007[140] Good	315	Short: NA	--	--	--	--	--
		Intermediate: 12	SBP↑ DBP: NR	TC↑ HDL↔	FBG↔	BMI↔	Composite CVD risk# ↑
		Long: NA	--	--	--	--	--
Physical activity–only interventions							
Green Prescription Programme (Walk to Heart, Health & Activity study), 2003[123] Fair	878	Short: NA	--	--	--	--	--
		Intermediate: 12	SBP¶¶¶↔ DBP¶¶¶↔	TC↔	NR	BMI↔	Composite CVD risk##↔
		Long: NA	--	--	--	--	--
NERS, 2012[109] Fair	2,160	Short: NA	--	--	--	--	--
		Intermediate: 12	NR	NR	NR	NR	NR
		Long: NA	--	--	--	--	--
PAC, 2011[122] Fair	120	Short: 6	NR	TC↔ LDL↔ HDL↔ TG↔	NR†††	NR†††	NR
		Intermediate: NA	--	--	--	--	--
		Long: NA	--	--	--	--	--
PACE, 2005[131] Fair	771	Short: 6	NR	NR	NR	NR	NR
		Intermediate: 12	NR	NR	NR	Weight↔ BMI↔	NR
		Long: NA	--	--	--	--	--

Table 15. Behavioral Counseling Trials in Persons With Mixed Cardiovascular Risk Factors: Key Question 2 Outcomes

Study, Year Quality	N	Followup Time, Mo	BP, mm Hg	Lipids, mg/dL	Glucose (FBG/GTT/HbA1c)	Weight (lb/BMI)	Other Intermediate Outcomes
Kallings, 2009[141] Good	101	Short: 6	SBP↔ DBP↔	TC↑ LDL↔ HDL↔ TG↔	FBG↔ A1c↑	Weight↑ BMI↑	NR
		Intermediate: NA	--	--	--	--	--
		Long: NA	--	--	--	--	--
LIFE, 2010[130] Fair	186	Short: 6	SBP↔ DBP↔	TC↔ LDL↔ HDL↔	FBG↔	Weight↔ BMI↔	NR
		Intermediate: NA	--	--	--	--	--
		Long: NA	--	--	--	--	--

* 10-year CVD risk based on SCORE.
† Poor-quality trials not abstracted.
‡ Based on DASS-21 scale.
§ Based on CES-D.
¶ Visual analogue scale.
# 10-year CVD risk using FRS.
** SF-36.
†† Using GHQ-30.
‡‡ A1c only reported for persons with DM.
§§ Based on SF-8, PCS and MCS both ↔.
‖‖ SF-36 used but PCS and MCS NR.
¶¶ Only reported for subgroup ages 65 to 79 years.
4-year CVD risk using FRS.
*** Based on SF-12, PCS and MCS.
††† Only 13-week outcomes reported, assume 24-week outcomes were not significant.
‡‡‡ More patients started angiotensin-converting enzyme inhibitors and statins in IG vs. CG, perhaps accounting for increase in persons meeting BP and lipid goals.
§§§ Subgroup analysis: ↑ for men, ↔ for women.
‖‖‖ ↑ at 36 months.
¶¶¶ P=0.051.
More persons in IG started lipid medications (p=NR).
**** 36-month outcomes.
†††† Based on 5-year CVD risk; risk score that was used NR.

Abbreviations: BMI = body mass index; BP = blood pressure; CVD = cardiovascular disease; DBP = diastolic blood pressure; DM = diabetes mellitus; FBG = fasting blood glucose; GOAL = Groningen Overweight and Lifestyle Study; GTT = glucose tolerance test; HbA1c = glycated hemoglobin; HDL = high-density lipoprotein; HIPS = Health Improvement and Prevention Study; HTN = hypertension; IMPALA = Improving Patient Adherence to Lifestyle Advice; LDL = low-density lipoprotein; LIFE = Lifestyle Interventions and Independence for Elder; meds = medications; N = study population; NA = not available; NERS = National Exercise Referral Scheme; NR = not reported; PACE = Physical Activity Counseling; PAC = Physician-based Assessment and Counseling for Exercise; PEGASE = Pan European Grid Advanced Simulation and State Examination; PHPP = Physician-motivated Health Promotion Program; RIS = Risk Factor Intervention Study; SBP = systolic blood pressure; SPRING = Self-monitoring and Prevention of Risk Factors; TC = total cholesterol; TG = triglycerides.

Table 16. Pooled Effect Sizes for Intermediate Health Outcomes in Persons With Dyslipidemia

Followup, months	Cholesterol			Cholesterol and Mixed		
	Effect Size (95% CI)	K	I^2	Effect Size (95% CI)	K	I^2
Total cholesterol, mg/dL						
<12	-4.18 (-8.53 to 0.18)	5	38	-4.52 (-7.92 to -1.13)	9	34
12–24	-3.31 (-5.98 to -0.64)	9	24	-5.11 (-7.77 to -2.45)	22	68
>24	NR	--	--	-19.31 (-25.36 to -13.25)	1	NA
Low-density lipoprotein cholesterol, mg/dL						
<12	-1.33 (-5.06 to 2.40)	5	43	-2.14 (-4.94 to 0.66)	9	24
12–24	-3.93 (-7.23 to -0.62)	8	34	-3.74 (-6.39 to -1.09)	17	53
>24	NR	--	--	-15.44 (-21.50 to -9.39)	1	NA
High-density lipoprotein cholesterol, mg/dL						
<12	-0.20 (-1.52 to 1.12)	2	0	0.13 (-0.98 to 1.24)	4	0
12–24	-0.29 (-1.62 to 1.04)	3	0	0.74 (-0.24 to 1.72)	11	51
>24	NR	--	--	0.77 (-0.74 to 2.29)	1	NA
Triglycerides, mg/dL						
<12	NR	--	--	-10.82 (-26.23 to 4.64)	2	34
12–24	-17.86 (-33.10 to -2.62)	3	0	-13.35 (-20.34 to -6.35)	6	0.0
>24	NR	--	--	-19.47 (-31.61 to -7.33)	1	NA
Systolic blood pressure, mm Hg						
<12	NR	--	--	0.12 (-3.44 to 3.68)	3	60
12–24	-0.19 (-0.53 to -0.14)	3	73	-1.83 (-3.19 to -0.47)	17	57
>24	NR	--	--	-2.00 (-4.80 to 0.80)	1	NA
Diastolic blood pressure, mm Hg						
<12	NR	--	--	-0.54 (-3.07 to 1.99)	3	69
12–24	-0.32 (-0.55 to -0.08)	2	0	-1.35 (-2.08 to -0.62)	14	34
>24	NR	--	--	-1.00 (-2.29 to 0.29)	1	NA
Fasting glucose, mg/dL						
<12	NR	--	--	-1.72 (-4.26 to 0.83)	2	0
12–24	-0.82 (-1.67 to 0.4)	3	96	-2.50 (-4.40 to -0.59)	10	76
>24	NR	--	--	-3.60 (-7.84 to 0.63)	1	NA
Diabetes incidence, RR						
<12	NR	--	--	NR	--	--
12–24	NR	--	--	0.26 (0.09 to 0.76)	2	0
>24	NR	--	--	1.03 (0.67 to 1.59)	1	NA
Adiposity, Hedges g						
<12	-0.20 (-0.38 to -0.02)	5	41	-0.20 (-0.32 to -0.08)	9	26
12–24	-0.38 (-0.78 to 0.03)	6	90	-0.22 (-0.35 to -0.10)	18	80
>24	NR	--	--	-0.23 (-0.52 to 0.06)	2	76

Abbreviations: CI = confidence interval; NR = not reported; NA = not available; RR = relative risk.

Table 17. Pooled Effect Sizes for Intermediate Health Outcomes in Persons With Hypertension

Followup, months	Hypertension Effect Size (95% CI)	K	I^2	Hypertension and Mixed Effect Size (95% CI)	K	I^2
Total cholesterol, mg/dL						
<12	-6.15 (-15.03 to 2.73)	1	NA	-5.37 (-10.22 to -0.53)	5	25
12–24	-3.43 (-5.78 to -1.08)	4	0	-5.77 (-8.73 to -2.80)	17	71
>24	-3.86 (-11.50 to 3.78)	1	NA	-11.77 (-26.90 to 3.36)	2	90
Low-density lipoprotein cholesterol, mg/dL						
<12	NR	--	--	-4.22 (-8.82 to 0.38)	4	0
12–24	-5.29 (-7.53 to -3.05)	2	0	-4.20 (-7.07 to -1.33)	11	58
>24	NR	--	--	-15.44 (-21.50 to -9.39)	1	NA
High-density lipoprotein cholesterol, mg/dL						
<12	NR	--	--	0.92 (-1.12 to 2.97)	2	0
12–24	-0.24 (-4.41 to 3.93)	2	55	1.00 (-0.02 to 2.01)	10	50
>24	-0.77 (-2.50 to 0.96)	1	NA	0.06 (-1.45 to 1.57)	2	42
Triglycerides, mg/dL						
<12	NR	--	--	-10.82 (-26.29 to 4.64)	2	34
12–24	-0.54 (-5.92 to 4.83)	2	0	-5.62 (-12.08 to 0.84)	5	45
>24	NR	--	--	-19.47 (-31.61 to -7.33)	1	NA
Systolic blood pressure, mm Hg						
<12	-4.47 (-7.91 to -1.04)	5	80	-2.73 (-5.44 to -0.01)	8	79
12–24	-2.29 (-3.81 to -0.76)	6	20	-1.99 (-3.15 to -0.83)	20	50
>24	-2.00 (-4.97 to 0.97)	1	NA	-2.00 (-4.04 to 0.04)	2	0.0
Diastolic blood pressure, mm Hg						
<12	-2.33 (-5.02 to -0.36)	3	62	-1.39 (-3.09 to 0.30)	6	64
12–24	-1.22 (-2.53 to 0.08)	4	38	-1.24 (-1.91 to -0.56)	16	36
>24	-1.00 (-3.22 to 1.22)	1	NA	-1.00 (-2.12 to 0.12)	2	0
Fasting glucose, mg/dL						
<12	-1.80 (-15.29 to 11.68)	1	NA	-1.72 (-4.22 to 0.78)	3	0
12–24	-0.18 (-1.20 to 0.84)	1	NA	-1.59 (-3.92 to 0.74)	8	76
>24	0.0 (-2.72 to 2.72)	1	NA	-1.42 (-4.87 to 2.03)	2	49
Diabetes incidence, RR						
<12	NR	--	--	NR	--	--
12–24	NR	--	--	0.26 (0.09 to 0.76)	2	0
>24	NR	--	--	1.03 (0.67 to 1.59)	1	NA
Adiposity, Hedges g						
<12	-0.45 (-0.88 to -0.02)	5	87	-0.35 (-0.61 to -0.09)	9	81
12–24	-0.37 (-0.93 to 0.19)	4	93	-0.21 (-0.34 to -0.08)	16	81
>24	-0.08 (-0.33 to 0.17)	1	NA	-0.19 (-0.40 to 0.02)	3	64

Abbreviations: CI = confidence interval; NA = not available; NR = not reported; RR = relative risk.

Table 18. Pooled Effect Sizes for Intermediate Health Outcomes in Persons With Impaired Fasting Glucose or Impaired Glucose Tolerance

Followup, months	Impaired Fasting Glucose/Tolerance			Impaired Fasting Glucose/Tolerance and Mixed		
	Effect Size (95% CI)	K	I^2, %	Effect Size (95% CI)	K	I^2, %
Total cholesterol, mg/dL						
<12	-5.01 (-17.45 to 7.42)	2	50	-5.04 (-10.22 to 0.14)	6	31
12–24	-2.62 (-5.43 to 0.91)	8	0	-5.21 (-8.264 to -2.15)	21	68
>24	-2.05 (-14.46 to 10.36)	2	77	-7.93 (-20.31 to 4.46)	3	89
Low-density lipoprotein cholesterol, mg/dL						
<12	-4.15 (-8.39 to 0.09)	3	0	-4.18 (-7.30 to -1.07)	7	0
12–24	0.04 (-3.45 to 3.54)	6	0	-2.57 (-5.70 to 0.55)	15	55
>24	4.63 (-4.68 to 13.94)	1	NA	-5.73 (-25.40 to 13.94)	2	92
High-density lipoprotein cholesterol, mg/dL						
<12	0.46 (-2.38 to 3.30)	3	56	0.88 (-0.78 to 2.53)	5	26
12–24	0.38 (-0.28 to 1.04)	6	16	0.90 (-0.14 to 1.65)	14	55
>24	0.22 (-0.93 to 1.38)	2	32	0.17 (-0.46 to 0.80)	3	20
Triglycerides, mg/dL						
<12	-20.27 (-34.27 to -6.26)	3	0	-15.28 (-24.56 to -6.01)	5	0
12–24	-12.46 (-19.96 to 4.97)	6	0	-12.31 (-17.74 to -6.88)	9	0
>24	-8.85 (-20.76 to 3.06)	1	NA	-14.09 (-24.50 to -3.68)	2	33
Systolic blood pressure, mm Hg						
<12	-1.10 (-6.42 to 4.22)	3	59	-0.23 (-2.85 to 2.39)	6	51
12–24	-2.42 (-4.02 to -0.82)	8	35	-1.96 (-3.10 to -0.82)	22	54
>24	-2.10 (-4.68 to 0.48)	2	26	-2.41 (-3.63 to -1.20)	3	0
Diastolic blood pressure, mm Hg						
<12	-4.90 (-9.76 to -0.04)	1	NA	-1.19 (-3.58 to 1.19)	4	65
12–24	-1.50 (-2.64 to -0.35)	6	43	-1.33 (-2.01 to -0.65)	18	48
>24	-1.88 (-2.68 to -1.08)	2	0	-1.63 (-2.32 to -0.95)	3	0
Fasting glucose, mg/dL						
<12	-1.69 (-3.82 to 0.45)	5	59	-1.51 (-3.15 to 0.13)	7	45
12–24	-2.05 (-3.86 to -0.24)	11	74	-2.04 (-3.58 to -0.50)	18	74
>24	-2.53 (-5.09 to 0.03)	2	16	-2.63 (-4.54 to -0.71)	3	0
Diabetes incidence, RR						
<12	1.70 (0.76 to 3.81)	1	NA	1.70 (0.76 to 3.81)	1	NA
12–24	0.65 (0.42 to 1.02)	6	34	0.58 (0.37 to 0.89)	8	32
>24	0.55 (0.46 to 0.67)	5	27	0.61 (0.46 to 0.79)	6	61
Adiposity, Hedges g						
<12	-0.26 (-0.44 to 0.08)	6	54	-0.23 (-0.36 to -0.11)	10	40
12–24	-0.26 (-0.39 to -0.13)	12	64	-0.21 (-0.29 to -0.13)	24	63
>24	-0.63 (-1.21 to -0.04)	3	94	-0.46 (-0.84 to -0.09)	5	93

Abbreviations: CI = confidence interval; NA = not available; RR = relative risk.

Table 19. Pooled Effect Sizes for Intermediate Health Outcomes in Persons in All Risk Groups

Followup, months	All Risk Groups		
	Effect Size (95% CI)	K	I^2
Total cholesterol, mg/dL			
<12	-4.58 (-7.44 to -1.73)	12	23
12–24	-4.48 (-6.36 to -2.59)	34	56
>24	-7.03 (-16.46 to 2.40)	4	85
Low-density lipoprotein cholesterol, mg/dL			
<12	-2.53 (-4.74 to -0.32)	12	10
12–24	-3.43 (-5.37 to -1.49)	25	47
>24	-5.73 (-25.40 to 13.94)	2	92
High-density lipoprotein cholesterol, mg/dL			
<12	0.38 (-0.72 to 1.49)	7	17
12–24	0.69 (0.09 to 1.30)	19	46
>24	0.02 (-0.40 to 0.44)	4	8
Triglycerides, mg/dL			
<12	-15.28 (-24.56 to -6.01)	5	0
12–24	-8.85 (-13.91 to -3.78)	14	32
>24	-14.09 (-24.50 to -3.68)	2	33
Systolic blood pressure, mm Hg			
<12	-2.36 (-4.78 to 0.06)	11	77
12–24	-2.03 (-2.91 to -1.15)	31	48
>24	-2.35 (-3.48 to -1.23)	4	0
Diastolic blood pressure, mm Hg			
<12	-1.67 (-3.30 to -0.04)	7	61
12–24	-1.38 (-1.92 to -0.84)	24	41
>24	-1.58 (-2.23 to -0.93)	4	0
Fasting glucose, mg/dL			
<12	-1.44 (-2.97 to 0.09)	8	36
12–24	-2.08 (-3.29 to -0.88)	22	80
>24	-1.89 (-3.73 to -0.04)	4	22
Diabetes incidence, RR			
<12	1.70 (0.76 to 3.81)	1	NA
12–24	0.58 (0.37 to 0.89)	8	32
>24	0.61 (0.46 to 0.79)	6	61
Adiposity, Hedges g			
<12	-0.30 (-0.42 to -0.17)	20	71
12–24	-0.26 (-0.35 to -0.16)	34	80
>24	-0.40 (-0.73 to -0.07)	6	92

Abbreviations: CI = confidence interval; NA = not available; RR = relative risk.

Table 20. Pooled Effect Sizes for Intermediate Health Outcomes by Intervention Type

Followup, months	Healthy Diet + Physical Activity Effect Size (95% CI)	K	I^2, %	Healthy Diet Only Effect Size (95% CI)	K	I^2, %	Physical Activity Only Effect Size (95% CI)	K	I^2, %
Total cholesterol, mg/dL									
<12	-4.01 (-7.97 to -0.05)	4	0	-4.18 (-8.53 to 0.18)	5	38	-8.53 (-21.39 to 4.33)	3	51
12–24	-5.43 (-7.97 to -2.89)	22	61	-3.75 (-6.50 to -1.01)	9	24	0.25 (-3.80 to 4.31)	3	20
>24	-7.03 (-16.46 to 2.40)	4	85	NR	--	--	NR	--	--
Low-density lipoprotein cholesterol, mg/dL									
<12	-2.53 (-5.43 to 0.38)	6	0	-2.34 (-6.65 to 1.96)	4	44	-3.18 (-16.97 to 10.61)	2	38
12–24	-3.69 (-5.98 to -1.40)	17	43	-4.27 (-7.84 to -0.70)	7	40	3.90 (-2.05 to 9.85)	1	NA
>24	-5.73 (-25.40 to 13.94)	2	92	NR	--	--	NR	--	--
High-density lipoprotein cholesterol, mg/dL									
<12	1.13 (-0.69 to 2.95)	3	30	-0.20 (-1.52 to 1.12)	2	0	0.48 (-4.65 to 5.61)	2	50
12–24	0.98 (0.25 to 1.70)	14	56	-0.85 (-2.64 to 0.94)	3	0	-0.17 (-1.66 to 1.32)	2	0
>24	0.02 (-0.40 to 0.44)	4	8	NR	--	--	NR	--	--
Triglycerides, mg/dL									
<12	-13.99 (-28.40 to 0.42)	3	20	NR	--	--	-16.98 (-30.57 to -3.38)	2	0
12–24	-8.33 (-13.80 to -2.86)	10	38	-17.86 (-33.10 to -2.62)	3	0	2.66 (-21.63 to 26.94)	1	NA
>24	-14.09 (-24.50 to -3.68)	2	33	NR	--	--	NR	--	--
Systolic blood pressure, mm Hg									
<12	-2.20 (-4.39 to -0.02)	8	67	NR	--	--	-2.12 (-11.82 to 7.57)	3	90
12–24	-2.06 (-3.03 to -1.08)	27	50	-3.34 (-7.48 to 0.80)	2	67	-0.54 (-3.64 to 2.56)	2	23
>24	-2.35 (-3.48 to -1.23)	4	0	NR	--	--	NR	--	--
Diastolic blood pressure, mm Hg									
<12	-1.82 (-3.67 to 0.03)	5	69	NR	--	--	-1.10 (-5.58 to 3.38)	2	45
12–24	-1.30 (-1.93 to -0.68)	21	48	-1.90 (-3.35 to -0.46)	2	0	-1.40 (-3.36 to 0.56)	1	NA
>24	-1.58 (-2.23 to -0.93)	4	0	NR	--	--	NR	--	--
Fasting glucose, mg/dL									
<12	-0.98 (-2.85 to 0.89)	4	47	NR	--	--	-2.47 (-4.70 to -0.24)	4	0
12–24	-1.86 (-3.24 to -0.49)	18	74	-3.65 (-4.35 to -2.94)	2	0	-1.80 (-6.88 to 3.28)	2	62
>24	-1.89 (-3.73 to -0.04)	4	22	NR	--	--	NR	--	--
Adiposity, Hedges g									
<12	-0.36 (-0.56 to -0.16)	10	84	-0.20 (-0.36 to -0.05)	6	29	-0.24 (-0.51 to 0.03)	4	0
12–24	-0.24 (-0.35 to -0.14)	25	77	-0.44 (-0.87 to -0.01)	6	88	-0.05 (-0.16 to 0.06)	3	0
>24	-0.40 (-0.73 to -0.07)	6	92	NR	--	--	NR	--	--
Diabetes incidence, RR									
<12	1.70 (0.76 to 3.81)	1	NA	NR	--	--	NR	--	--
12–24	0.54 (0.34 to 0.88)	6	40	NR	--	--	0.66 (0.11 to 4.11)	2	38
>24	0.61 (0.46 to 0.79)	6	61	NR	--	--	NR	--	--

Abbreviations: CI = confidence interval; NA = not available; NR = not reported; RR = relative risk.

Table 21. Behavioral Counseling Trials in Persons With Dyslipidemia or Elevated Cholesterol: Key Question 3 Outcomes

Study, Year Quality	N	Followup Time, months	Fat Intake	Saturated Fat Intake	Cholesterol Intake	Fiber	Other Behavioral Outcomes
Healthy diet and physical activity interventions							
CouPLES, 2013[67] Fair	255	Short: 11	g/d ↑ % Fat ↑	g/d ↑ %SF ↔	Mg/d ↔	g/d ↔	Total energy (kcal/d) ↑ Frequency of moderate PA/wk ↔ Duration of moderate-intensity PA/wk ↔
		Intermediate: NA	--	--	--	--	--
		Long: NA	--	--	--	--	--
PRO-FIT, 2012[68]	340	Short: NA	--	--	--	--	--
		Intermediate: 12	NR	g/d ↔	NR	NR	Fruit intake (servings/d) ↔ Vegetable intake (g/d) ↔ Moderate-/vigorous-intensity PA (min/wk) ↔
		Long: NA	--	--	--	--	--
RHPP Trial, 1993[69] Fair	1,197	Short: NA	--	--	--	--	--
		Intermediate: NA	--	--	--	--	--
		Long: 30	NR	NR	NR	NR	NR
Healthy diet–only interventions							
Anderson, 1992[70] Fair	177	Short: NA	--	--	--	--	--
		Intermediate: 12	% Fat ↑	% SF ↑	Mg/d ↔	g/d ↑	Total energy (kJ/d) ↔ % MUFA ↑ % PUFA ↔ % Protein ↔ % Carbohydrates (no difference) Exercise, total energy (kJ*kg/lb*d) ↑
		Long: NA	--	--	--	--	--
Ammerman, 2003[74] Keyserling, 1999[174] Fair	468	Short: 6	NR	NR	NR	NR	NR
		Intermediate: 12	NR	NR	NR	NR	DRA score ↑
		Long: NA	--	--	--	--	--
Bloemberg, 1991[75] Fair	80	Short: 6	% Fat ↑	% SF ↑	Mg/mJ ↑	g/mJ ↑	% Protein ↔ % MUFA ↑ % PUFA ↑ % Carbohydrates: increase
		Intermediate: NA	--	--	--	--	--
		Long: NA	--	--	--	--	--
DEER, 1998[71]	189	Short: NA	--	--	--	--	--
		Intermediate: 12*	% Fat ↑	% SF ↑	Mg/d ↑	NR	Total energy (kcal/d) ↑ % Carbohydrates: increase % MUFA ↑ % PUFA ↔
		Long: NA	--	--	--	--	--

Table 21. Behavioral Counseling Trials in Persons With Dyslipidemia or Elevated Cholesterol: Key Question 3 Outcomes

Study, Year Quality	N	Followup Time, months	Fat Intake	Saturated Fat Intake	Cholesterol Intake	Fiber	Other Behavioral Outcomes
Delahanty, 2001[72] Good	90	Short: 6	% Fat ↑	% SF ↑	Mg/dL ↑	g/d ↔	Total energy (kcal/d) ↔ % MUFA ↑ % PUFA ↔ Total PA (min/week) ↔
		Intermediate: 12	% Fat ↔	% SF ↔	Mg/dL ↔	g/d ↔	Total energy (kcal/d) ↔ % MUFA ↔ % PUFA ↔ Total PA (min/week) ↔
		Long: NA	--	--	--	--	--
Hyman, 1998[76] Fair	123	Short: 6	Fat intake score† ↔	NR	NR	NR	NR
		Intermediate: NA	--	--	--	--	--
		Long: NA	--	--	--	--	--
Johnston, 1995[77] Fair	179	Short: 6	NR	NR	NR	NR	NR
		Intermediate: NA	--	--	--	--	--
		Long: NA	--	--	--	--	--
Moy, 2001[73] Fair	235	Short: NA	--	--	--	--	--
		Intermediate: 24	g/d ↑ % Fat ↑	g/d ↑ % SF ↑	Mg/d ↑	NR	Total energy (kcal) ↑
		Long: NA	--	--	--	--	--
Neil, 1995[78] Fair	309	Short: 6	NR	NR	NR	NR	NR
		Intermediate: NA	--	--	--	--	--
		Long: NA	--	--	--	--	--
NFPMP, 2002[79] Fair	143	Short: 6	% Fat ↑	% SF ↑	Mg/d ↑	NR	Total energy (MJ/d) ↑ % MUFA ↑ % Un-SF ↔ % no exercise, % <3 times/wk, % exercise >3 times/wk ↔
		Intermediate: 12	% Fat ↑	% SF ↑	Mg/d ↑	NR	Total energy (MJ/d) ↑ % MUFA ↑ % Un-SF ↔ % no exercise, % <3 times/wk, % exercise >3 times/wk ↔
		Long: NA	--	--	--	--	--
ODES, 1995[80] Fair	98	Short: NA	--	--	--	--	--
		Intermediate: 12	% Fat ↑ g/d ↑‡	% SF ↑ g/d ↑‡	Mg/d ↑‡	NR	Total energy (kJ/d) ↑ Protein (g/d) ↑‡ Carbohydrates (g/d): increase‡ Sugar (g/d) ↑‡ MUFA (g/d) ↑‡ PUFA (g/d) ↑‡
		Long: NA	--	--	--	--	--

Table 21. Behavioral Counseling Trials in Persons With Dyslipidemia or Elevated Cholesterol: Key Question 3 Outcomes

Study, Year Quality	N	Followup Time, months	Fat Intake	Saturated Fat Intake	Cholesterol Intake	Fiber	Other Behavioral Outcomes
Southeast Cholesterol Project, 1997[81] Fair	372	Short: 7	NR	NR	NR	NR	NR
		Intermediate: 12	NR	NR	NR	NR	DRA score ↑
		Long: NA	--	--	--	--	--
Stevens, 2003[82] Fair	616	Short: NA	--	--	--	--	--
		Intermediate: 12	% Fat ↑ Kristal fat score ↑	% SF ↑	NR	NR	Number of fruit/vegetable servings ↑ % MUFA ↑ % PUFA ↑
		Long: NA	--	--	--	--	--
Tomson, 1995[83] Tomson, 1994[175] Fair	92	Short: NA	--	--	--	--	--
		Intermediate: 12	NR	NR	NR	NR	NR
		Long: NA	--	--	--	--	--

* Outcomes reported by sex; no differences between sexes.
† 9-item research scale.
‡ Men-only subgroup analysis.

Abbreviations: CouPLES = Couples Partnering for Lipid Enhancing Strategies; DEER = Diet and Exercise for Elevated Risk; DRA = Developmental Reading Assessment; MUFA = monounsaturated fatty acid; N = study population; NA = not available; NFPMP = Nijmegen Family Practices Monitoring Program; NR = not reported; PA = physical activity; PUFA = polyunsaturated fatty acid; SF = saturated fat; Un-SF = unsaturated fat.

Table 22. Behavioral Counseling Trials in Persons With Hypertension: Key Question 3 Outcomes

Study, Year Quality	N	Followup Time, months	Urinary Sodium or Sodium Intake	PA Outcomes	Other Behavioral Outcomes
Healthy diet and physical activity interventions					
ADAPT, 2006[138] Fair	241	Short: NA	--	--	--
		Intermediate: 12	g/d ↑	At least moderate-intensity exercise (mean hr/wk) ↔	Total energy (MJ) ↑ % Fat ↑ % SF ↑ % PUFA ↔ % MUFA ↑ Cholesterol (mg/d) ↔ Fiber (g/d) ↑ % Protein ↑ % Carbohydrates: increase Servings per day of low-fat dairy ↔ Servings per day of fish ↔ Servings per day of meat ↔ Servings per day of fruits/vegetables ↔
		Long: 36	g/d ↔	At least moderate-intensity exercise (mean hr/wk) ↑	Total energy (MJ) ↔ % Fat ↔ % SF ↑ % PUFA ↔ % MUFA ↔ Cholesterol (mg/d) ↔ Fiber (g/d) ↔ % Protein ↔ % Carbohydrates: no difference Servings per day of fish ↑ Servings per day of fruits ↔ Servings per day of vegetables ↑
Applegate, 1992[127] Fair	56	Short: 6	NR	NR	NR
		Intermediate: NA	--	--	--
		Long: NA	--	--	--
Arroll, 1995[128] Fair (Also arms in HD- & PA-only sections)	208	Short: 6	Salt frequency score ↑ 24-hr urinary sodium ↑	Total PA (kJ/kg/d) ↑ Moderate PA (kJ/kg/d) ↑	NR
		Intermediate: NA	--	--	--
		Long: NA	--	--	--
Bosworth, 2009[84] Fair	477	Short: NA	--	--	--
		Intermediate: 12	NR	NR	NR
		Long: 24	NR	NR	NR

Table 22. Behavioral Counseling Trials in Persons With Hypertension: Key Question 3 Outcomes

Study, Year Quality	N	Followup Time, months	Urinary Sodium or Sodium Intake	PA Outcomes	Other Behavioral Outcomes
HIP, 2009[136] Fair	574	Short: 6*	24-hr urinary sodium: MD ↔, Pt ↔	Moderate to vigorous PA (min/wk): MD ↔, Pt ↔	Total energy (kcal): MD ↔, Pt ↑ % Fat ↑ % SF ↑ Cholesterol (mg/d): MD ↔, Pt ↑ Servings of fruits/vegetables ↑ Fiber (g/d): MD ↔, Pt ↑ % Protein: MD ↔, Pt ↑ % Carbohydrates: increase Servings of dairy: MD ↔, Pt ↑
		Intermediate: 18*	24-hr urinary sodium: MD ↑, Pt ↔	Moderate to vigorous PA (min/wk): MD ↔, Pt ↔	Total energy (kcal) ↔ % Fat ↔ % SF: MD ↔, Pt ↑ Cholesterol (mg/d) ↔ Servings of fruits/vegetables: MD ↔, Pt ↑ Fiber (g/d) ↔ % Protein ↔ % Carbohydrates: increase Servings of dairy ↔
		Long: NA	--	--	--
HTTP, 1993[134] Fair	200	Short: NA			
		Intermediate: 18	NR	NR	NR
		Long: NA			
Hyman, 2007[135] Fair	281	Short: 6	24-hr urinary sodium ↔	Pedometer steps per day ↔	% current smoker (urine cotinine) ↔
		Intermediate: 18	24-hr urinary sodium ↔	Pedometer steps per day ↔	% current smoker (urine cotinine) ↔
		Long: NA	--	--	--
LIHEF, 2002[137] Fair	715	Short: NA			
		Intermediate: 12 + 24‡	Mg/dL ↑	% Participating in moderate PA at least 3 times/wk for 30 min ↑	Total energy (kcal) ↔ % Fat ↑ % SF ↑ % MUFA ↑ % PUFA ↔ Cholesterol (mg) ↑ Fiber (g) ↑¶
		Long: NA			--

Table 22. Behavioral Counseling Trials in Persons With Hypertension: Key Question 3 Outcomes

Study, Year Quality	N	Followup Time, months	Urinary Sodium or Sodium Intake	PA Outcomes	Other Behavioral Outcomes
Migneault, 2012[126] Fair	337	Short: 8	NR	Moderate or greater PA (min/wk) ↔ >150 min/wk of moderate or greater PA (%) ↔ Total energy expenditure (kcal/d) ↑	Composite diet score§ ↑
		Intermediate: 12	NR	Moderate or greater PA (min/wk) ↔ >150 min/wk of moderate or greater PA (%) ↔ Total energy expenditure (kcal/d) ↔	Composite diet score§ ↔
		Long: NA			
PREMIER, 2003[116] Good	304	Short: 6	24-hr urinary sodium ↔	Fitness (heart rate at stage 2 or last available heart rate at stage 1) ↔	% SF ↔ % Low-fat dairy ∥ ↔ Servings of fruits/vegetables ↑ Servings of dairy ↔
		Intermediate: 18	NR	NR	NR
		Long: NA			
Rodriguez, 2012[113] Fair (poor for diet)	533	Short: 6	NR	PA hr/wk ↔	NR
		Intermediate: 12	NR	PA hr/wk ↔	NR
		Long: NA			
TONE, 1998[117] Good (Also arm in HD-only section)	975	Short: 9	24-hr urinary sodium ↑	NR	NR
		Intermediate: 18	24-hr urinary sodium ↑	NR	NR
		Long: 36	24-hr urinary sodium ↑	NR	NR
Vitalum[105] Fair	1,629	Short: 6	NR	PA hr/wk: IG1 ↑ IG2 ↔ IG3 ↑	Servings per day of fruits, vegetables: IG1 ↑, ↑ IG2 ↑, ↑ IG3 ↑, NR
		Intermediate: 18	NR	PA hr/wk: IG1 ↔ IG2 ↔ IG3 ↑	Servings per day of fruits, vegetables: IG1 ↑, ↑ IG2 ↑, ↑ IG3 ↑, ↔
		Long: NA			
Healthy diet–only interventions					
Arroll, 1995[128] Fair (Also arms in HD+PA & PA-only sections)	208	Short: 6	Salt frequency score ↑ 24-hr urinary sodium ↑	Total PA (kJ/kg/d) ↔ Moderate PA (kJ/kg/d) ↔	NR
		Intermediate: NA			
		Long: NA			

Table 22. Behavioral Counseling Trials in Persons With Hypertension: Key Question 3 Outcomes

Study, Year Quality	N	Followup Time, months	Urinary Sodium or Sodium Intake	PA Outcomes	Other Behavioral Outcomes
Beckman, 1995[111] Fair	64	Short: 6	24-hr urinary sodium ↑	NR	NR
		Intermediate: 12	24-hr urinary sodium ↑	NR	NR
		Long: NA	--	--	--
TONE, 1998[117] Good (Also arm in HD+PA section)	975	Short: 9	24-hr urinary sodium ↑	NR	NR
		Intermediate: 18	24-hr urinary sodium ↑	NR	NR
		Long: 30	24-hr urinary sodium ↑	NR	NR
Physical activity–only interventions					
Arroll, 1995[128] Fair (Also arms in HD+PA & HD-only sections)	208	Short: 6	Salt frequency score ↔ 24-hr urinary sodium ↔	Total PA (kJ/kg/d) ↑ Moderate PA (kJ/kg/d) ↑	NR
		Intermediate: NA	--	--	--
		Long: NA	--	--	--
Moreau, 2001[104] Fair	24	Short: 6	NR	Pedometer steps per day ↑	Total energy (kcal) ↔
		Intermediate: NA	--	--	--
		Long: NA	--	--	--

* Results are for both physicians and patients unless otherwise noted.
† Only reported at 3 to 24 weeks (composite), did not collect data on control group.
‡ Outcomes for 12 and 24 months unless otherwise noted.
§ Based on fat, saturated fat, fiber, fruit/vegetable, and salt intake.
|| METs group only.
¶ Significant at 24 months, not significant at 12 months.

Abbreviations: ADAPT = Activity Diet and Blood Pressure Trial; HD = healthy diet; HIP = Hypertension Improvement Project; HTTP = Hypertension Teaching and Treatment Programme; IG = intervention group; LIHEF = Lifestyle Intervention against Hypertension in Eastern Finland; MD = physician; MUFA = monounsaturated fatty acid; N = study population; NA = not available; NR = not reported; PA = physical activity; pt = patient; PUFA = polyunsaturated fatty acid; SF = saturated fat; TONE = Trial of Non-Pharmacological Interventions in the Elderly.

Table 23. Behavioral Counseling Trials in Persons With Impaired Fasting Glucose or Impaired Glucose Tolerance: Key Question 3 Outcomes

Study, Year Quality	N	Followup Time, months	Fat Intake	Saturated Fat Intake	Cholesterol Intake	PA Outcomes	Other Behavioral Outcomes
Healthy diet and physical activity interventions							
APHRODITE, 2011[88] Fair	925	Short term: 6	↔	↑	NR	Total PA (min/wk) ↑ Average- to high-intensity activity (min/wk) ↔	Total energy intake (kcal/d) ↔ Fiber intake (g/MJ) ↑
		Intermediate: 18	↔	↑	NR	Total PA (min/wk) ↑ Average to high intensity activity (min/wk) ↔	Total energy intake (kcal/d) ↔ Fiber intake (g/MJ) ↑
		Long term: NA	--	--	--	--	--
DPP, 2002[89] Good	2,161	Short term: NA	--	--	--	--	--
		Intermediate: 12 + 24 months§	↑	↑	NR	PA (MET-hr/wk) ↑	Total energy ↑ % PUFA ↑ % Carbohydrates: increase Fiber (g/d) ↑ Fruits (servings/d) ↑ Vegetables (servings/d) ↔ Fish (servings/d) ↔ Red meat (servings/d) ↑ Dairy (servings/d) ↑ Sweets (servings/d) ↑
		Long term: 36	NR	NR	NR	PA (MET-hr/wk) ↑	NR
EDIPS, 2001[90] Fair	78	Short term: 6	↑	↔	NR	Vigorous activity >3 times/wk ↑ Vigorous activity ≥1 times/wk ↑	Total energy (kcal/d) ↔ MUFA (g/d) ↑ PUFA (g/d) ↑ Sucrose (g/d) ↔ Fiber (g/d) ↔
		Intermediate: 24	↑	NR	NR	Regular activity ≥1 times/wk ↑ Vigorous activity ≥1 times/wk ↑	Fiber (g/d) ↔
		Long term: NA	--	--	--	--	--
EDIPS-Newcastle, 2009[91] Fair	102	Short term: NA	--	--	--	--	--
		Intermediate: 12	↔	NR	NR	Physical activity score† ↔	% Carbohydrates: no difference % Fiber ↔
		Long term: 36‡	↔	NR	NR	Physical activity score† ↔	% Carbohydrates: no difference % Fiber ↔
E-LITE, 2013[87] Good	162	Short: 6	NR	NR	NR	NR	NR
		Intermediate: 15	NR	NR	NR	NR	NR
		Long: NA	--	--	--	--	--
FDPS, 2001[118] Good	522	Short term: 12	↑	↑	↑	Increased PA ↑ Meeting goal of PA >4 hr/wk ↑ Total PA (min/wk) ↔ Moderate to vigorous PA (min/wk) ↑	Increased consumption of vegetables ↑ Decreased consumption of sugar ↑ Decreased consumption of salt† Total energy intake ↑ % MUFA ↑ % PUFA ↔ Fiber (g) ↔ Fiber (g/1,000 kcal) ↑

Table 23. Behavioral Counseling Trials in Persons With Impaired Fasting Glucose or Impaired Glucose Tolerance: Key Question 3 Outcomes

Study, Year Quality	N	Followup Time, months	Fat Intake	Saturated Fat Intake	Cholesterol Intake	PA Outcomes	Other Behavioral Outcomes
HLC, 2011[92] Fair	307	Short: 6	NR	NR	NR	NR	NR
		Intermediate: 24	NR	NR	↔	Total PA (min/wk) ↔ Moderate to vigorous PA (min/wk) ↑	Total energy intake ↑ % Carbohydrates: increase % MUFA ↑ % PUFA ↔ Fiber (g) ↔ Fiber (g/1,000 kcal) ↑
		Long term: 36	↑	↑			
Kosaka, 2005[93] Fair	NR	Short term: 12	NR	NR	NR	Total PA (min/wk) ↔	Composite diet measure* ↑
		Intermediate: 24	NR	NR	NR	--	--
		Long term: 48	NR	NR	NR	--	NR
Live Well, Be Well, 2012[86] Good	238	Short: 6	g/d ↑	NR	NR	Total PA (hr/wk) ↔ Total PA (MET-hr/wk) ↔ Walking (hr/wk) ↔	Total energy (kcal/d) ↔ Fiber (g/d) ↔ Daily frequency of fruit and vegetables ↑
		Intermediate: 12	g/d ↔	NR	NR	Total PA (hr/wk) ↔ Total PA (MET-hr/wk) ↔ Walking (hr/wk) ↔	Total energy (kcal/d) ↔ Fiber (g/d) ↔ Daily frequency of fruit and vegetables ↑
		Long: NA	--	--	--	--	--
LLDP[94] Good	312	Short: NA	--	--	--	--	--
		Intermediate: 12	% ↑	% ↔	NR	Leisure time PA (min/wk) ↔	Total energy (kcal/d) ↔ % Carbohydrates: no difference % Protein ↔ Fiber (g/d) ↔
		Long: NA	--	--	--	--	--
Melbourne DPS, 2012[85] Fair	92	Short: NA	--	--	--	--	--
		Intermediate: 12	% ↔	% ↑	NR	% meeting goal of moderate PA for 30 min/d ↔	Fiber (g/d) ↑
		Long: NA	--	--	--	--	--
PREDIAS, 2009[95] Fair	182	Short term: NA	--	--	--	--	--
		Intermediate: 12	NR	NR	NR	PA (min/wk) ↑	NR
		Long term: NA	--	--	--	--	--
SLIM[149] Fair	147	Short term: NA	--	--	--	--	--
		Intermediate: 12 + 24‖	↑	↑	NR	VO$_2$max (l/min) ↑	Total energy ↔¶ % CHO: Increase % MUFA ↑# % PUFA ↔# % Protein ↔ Fiber ↔¶
		Long term: 36–72	↑	↑	NR	PA d/wk ↔	Fiber ↑
Healthy diet–only interventions							
Watanabe, 2003[97] Fair	173	Short term: NA	--	--	--	--	--
		Intermediate: 12	NR	NR	NR	NR	Total energy ↑**
		Long term: NA	--	--	--	--	--

Table 23. Behavioral Counseling Trials in Persons With Impaired Fasting Glucose or Impaired Glucose Tolerance: Key Question 3 Outcomes

Study, Year Quality	N	Followup Time, months	Fat Intake	Saturated Fat Intake	Cholesterol Intake	PA Outcomes	Other Behavioral Outcomes
Physical activity–only interventions							
Enhanced Fitness Trial, 2012[98] Fair	302	Short term: NA	--	--	--	--	--
		Intermediate: 12	NR	NR	NR	Endurance (min/wk) ↑ Strength (min/wk) ↔ % Meeting goal of 150 min/wk ↑ Cardiorespiratory fitness ↔††	NR
		Long term: NA	--	--	--	--	--
Prepare Trial, 2009[99] Fair	98	Short term: 6‡‡	NR	NR	NR	Steps per day ↑§§ Self-reported walking (MET-min/wk) ↑§§ Moderate to vigorous PA (MET-min/wk) ↑§§	NR
		Intermediate: 12	NR	NR	NR	Steps per day ↑§§ Self-reported walking (MET-min/wk) ↑ Moderate to vigorous PA (MET-min/wk) ↑§§	NR
		Long term: NA	--	--	--	--	--

* Based on 16-item Food Choices Questionnaire.
† Score based on METs per activity using 3-day PA diaries.
‡ Mean followup.
§ Dietary behavioral outcomes only at 12 months, PA behavioral outcomes at 12 and 24 months.
‖ For 12 and 24 months unless otherwise noted.
¶ ↑ at 12 months.
# Only reported for 12 months.
** Overintake/underintake fraction.
†† Measured by 6 minute walk test.
‡‡ For IG1 and IG2 unless otherwise noted.
§§ ↔ for IG1.

Abbreviations: APHRODITE = Active Prevention in High-Risk Individuals of Diabetes Type 2 in and Around Eindhoven; DPP = Diabetes Prevention Program; DPS = Diabetes Prevention Study; EDIPS = European Diabetes Prevention Study; E-LITE = Evaluation of Lifestyle Interventions to Treat Elevated Cardiometabolic Risk in Primary Care; FDPS = Finnish Diabetes Prevention Study; HLC = Healthy Living Course; LLDP = Lawrence Latino Diabetes Prevention Project; MET = metabolic equivalent; MUFA = monounsaturated fatty acid; N = study population; NA = not available; NR = not reported; PA = physical activity; PREDIAS = Prevention of Diabetes Self-Management Program; PUFA = polyunsaturated fatty acid; SLIM = Study on Lifestyle Intervention and IGT Maastricht.

Table 24. Behavioral Counseling Trials in Persons With Mixed Cardiovascular Risk Factors: Key Question 3 Outcomes

Study, Year	Quality	N	Followup Time, months	Healthy Diet Behavioral Outcomes	Physical Activity Outcomes
Healthy diet and physical activity interventions					
Bo, 2007[146]	Fair	375	Short: NA	--	--
			Intermediate: 12	Total energy (kcal/d) ↔ % Fat ↑ % SF ↑ % PUFA ↑ % Carbohydrates: increase % Protein ↔ % Fiber ↑	Metabolic equivalent of activity (hr/wk) ↑
			Long: NA	--	--
Cochrane, 2012[102]	Fair	601	Short: NA	--	--
			Intermediate: 12	Primary Prevention Toolkit Diet Score ↔	Primary Prevention Toolkit PA Score ↔
			Long: NA	--	--
Edelman, 2006[129]	Fair	154	Short: 10	NR	Total PA (d/wk) ↑
			Intermediate: NA	--	--
			Long: NA	--	--
EUROACTION, 2008[106]	Fair	2,384	Short: NA	--	--
			Intermediate: 12	% Eating oily fish (≥3 times/wk) ↔ % Eating fish (≥20 g/d) ↔ % Eating fruits/vegetables (≥400 g/d) ↑	% Participating in PA (≥30 min ≥4 times/wk) ↑ % with PA change ↑
			Long: NA	--	--
GOAL, 2009[139]	Good	457	Short: NA	--	--
			Intermediate: 12	Total energy (kcal) ↔ % Fat ↔ % SF ↔ % Protein ↔ Cholesterol (mg) ↔ Vegetables (g) ↔ Fruits (g) ↔	Total PA (min/wk) ↔ Moderate- to heavy-intensity PA (min/wk) ↔
			Long: 36	Total energy (kcal) ↔ % Fat ↔ % SF ↔ % Protein ↔ Cholesterol (mg) ↔ Vegetables (g) ↔ Fruits (g) ↔	Total PA (min/wk) ↔ Moderate- to heavy-intensity PA (min/wk) ↔ % Meeting recommended 150 min/wk PA ↔ % Meeting recommended 60 min/wk vigorous PA ↔
Hardcastle, 2008[168]	Fair	334	Short: 6	% Fat ↑ Fruits/vegetables per day ↔	PA MET-min/wk ↑ Vigorous PA MET-min/wk ↔ Moderate PA MET-min/wk ↔ Walking MET-min/wk ↑
			Intermediate: 18	% Fat ↑ Fruits/vegetables per day ↔	PA MET-min/wk ↔ Moderate PA MET-min/wk ↔ Walking MET-min/wk ↑
			Long: NA	--	--

Table 24. Behavioral Counseling Trials in Persons With Mixed Cardiovascular Risk Factors: Key Question 3 Outcomes

Study, Year	Quality	N	Followup Time, months	Healthy Diet Behavioral Outcomes	Physical Activity Outcomes
HIPS, 2012[103]	Fair	814	Short: 6	Portions fruits/vegetables per day ↑	PA Score‡‡ ↑
			Intermediate: 12	Portions fruits/vegetables per day ↔	PA Score‡‡ ↑
			Long: NA	--	--
Hoorn, 2013[132]	Fair	622	Short: 6	Fruits (pieces/d) ↔ Met recommended fruit intake (2 pieces/d) ↑ Vegetables (g/d) ↔ Met recommended vegetable intake (200 g/d) ↑	Vigorous PA MET-min/wk ↔ Moderate PA MET-min/wk ↔ % Meeting recommended PA levels (150 min/wk moderate PA) ↑
			Intermediate: 12	Fruit (pieces/d) ↔ Vegetables (g/d) ↔ Met recommended vegetable intake (200 g/d) ↑	Vigorous PA MET-min/wk ↔ Moderate PA MET-min/wk ↔ % Meeting recommended PA levels (150 min/wk moderate PA) ↑
			Long: NA	--	--
IMPALA, 2009[133]	Fair	615	Short: NA		
			Intermediate: 12	Fat score ↑ Met recommended fat intake ↔ Fruit (pieces/wk) ↔ Met recommended fruit intake (200 g/d) ↔ Vegetables (Tbsp/d) ↔ Met recommended vegetable intake (200 g/d) ↑	Total PA (min/wk) ↔ Met recommended PA levels ↔
			Long: NA	--	--
Inter99 2008[107]	Fair	4,053	Short: NA		
			Intermediate: 12**	% SF: men ↑, women ↔ Total energy (kJ/d) ↔ Un-SF fat ratio ↑ Fish intake (g/d) ↔ Fruit intake (women) ↓	Total PA (min/wk): men ↑↑↑, women ↔††
			Long: 60*	% SF ↔ Un-SF fat ratio ↑ Fish intake (g/d) ↑ Fruit intake (women) ↔	Total PA at 36 months (min/wk) ↔
Logan Healthy Living, 2009[114]	Fair	434	Short: 12	% Fat ↔ % SF ↑ Fiber (g/d) ↑ Fruit/vegetable intake (servings/d) ↑	Total PA (min/wk) ↔ Moderate to vigorous PA sessions/wk ↔ % Meeting PA guidelines (≥150 min, ≥5 sessions/wk) ↔††
			Intermediate: 18	% Fat ↑ % SF ↑ Fiber (g/d) ↑ Fruit/vegetable intake (servings/d) ↑	Total PA (min/wk) ↔ Moderate to vigorous PA sessions/wk ↔
			Long: NA	--	--

Table 24. Behavioral Counseling Trials in Persons With Mixed Cardiovascular Risk Factors: Key Question 3 Outcomes

Study, Year	Quality	N	Followup Time, months	Healthy Diet Behavioral Outcomes	Physical Activity Outcomes
Nilsson, 1992[119]	Fair	63	Short: NA	--	--
			Intermediate: 12	Total energy (kcal) ↑ Protein (g) ↔ Carbohydrates (g) (no difference) Fat (g) ↑ Fiber (g) ↑ SF (g) ↑ MUFA (g) ↑ PUFA (g) ↔ Cholesterol (mg) ↑ Change in dietary habits‡ ↑	Change in PA‡ ↑↑↑
			Long: NA	--	--
PEGASE, 2008[120]	Fair	640	Short: 6	NR§	NR§
			Intermediate: NA	--	--
			Long: NA	--	--
PHPP, 2007[121]	Fair-	99	Short: NA	--	--
			Intermediate: 12	Total energy (kcal/d) ↔ Meals/d with vegetable ↑	Steps/d ↑
			Long: NA	--	--
RIS, 1994[115]	Good KQ1 Fair KQ2	508	Short: NA	--	--
			Intermediate: 12	NR	NR
			Long: 79	NR	NR
Rodriguez-Cristobal, 2012[173]	Fair	436	Short: NA	--	--
			Intermediate: 24	NR	NR
			Long: NA	--	--
SPRING, 2012[100]	Fair	201	Short: NA	--	--
			Intermediate: 12	NR	% Physically inactive ↔
			Long: NA	--	--
WISEWOMAN California, 2010[108]	Fair	1093	Short: NA	--	--
			Intermediate: 12	NR	Level of exercise, moderate or vigorous ↑↑↑
			Long: NA	--	--
WISEWOMAN NC, 2008[110]	Fair	236	Short: 6	Composite Diet Score‖ ↑	Moderate PA (min/d) ↔ PA assessment, moderate ↑ PA assessment, vigorous ↑ PA assessment, all activity ↑
			Intermediate: 12	Composite Diet Score‖ ↑	Moderate PA min/d ↔ PA assessment, moderate ↑ PA assessment, vigorous ↔ PA assessment, all activity ↔
			Long: NA	--	--
Wister, 2007[140]	Good	315	Short: NA	--	--
			Intermediate: 12	Composite diet score¶ ↑	Composite PA score¶ ↔
			Long: NA	--	--

Table 24. Behavioral Counseling Trials in Persons With Mixed Cardiovascular Risk Factors: Key Question 3 Outcomes

Study, Year	Quality	N	Followup Time, months	Healthy Diet Behavioral Outcomes	Physical Activity Outcomes
Physical activity–only interventions					
Green Prescription Programme (Walk to Heart, Health & Activity study), 2003[123]	Fair	878	Short: NA Intermediate: 12 Long: NA	-- NR --	Total energy expenditure (kcal/kg/wk) ↑ Leisure PA expenditure (kcal/kg/wk) ↑ Moderate or vigorous exercise (min/wk) ↑ % Meeting recommended PA levels (2.5 hr/wk moderate or vigorous PA) ↑
NERS, 2012[109]	Fair, poor for QOL	2,160	Short: NA Intermediate: 12 Long: NA	-- NR --	Total PA (min/wk)# ↑
PAC, 2011[122]	Fair	120	Short: 6 Intermediate: NA Long: NA	NR -- --	Leisure-time activity score ↑ Total leisure activity ↔ Total activity counts/min ↔ Moderate or vigorous activity (min/d) ↔ VO_2 peak (LO_2min-1) ↔
PACE, 2005[131]	Fair	771	Short: 6 Intermediate: 12 Long: NA	NR NR --	NR†† Total PA (min/wk) ↔ Leisure PA (min/wk) ↔ Met ACSM/CDC guidelines ↔
Kallings, 2009[141]	Good	101	Short: 6 Intermediate: NA Long: NA	NR -- --	Total PA (steps/d) ↔ Increase of ≥3,000 steps/d ↔ Moderate-intensity PA ≥30 min 5 times/wk ↑ Vigorous-intensity PA ≥20 min 3 times/wk ↑ Muscle strengthening ≥2 times/wk on moderate-high intensity ↔ Sessions/wk of at least moderate PA ↑ Min/wk of at least moderate PA ↑
LIFE, 2010[130]	Fair	186	Short: 11 Intermediate: NA Long: NA	NR -- --	VO_2max (mL/kg/min) ↔ Objective measure of muscle fitness ↔ Objective measure of muscle strength ↔ Objective measure of muscle endurance ↑

* Based on 16-item Food Choices Questionnaire.
‡ Visual Analogue Scale.
§ Not abstracted because of poor quality.
|| Based on Dietary Risk Assessment.
¶ Based on meeting ACSM guidelines.
# Text states "borderline statistical significance"; p=NR.

Table 24. Behavioral Counseling Trials in Persons With Mixed Cardiovascular Risk Factors: Key Question 3 Outcomes

** Outcomes for men and women unless otherwise noted.
†† Only raw data reported; p=NR.
‡‡ Based on self-reported questionnaire; combined assessment of duration of vigorous and moderate PA.

Abbreviations: ACSM = American College of Sports Medicine; CDC = Centers for Disease Control and Prevention; GOAL = Groningen Overweight and Lifestyle Study; HD = healthy diet; HIPS = Health Improvement and Prevention Study; IMPALA = Improving Patient Adherence to Lifestyle Advice; LIFE = Lifestyle Interventions and Independence for Elder; MUFA = monounsaturated fatty acid; N = study population; NA = not available; NERS = National Exercise Referral Scheme; NR = not reported; PA = physical activity; PAC = Physical Activity Counseling; PACE = Physician-based Assessment and Counseling for Exercise; PEGASE = Pan European Grid Advanced Simulation and State Examination; PHPP = Physician-motivated Health Promotion Program; PUFA = polyunsaturated fatty acid; QOL = quality of life; RIS = Risk Factor Intervention Study; SF = saturated fat; SPRING = Self-monitoring and Prevention of Risk Factors; Un-SF = unsaturated fat; VO_2 = oxygen consumption.

Table 25. Overall Summary of Evidence by Key Question

Trials (k), Participants (n)	Overall quality	Consistency	Applicability	Summary of findings
Key Question 1. Health outcomes				
k=16 n=7,053	Fair: sparse reporting of health outcomes or use of clinically important self-reported health outcomes (i.e., QOL); generally low CVD event rates; variation in QOL instruments used	Generally consistent findings of no benefit on reduction of CVD events, mixed findings for benefit on QOL	Persons with any number of CVD risk factors, no major limitations in populations studied; mainly high-intensity combined lifestyle counseling interventions	Generally no reduction in CVD events (including mortality) at 6 to 79 months and at 10 years (k=4); no reduction in depression symptoms at 6 to 12 months (k=4); mixed findings on self-reported measures of QOL at 6 to 12 months (k=7). One earlier trial found a reduction in CVD events at 6.6 years (RR, 0.71 [95% CI, 0.51 to 0.99]) using a high-intensity intervention including a protocol to initiate medication in Swedish men at high risk for CVD (including 29% smokers, 22% with diabetes).
Key Question 2. Intermediate outcomes				
k=71 n=32,734	Fair to good: high statistical heterogeneity for fasting glucose and weight outcomes; sparse reporting of outcomes beyond 24 months; limited number of trials with significant clinical heterogeneity among physical activity–only counseling trials	Consistent findings of benefit across intermediate health outcomes; trials not included in meta-analyses generally consistent with trials that could be included	Persons with any number of CVD risk factors, no major limitations in populations studied. Medium- to high-intensity combined lifestyle counseling; diet-only counseling mostly in persons with dyslipidemia not yet taking medications	Across all trials reporting each specific outcome, at 12 to 24 months, overall reduction in: • Total cholesterol (k=34) by 4.48 mg/dL (95% CI, 6.36 to 2.59) • LDL cholesterol (k=25) by 3.43 mg/dL (95% CI, 5.37 to 1.49) • SBP (k=31) by 2.03 mm Hg (95% CI, 2.91 to 1.15) • DBP (k=24) by 1.38 mm Hg (95% CI, 1.92 to 0.84) • Fasting glucose (k=22) by 2.08 mg/dL (95% CI, 3.29 to 0.88) • Diabetes incidence (k=8) by RR of 0.58 (95% CI, 0.37 to 0.89) • Weight outcomes (k=34) by SMD of 0.26 (95% CI, 0.35 to 0.16) Overall evidence for longer-term (>24 months) findings are limited, except for reduction in diabetes incidence in persons with impaired fasting glucose or glucose tolerance (k=5) (RR, 0.55 [95% CI, 0.45 to 0.67]). No consistent finding of benefit on intermediate health outcomes for physical activity–only counseling interventions.
Key Question 3. Behavioral outcomes				
k=61 n=31,751	Fair: heterogeneity in dietary and physical activity outcome measures, mainly use of self-reported outcomes	Generally consistent with intermediate outcome findings	Persons with any number of CVD risk factors, no major limitations in populations studied. Medium- to high-intensity combined lifestyle counseling and diet-only counseling	Generally findings of improvement, or lack of improvement, in behavioral outcomes consistent with findings on intermediate health outcomes. Overall improved dietary intake and physical activity outcomes in trials of persons taking lipid- or blood pressure-lowering medications, which did not demonstrate a benefit on intermediate health outcomes (k=6). Trials only reporting behavioral outcomes (no intermediate outcomes) found small but statistically significant improvements in diet (fat, saturated fat, fiber, fruits/vegetables) and total physical activity (~35–50 minutes more per week) at 12 to 18 months (k=3).
Key Question 4. Adverse effects				
k=10 n=6,381	Fair: sparse reporting of harms	Generally consistent findings of no significant harms	Finding of serious harm applicable to high-intensity physical activity counseling in older adult VA population	Generally no findings of serious harms (i.e., requiring unexpected or unwanted medical attention), except in one trial (n=302) targeting older adults (2 persons with serious adverse events attributed to physical activity). Generally no findings of paradoxical changes in intermediate or behavioral outcomes. Increased self-reported carbohydrate intake accompanied by dietary improvements in fat/saturated fat, fiber, fruits/vegetables without an overall increase in energy intake (k=9).

Appendix A. Literature Search Strategies

Databases searched:
MEDLINE
Cochrane Database of Systematic Reviews (CDSR)
Cochrane Central Register of Controlled Trials (CENTRAL)
Database of Abstracts of Reviews of Effects (DARE)
PsycInfo
PubMed

Key:
/ = MeSH subject heading
$ = truncation
ti = word in title
ab = word in abstract
adj# = adjacent within x number of words
pt = publication type
* = truncation
md = methodology
kw = keyword
id = key phrase identifier
hw = subject heading word
up = update code

Ovid Medline
Database: Ovid MEDLINE without Revisions <1996 to January Week 5 2013>, Ovid MEDLINE Daily Update <February 06, 2013>, Ovid MEDLINE In-Process & Other Non-Indexed Citations <February 06, 2013>
Search Strategy:
----
1   Diet, Reducing/ (4116)
2   Diet, Fat-Restricted/ (2322)
3   Diet, Mediterranean/ (1170)
4   Diet, Sodium-Restricted/ (1671)
5   Diet, Carbohydrate-Restricted/ (658)
6   Caloric Restriction/ (3011)
7   Fruit/ (17529)
8   Vegetables/ (8398)
9   Diet Therapy/ (1386)
10   Food Habits/ (12503)
11   Exercise/ (49022)
12   Exercise Therapy/ (14088)
13   Motor Activity/ (42897)
14   Physical Fitness/ (12137)
15   Walking/ (15439)
16   (diet or dietary).ti. (50362)
17   (fruit$ or vegetable$).ti. (13806)
18   (exercise or physical activity).ti. (52839)

Appendix A. Literature Search Strategies

19   walking.ti. (6115)
20   1 or 2 or 3 or 4 or 5 or 6 or 7 or 8 or 9 or 10 or 11 or 12 or 13 or 14 or 15 or 16 or 17 or 18 or 19 (224973)
21   Counseling/ (14120)
22   Directive Counseling/ (975)
23   "Behavior-Therapy"/ (9261)
24   Cognitive Therapy/ (12320)
25   "Referral and Consultation"/ (28304)
26   Persuasive Communication/ (1910)
27   Social Control, Informal/ (1702)
28   Risk Reduction Behavior/ (5842)
29   Life Style/ (28852)
30   Motivation/ (27011)
31   Social Support/ (36654)
32   Feedback, Psychological/ (1895)
33   Self Efficacy/ (10309)
34   Health Knowledge, Attitudes, Practice/ (57028)
35   Health Behavior/ (25308)
36   Health Education/ (22824)
37   Health Promotion/ (36905)
38   Patient Education as Topic/ (45924)
39   counsel$.ti,ab. (43803)
40   advice.ti,ab. (21419)
41   (behavio$ adj (therap$ or chang$ or modification$)).ti,ab. (22790)
42   referral.ti,ab. (41636)
43   (life style or lifestyle).ti,ab. (40855)
44   motivation$.ti,ab. (32949)
45   health behavio$.ti,ab. (8461)
46   health education.ti,ab. (10316)
47   health promotion.ti,ab. (13023)
48   patient education.ti,ab. (7409)
49   nonpharmacologic intervention$.ti,ab. (412)
50   non pharmacologic intervention$.ti,ab. (79)
51   21 or 22 or 23 or 24 or 25 or 26 or 27 or 28 or 29 or 30 or 31 or 32 or 33 or 34 or 35 or 36 or 37 or 38 or 39 or 40 or 41 or 42 or 43 or 44 or 45 or 46 or 47 or 48 or 49 or 50 (433088)
52   20 and 51 (34659)
53   limit 52 to (clinical trial or controlled clinical trial or meta analysis or randomized controlled trial) (5261)
54   clinical trials as topic/ or controlled clinical trials as topic/ or randomized controlled trials as topic/ (155819)
55   Meta-Analysis as Topic/ (10422)
56   (control$ adj3 trial$).ti,ab. (109522)
57   random$.ti,ab. (498170)
58   clinical trial$.ti,ab. (152619)
59   54 or 55 or 56 or 57 or 58 (699757)
60   52 and 59 (6940)

Appendix A. Literature Search Strategies

61 53 or 60 (8350)
62 limit 61 to "all child (0 to 18 years)" (2185)
63 limit 61 to "all adult (19 plus years)" (5666)
64 62 not 63 (1164)
65 61 not 64 (7186)
66 limit 65 to animals (153)
67 limit 65 to humans (6939)
68 66 not 67 (46)
69 65 not 68 (7140)
70 limit 69 to english language (6828)
71 limit 70 to yr="2009 - 2013" (2780)
72 (harm or harms or harmful or harmed).ti,ab. (43331)
73 (risky behavior$ or risky behaviour$).ti,ab. (1462)
74 (adverse effects or mortality).fs. (937883)
75 Mortality/ (14354)
76 Morbidity/ (11716)
77 death/ (3972)
78 Athletic injuries/ (10205)
79 Malnutrition/ (5670)
80 nutritional defici$.ti,ab. (2107)
81 (death or deaths).ti,ab. (355179)
82 fracture$.ti,ab,hw. (110433)
83 72 or 73 or 74 or 75 or 76 or 77 or 78 or 79 or 80 or 81 or 82 (1355651)
84 52 and 83 (4148)
85 case-control studies/ or cohort studies/ or longitudinal studies/ or follow-up studies/ or prospective studies/ (756491)
86 case control$.ti,ab. (57859)
87 cohort.ti,ab. (184566)
88 longitudinal.ti,ab. (92373)
89 (follow-up or followup).ti,ab. (423455)
90 prospective$.ti,ab. (311455)
91 (comparison group$ or CG$).ti,ab. (200550)
92 observational.ti,ab. (58624)
93 retrospective studies/ (347399)
94 retrospective$.ti,ab. (279868)
95 database$.ti,ab. (153517)
96 nonrandomi$.ti,ab. (6428)
97 population$.ti,ab. (721935)
98 85 or 86 or 87 or 88 or 89 or 90 or 91 or 92 or 93 or 94 or 95 or 96 or 97 (2204688)
99 84 and 98 (2060)
100 limit 99 to "all child (0 to 18 years)" (355)
101 limit 99 to "all adult (19 plus years)" (1484)
102 100 not 101 (128)
103 99 not 102 (1932)
104 limit 103 to animals (69)
105 limit 103 to humans (1901)

Appendix A. Literature Search Strategies

106   104 not 105 (10)
107   103 not 106 (1922)
108   limit 107 to english language (1794)
109   70 or 108 (8126)
110   limit 109 to yr="2009 - 2013" (3260)
111   remove duplicates from 110 (3257)

Cochrane Database of Systematic Reviews
#1   diet:ti from 2001 to 2013, in Cochrane Reviews (Reviews only)   15
#2   diets:ti from 2001 to 2013, in Cochrane Reviews (Reviews only)   15
#3   dietary:ti from 2001 to 2013, in Cochrane Reviews (Reviews only) 31
#4   exercis*:ti from 2001 to 2013, in Cochrane Reviews (Reviews only)   69
#5   "physical activity":ti,ab,kw from 2001 to 2013, in Cochrane Reviews (Reviews only) 52
#6   fruit*:ti,ab,kw from 2001 to 2013, in Cochrane Reviews (Reviews only)   21
#7   vegetable*:ti,ab,kw from 2001 to 2013, in Cochrane Reviews (Reviews only)   17
#8   (#1 or #2 or #3 or #4 or #5 or #6 or #7) from 2001 to 2013, in Cochrane Reviews (Reviews only)   169
#9   Counsel*:ti,ab,kw from 2001 to 2013, in Cochrane Reviews (Reviews only)   154
#10   (Behavio* next therap*):ti,ab,kw from 2001 to 2013, in Cochrane Reviews (Reviews only) 181
#11   (cognitive next therap*):ti,ab,kw from 2001 to 2013, in Cochrane Reviews (Reviews only) 61
#12   advice:ti,ab,kw from 2001 to 2013, in Cochrane Reviews (Reviews only)   135
#13   (Behavio* next chang*):ti,ab,kw from 2001 to 2013, in Cochrane Reviews (Reviews only) 134
#14   (Behavio* next modification*):ti,ab,kw from 2001 to 2013, in Cochrane Reviews (Reviews only)   22
#15   Referral:ti,ab,kw from 2001 to 2013, in Cochrane Reviews (Reviews only) 45
#16   "life style":ti,ab,kw from 2001 to 2013, in Cochrane Reviews (Reviews only)   12
#17   lifestyle:ti,ab,kw from 2001 to 2013, in Cochrane Reviews (Reviews only) 72
#18   (nonpharmacologic next intervention*):ti,ab,kw from 2001 to 2013, in Cochrane Reviews (Reviews only)   0
#19   ("non pharmacologic" next intervention*):ti,ab,kw from 2001 to 2013, in Cochrane Reviews (Reviews only)   4
#20   (#9 or #10 or #11 or #12 or #13 or #14 or #15 or #16 or #17 or #18 or #19) from 2001 to 2013, in Cochrane Reviews (Reviews only)   552
#21   (#8 and #20) from 2001 to 2013, in Cochrane Reviews (Reviews only)   53

CENTRAL
#1   diet:ti from 2001 to 2013, in Trials   1816
#2   diets:ti from 2001 to 2013, in Trials   1816
#3   dietary:ti from 2001 to 2013, in Trials   1641
#4   exercis*:ti from 2001 to 2013, in Trials   6805
#5   "physical activity":ti,ab,kw from 2001 to 2013, in Trials   3270
#6   fruit*:ti,ab,kw from 2001 to 2013, in Trials   1228

Appendix A. Literature Search Strategies

#7 vegetable*:ti,ab,kw from 2001 to 2013, in Trials   1115
#8 (#1 or #2 or #3 or #4 or #5 or #6 or #7) from 2001 to 2013, in Trials   13472
#9 Counsel*:ti,ab,kw from 2001 to 2013, in Trials   3856
#10 (Behavio* next therap*):ti,ab,kw from 2001 to 2013, in Trials   3394
#11 (cognitive next therap*):ti,ab,kw from 2001 to 2013, in Trials   3158
#12 advice:ti,ab,kw from 2001 to 2013, in Trials 1390
#13 (Behavio* next chang*):ti,ab,kw from 2001 to 2013, in Trials   952
#14 (Behavio* next modification*):ti,ab,kw from 2001 to 2013, in Trials   169
#15 Referral:ti,ab,kw from 2001 to 2013, in Trials   2235
#16 "life style":ti,ab,kw from 2001 to 2013, in Trials   1286
#17 lifestyle:ti,ab,kw from 2001 to 2013, in Trials   2224
#18 (nonpharmacologic next intervention*):ti,ab,kw from 2001 to 2013, in Trials   23
#19 ("non pharmacologic" next intervention*):ti,ab,kw from 2001 to 2013, in Trials   9
#20 (#9 or #10 or #11 or #12 or #13 or #14 or #15 or #16 or #17 or #18 or #19) from 2001 to 2013, in Trials 14027
#21 (#8 and #20) from 2001 to 2013, in Trials   2224

DARE (via CRD)
1 (diet*) OR (fruit*) OR (vegetable*) IN DARE WHERE PD FROM 01/01/2009 TO 02/07/2013
2 (physical adj activity) OR (exercise*) OR (walking) IN DARE WHERE PD FROM 01/01/2009 TO 02/07/2013
3 #1 OR #2
4 (counsel*) OR (advice) OR (advise*) OR (behavio* NEAR chang*) OR (behavio* NEAR modif*) IN DARE WHERE PD FROM 01/01/2009 TO 02/07/2013
5 (lifestyle) OR (life ADJ style) OR (behavio* NEAR intervention*) OR (behavio* NEAR therap*) OR (cognitive NEAR therap*) OR (referral) IN DARE WHERE PD FROM 01/01/2009 TO 02/07/2013
6 #4 OR #5
7 #3 AND #6

PsycINFO <1806 to January Week 5 2013>
Search Strategy:
----
1   Diets/ (8146)
2   Dietary Restraint/ (1236)
3   Eating Behavior/ (6300)
4   fruit$.ti,ab,id,hw. (11022)
5   vegetable$.ti,ab,id,hw. (2806)
6   Exercise/ (13063)
7   Physical Activity/ (7903)
8   Aerobic Exercise/ (1012)
9   Walking/ (2858)
10   or/1-9 (45307)
11   behavior therapy/ (11986)
12   cognitive behavior therapy/ (9346)
13   cognitive therapy/ (11261)

Appendix A. Literature Search Strategies

14 Cognitive Techniques/ (1461)
15 Behavior Modification/ (9825)
16 Behavior Change/ (8714)
17 Lifestyle Changes/ (788)
18 Lifestyle/ (6480)
19 Persuasive Communication/ (4312)
20 Motivation/ (33531)
21 Motivational Interviewing/ (968)
22 Self Efficacy/ (13055)
23 Health Knowledge/ (4845)
24 Health Behavior/ (14164)
25 Health Education/ (8945)
26 Health Promotion/ (12642)
27 Client Education/ (2813)
28 counseling/ (17861)
29 counseling.id. (37498)
30 counselling.id. (720)
31 advice.ti,ab,id,hw. (13481)
32 or/11-31 (189067)
33 10 and 32 (8659)
34 controlled trial$.ti,ab,id,hw. (17354)
35 clinical trial$.ti,ab,id,hw. (20489)
36 random$.ti,ab,id,hw. (116082)
37 treatment outcome clinical trial.md. (23389)
38 or/34-37 (139067)
39 33 and 38 (1573)
40 (harm or harms or harmful or harmed).ti,ab,id,hw. (24081)
41 (risky behavior$ or risky behaviour$).ti,ab,id,hw. (1922)
42 adverse effect$.ti,ab,id,hw. (9522)
43 mortality.ti,ab,id,hw. (22585)
44 morbidity.ti,ab,id,hw. (14902)
45 death.ti,ab,id,hw. (60424)
46 Nutritional Defici$.ti,ab,id,hw. (2290)
47 fracture$.ti,ab,id,hw. (2671)
48 cardiovascular.ti,ab,id,hw. (21923)
49 injur$.ti,ab,id,hw. (56183)
50 or/40-49 (187313)
51 33 and 50 (837)
52 case control$.ti,ab,id,hw. (5692)
53 cohort.ti,ab,id,hw. (30010)
54 longitudinal.ti,ab,id,hw. (68065)
55 (follow-up or followup).ti,ab,id,hw. (79721)
56 prospective$.ti,ab,id,hw. (38228)
57 (comparison group$ or CG$).ti,ab,id,hw. (60433)
58 observational.ti,ab,id,hw. (14926)
59 retrospective$.ti,ab,id,hw. (23785)

Appendix A. Literature Search Strategies

60 database$.ti,ab,id,hw. (3148452)
61 nonrandomi$.ti,ab,id,hw. (537)
62 population$.ti,ab,id,hw. (216217)
63 or/52-62 (3154437)
64 51 and 63 (829)
65 39 or 64 (2243)
66 limit 65 to (100 childhood <birth to age 12 yrs> or 120 neonatal <birth to age 1 mo> or 140 infancy <age 2 to 23 mo> or 160 preschool age <age 2 to 5 yrs> or 180 school age <age 6 to 12 yrs> or 200 adolescence <age 13 to 17 yrs>) (361)
67 limit 65 to ("300 adulthood <age 18 yrs and older>" or 320 young adulthood <age 18 to 29 yrs> or 340 thirties <age 30 to 39 yrs> or 360 middle age <age 40 to 64 yrs> or "380 aged <age 65 yrs and older>" or "390 very old <age 85 yrs and older>") (1607)
68 66 not 67 (228)
69 65 not 68 (2015)
70 limit 69 to english language (1985)
71 limit 70 to yr="2001 - 2013" (1634)
72 (200907$ or 200908$ or 200909$ or 20091$ or 2010$ or 2011$ or 2012$ or 2013$).up. (696356)
73 71 and 72 (780)

PubMed, publisher-supplied

#27	Search #23 AND #24 AND publisher[sb] Filters: English
#26	Search #23 AND #24 AND publisher[sb]
#25	Search #23 AND #24
#24	Search trial[tiab] OR trials[tiab] OR random*[tiab] OR metaanaly*[tiab] OR "meta analysis"[tiab] OR "meta analyses"[tiab] OR "meta analytic"[tiab] OR systematic[tiab]
#23	Search #5 AND #22
#22	Search #6 OR #7 OR #8 OR #9 OR #10 OR #11 OR #12 OR #13 OR #14 OR #15 OR #16 OR #17 OR #18 OR #19 OR #20 OR #21
#21	Search coronary[ti] OR cardiovascular[ti] OR hypertension[ti] OR "blood pressure"[ti]
#20	Search "patient education" [tiab]
#19	Search "health promotion" [tiab]
#18	Search "health education" [tiab]
#17	Search "health behaviours" [tiab]
#16	Search "health behaviour" [tiab]
#15	Search "health behaviors" [tiab]
#14	Search "health behavior" [tiab]
#13	Search motivation* [tiab]
#12	Search "life style"[tiab] OR lifestyle[tiab]
#11	Search referral[tiab]
#10	Search behavio*[tiab] AND modification*[tiab]
#9	Search behavio*[tiab] AND change[tiab]

Appendix A. Literature Search Strategies

#8	Search behavio*[tiab] AND therapy[tiab]
#7	Search advice[tiab]
#6	Search counsel*[tiab]
#5	Search #1 OR #2 OR #3 OR #4
#4	Search walking[ti]
#3	Search exercise[ti] OR "physical activity"[ti]
#2	Search fruit*[ti] OR vegetable*[ti]
#1	Search diet[ti] OR dietary[ti]

Appendix A Figure 1. Literature Flow Diagram

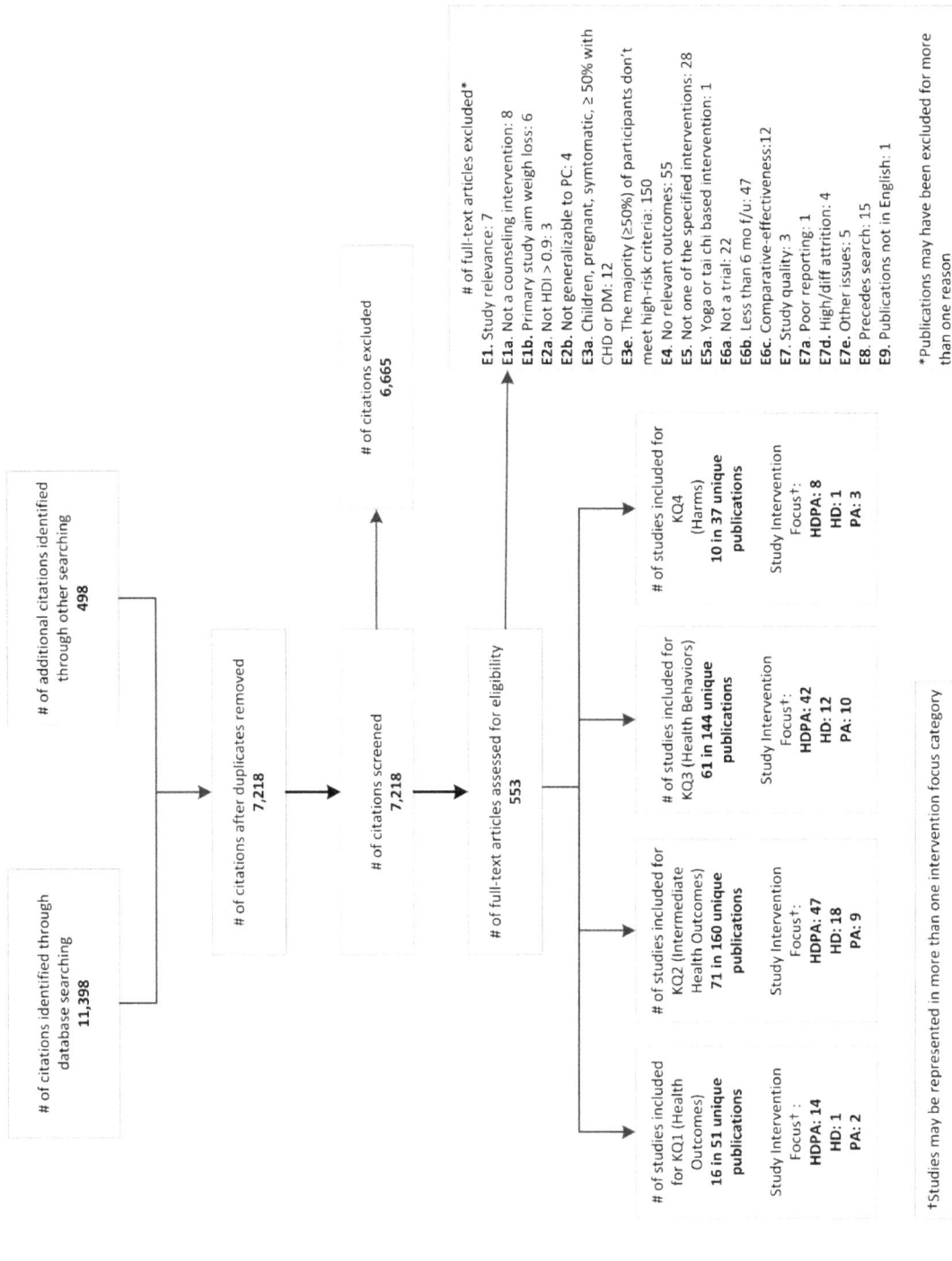

Appendix A Table 1. Inclusion and Exclusion Criteria

	Include	Exclude
Condition definition	Healthy diet is one designed to improve or maintain optimal health, which includes: • Appropriate energy (calorie) content • Balance of fats (consumption of mono and poly unsaturated fats, omega-3 fats, avoidance of excess saturated fat, avoidance of transfat) • Fruits and vegetables • Legumes • Lean proteins • Non- or low-fat dairy • Balance of carbohydrates (consumption of whole grain and fiber, avoidance of excess refined carbohydrates, including excess sweetened beverages) • Balance of sodium (avoidance of excess sodium) Physical activity may involve either: • Aerobic activities that involve repeated use of large muscles, such as walking, cycling, and swimming • Resistance training designed to improve physical strength	Aspects of a healthy diet that are out of scope include: • Dietary calcium and other vitamin, micronutrient, and antioxidant supplementation • Alcohol moderation Aspects of physical activity that are out of scope include: • Balance • Flexibility • Gait • Sedentary behaviors
Populations	Adults, at least 50% of whom have known CVD risk factors, including hypertension, metabolic syndrome, or impaired fasting glucose, such that >50% of the population is taking medication; mean systolic blood pressure of >140 mm Hg, diastolic blood pressure of >90 mm Hg, LDL cholesterol of >160 mg/dL or total cholesterol >200 mg/dL; or trial inclusion criteria specifies that population has one or more CVD risk factors	• Children and adolescents • Parents (if intended behavior change is directed toward children) • Persons with any acute disease (other than hypertension or dyslipidemia) • Persons with known CVD or diabetes mellitus, such that >50% of participants have known CVD, severe chronic kidney disease, or diabetes • Pregnant women with gestational diabetes • Persons in institutions • Persons with severe and persistent mental illness • Persons with cognitive impairment
Settings	• Primary care (including obstetrics/gynecology, internal medicine, family practice, military health clinics) or otherwise generalizable to primary care • Trials conducted in countries listed as "high" on the Human Development Index	Settings not generalizable to primary care (e.g., inpatient hospital units, emergency departments, nursing homes and other institutionalized settings, school-based programs, occupational settings, and other community-based settings); dental clinics

Appendix A Table 1. Inclusion and Exclusion Criteria

	Include	Exclude
Interventions	• Any behaviorally-based counseling intervention alone or as part of a larger multicomponent intervention on healthy diet and nutrition, physical activity, or both, including ≥1 of the following elements: assessment with feedback, advice, collaborative goal setting, assistance, or arranging further contacts • Either conducted in a primary care setting or judged to be feasible in primary care: 1) involves individual-level identification of being a patient or in need of intervention; 2) usually involves primary care physicians, other physicians, nurses, nurse practitioners, physician assistants, or other clinical staff (i.e., nutritionists, dieticians, physiotherapists, health educators), or the intervention will be seen as connected to the health care system by the participant • Or must be primary care referable, such that it is available for referral in most communities • Limited guided physical activity (i.e., 1 to 2 sessions) or provision of food samples allowed if intention is to teach or demonstrate healthy lifestyle principles • Optional or access to guided physical activity or exercises classes allowed	• Noncounseling interventions (e.g., use of incentives, supervised exercise with the goal of assessing effects of exercise) • Interventions providing controlled diets • Counseling interventions aimed at weight loss or weight maintenance, falls prevention, depression, cognitive functioning, or disease prevention other than CVD/diabetes mellitus • Prenatal or postnatal dietary counseling • Counseling interventions that are primarily community, nonreferral (e.g., occupational/ worksite or school-based); social marketing (e.g., media campaigns) • Policy (e.g., local or state public/health policy) • Interventions focused exclusively on reducing sedentary behavior (e.g., reduced television or screen time) • Interventions that use yoga or tai chi
Comparisons	• No intervention (e.g., wait-list control, usual care), minimal intervention (e.g., pamphlets, 1 annual session presenting information similar to usual care in a primary care setting), or attention control (e.g., similar format and intensity intervention on a different content area) • CG can receive 1 visit annually (limited to 45–60 min) or 2–3 brief sessions annually (limited to 15 min each), but no personalized prescription based on standardized assessment. CG may receive generic print materials twice yearly, but a more extensive print-based workbook would be considered comparative effectiveness and therefore excluded. CGs that received limited feedback on assessments were included	• Comparative effectiveness trials without a control (as defined above) • Physical activity only: studies in which the CG is instructed not to exercise
Outcomes	• KQ 1: Distal health outcomes (i.e., morbidity related to CVD, mortality) • KQ 2: Intermediate outcomes (i.e., blood pressure, hypertension, total cholesterol, LDL cholesterol or ratio of total/HDL cholesterol, serum fasting glucose or glucose tolerance, hemoglobin A1c, diabetes, weight, body mass index, hyperlipidemia) • KQ 3: Behavioral outcomes (i.e., physical activity, dietary intake or dietary patterns), self-reported or objectively measured • KQ 4: Adverse outcomes, including any harms requiring medical attention (e.g., nutritional deficiencies, musculoskeletal injuries, cardiovascular events)	• Knowledge, attitudes, self-efficacy, functioning, quality of life • Physical activity only: studies limited to balance or flexibility outcomes • Less than 6 months or 60% followup
Study Designs	• Fair- to good-quality studies • KQs 1–3: Systematic reviews, RCTs, CCTs (RCTs only before 2001) • KQ 4: Systematic reviews, RCTs, CCTs, comparative cohorts, population-based case-control studies	• Poor-quality studies • KQs 1–3: Any observational studies • KQ 4: Ecological studies, case-series, case reports

Appendix A Table 1. Inclusion and Exclusion Criteria

	Include	Exclude
Publication Date	Trials published from 1990 to present	Trials whose primary results were published before 1990, in which the interventions were generally conducted in the 1970s

Abbreviations: CCT = controlled clinical trial; CVD = cardiovascular disease; HDL = high-density lipoprotein; KQ = key question; LDL = low-density lipoprotein; RCT = randomized, controlled trial.

Appendix A Table 2. Quality Assessment Criteria

Design	USPSTF Quality Rating Criteria[60]	NICE Methodology Checklists[61]
Systematic reviews and meta-analyses	<ul><li>Comprehensiveness of sources considered/search strategy used</li><li>Standard appraisal of included studies</li><li>Validity of conclusions</li><li>Recency and relevance, especially for systematic reviews</li></ul>	<ul><li>Study addresses an appropriate and clearly focused question</li><li>Methodology is described</li><li>Literature search is sufficiently rigorous to identify all the relevant studies</li><li>Study quality is assessed and taken into account</li><li>There are enough similarities between the studies selected to make combining them reasonable</li></ul>
Randomized, controlled trials	<ul><li>Initial assembly of comparable groups employs adequate randomization, including first concealment and whether potential confounders were distributed equally among groups</li><li>Maintenance of comparable groups (includes attrition, crossovers, adherence, contamination)</li><li>Important differential loss to followup or overall high loss to followup</li><li>Measurements are equal, reliable, and valid (includes masking of outcome assessment)</li><li>Clear definition of the interventions</li><li>All important outcomes are considered</li></ul>	<ul><li>Study addresses an appropriate and clearly focused question</li><li>Assignment of subjects to treatment groups is randomized</li><li>Adequate concealment method is used</li><li>Subjects and investigators are kept blind about treatment allocation</li><li>Treatment and CGs are similar at the start of the trial</li><li>Only difference between groups is the treatment under investigation</li><li>All relevant outcomes are measured in a standard, valid, and reliable way</li><li>Percentage of individuals or clusters recruited into each treatment arm of the study that dropped out before the study was completed is reported</li><li>All the subjects are analyzed in the groups to which they were randomly allocated (often referred to as intention-to-treat analysis)</li><li>When the study is carried out at more than one site, results are comparable for all sites</li></ul>
Cohort studies	<ul><li>Initial assembly of comparable groups employs consideration of potential confounders, with either restriction or measurement for adjustment in the analysis; consideration of inception cohorts</li><li>Maintenance of comparable groups (includes attrition, crossovers, adherence, contamination)</li><li>Important differential loss to followup or overall high loss to followup</li><li>Measurements are equal, reliable, and valid (includes masking of outcome assessment)</li><li>Clear definition of the interventions</li><li>All important outcomes are considered</li></ul>	<ul><li>Study addresses an appropriate and clearly focused question</li><li>Two groups being studied are selected from source populations that are comparable in all respects other than the factor under investigation</li><li>Study indicates how many of the people asked to take part did so, in each of the groups being studied</li><li>Likelihood that some eligible subjects might have the outcome at the time of enrollment is assessed and taken into account in the analysis</li><li>Percentage of individuals or clusters recruited into each treatment arm of the study that dropped out before the study was completed is reported</li><li>Comparison is made between full participants and those lost to followup, by exposure status</li><li>Outcomes are clearly defined</li><li>Assessment of outcome is made blind to exposure status</li><li>When blinding is not possible, there is some recognition that knowledge of exposure status could have influenced the assessment of outcome</li><li>Measure of assessment of exposure is reliable</li><li>Evidence from other sources is used to demonstrate that the method of outcome assessment is valid and reliable</li><li>Exposure level or prognostic factor is assessed more than once</li><li>Main potential confounders are identified and taken into account in the design and analysis</li><li>Confidence intervals are provided</li></ul>

Appendix B. Ongoing or Recently Completed Studies

Investigator, Study Name, Location	Number of Participants	Intervention	Outcomes	2013 Status
Dr. Sheldon Tobe HBPS Canada (Heart and Stroke Foundation of Ontario)	5,000	Integrated model in which doctors, nurse practitioners, and pharmacists work together through use of evidence-informed tools, including a patient toolkit addressing lifestyle change information, to control BP in 11 family practice sites	BP	Ongoing
Göteborgs University (no named PI) DIAVIP Sweden	2,000	Diabetes prevention in primary health care, with emphasis on low- vs. high-intensity PA compared with no intervention	HOMA IR	Not yet enrolling
Dr. Denis Pouchain ESCAPE France (College National des Generalistes Enseignants)	1,836	General practice–delivered prevention consultations, focused on diet and exercise, to reduce CVD risk factors in patients with HTN	LDL, HbA1c, BP, PA, diet, QoL, number of targets reached	Completed
Region Skåne (no named PI) The MEDIM Study Sweden	1,244	Lifestyle intervention including group counseling and PA for Iraqi immigrants with prediabetes	FBG, QALY	Not yet enrolling
Dr. Olugbenga Ogedegbe CAATCH Columbia University	1,039	Counseling patients to control HTN using a multicomponent intervention aimed at patients and providers within Community Health Centers	SBP, DBP, cost effectiveness	Completed
Dr. Nancy Kressin Boston University, Boston Medical Center	870	Patient-centered counseling for HTN, with or without cultural competency training for physicians, compared with usual care, to improve control of HTN	BP, % with controlled HTN, medication adherence	Ongoing
Dr. Melanie Davies UK (University Hospitals, Leicester)	804	Group educational program to increase PA and reduce risk for developing diabetes in adults at high risk for diabetes (based on "risk score")	PA, FBG, HbA1c, adiposity (subset)	Recruiting
Dr. Melanie Davies PREVENTION UK (University Hospitals, Leicester)	748	Educational program focusing on lifestyle, PA, and food choices in individuals at high risk for diabetes	Diabetes incidence, FBG, METS, CVD risk, HbA1c	Enrolling
Dr. Esperanza Escortell EDUCORE Spain (Servicio Madrileno de Salud)	736	Use of the EDUCORE program, a visual aid educational intervention, to improve blood pressure control in patients with hypertension in 22 primary health care centers in Madrid	SBP, DBP, BP control, CVD risk score, TC	Completed
Dr. Beti Thompson Fred Hutchinson Cancer Research Center	430	Education-based, lay health educator-led intervention designed to educate participants with elevated HbA1c levels about diabetes and diet and lifestyle changes	PA, diet, HbA1c	Completed
Dr. Robert Reid FHHP-RCT Canada (University of Ottawa Heart Institute)	426	12-week lifestyle change program for increased exercise and improved nutrition and weight management, with telephone-based motivational counseling in high-risk adults	SBP, TC, HDL, LDL, PA, diet, body composition	Completed
Dr. Robert Nolan I-START Canada (University Health Network, Toronto)	387	Internet-based behavioral counseling for adaptive lifestyle change for subjects diagnosed with hypertension (I-START)	SBP, DBP, PA, diet, vagal-heart rate	Completed

Appendix B. Ongoing or Recently Completed Studies

Investigator, Study Name, Location	Number of Participants	Intervention	Outcomes	2013 Status
Dr. Andrea Kriska Healthy Lifestyle Project University of Pittsburgh	351	DPP-adapted program delivered in a community-based setting. In person vs. DVD session for group lifestyle education focused on weight loss and increasing PA levels for individuals at high risk for diabetes	Weight, BP, FBG, lipids, PA, QoL	Recruiting
Dr. Prabath Nanayakkara WISH The Netherlands (Vrije University Medical Center)	300	Tailored lifestyle advice through Web-based feedback system for adults with hypertension	SBP, DBP	Recruiting
Dr. Gladys Block ALIVE-PD Kaiser Permanente-Northern California, Berkeley Analytics	268	Lifestyle intervention with multichannel delivery, including email/Web goal setting to improve PA, diet and weight loss for patients with prediabetes	FBG, HbA1c, weight, PA, diet	Not yet enrolling
Dr. Robert Zweiker Austria (Medical University of Graz)	256	Structured educational program, including lifestyle and dietary habits, for patients with hypertension	BP, morbidity associated with CVD events	Completed
Dr. Olugbenga Ogedegbe COACH New York University School of Medicine	250	Comprehensive therapeutic lifestyle intervention delivered through group-based counseling and motivational interviewing in seniors with hypertension age 60 years and older	SBP, DBP, PA, weight, diet	Ongoing
Dr. Olugbenga Ogedegbe TLC-Clinic New York University School of Medicine	200	Primary care practice-based lifestyle intervention delivered through group-based counseling and motivational interviewing and focused on PA, diet, and weight management for hypertension	SBP, DBP, PA, diet, weight, sodium	Ongoing
Dr. Antti Jula Finland (National Institute for Health and Welfare)	144	Comprehensive intervention on blood pressure control in a primary care setting, with a focus on lifestyle guidance	SBP, DBP	Completed
Dr. Lena Holm Sweden (Karolinksa Institutet)	141	Group seminars and motivational interviewing to change lifestyle factors, including PA and diet, in patients with high blood pressure	BP, PA, diet, BMI, abdominal circumference	Completed
Dr. Theodore Kotchen Medical College of Wisconsin	120	Lifestyle counseling focusing on behavior change for diet and PA to reduce BP in patients with hypertension	SBP, DBP	Recruiting
Dr. Robert Ackermann Northwestern University	92	Group-based adaptation of DPP, delivered by DPP-trained YMCA staff in YMCA facilities	Weight loss, PA, diet	Completed
Dr. Devin Mann ADAPT Mt. Sinai Medical Center, Boston University	80	Use of electronic medical records to enhance lifestyle behavior change counseling in a primary care setting	PA, HbA1c	Recruiting
Dr. Kamlesh Khunti TRIMS UK (University of Leicester)	80	Group education program for individuals with diagnosable METS based on lifestyle changes (diet and increased PA) to decrease risk for diabetes or CVD	METS prevalence, FBG, HDL, BP, PA, Diet, QoL, Framingham risk score	Completed

Appendix B. Ongoing or Recently Completed Studies

Investigator, Study Name, Location	Number of Participants	Intervention	Outcomes	2013 Status
Dr. Namratha Kandula Northwestern University	60	Heart disease prevention group sessions focusing on PA, diet, weight, and stress for adults with at least one CHD risk factor	PA, diet, SBP, DBP, lipids, weight	Recruiting
Dr. Marie-France Longlois Canada (Université de Sherbrooke)	60	Use of interdisciplinary treatment program, including nurse, endocrinologist, nutritionist, and psychologist to discuss diet, PA, and psychological and medication-related issues	METS, weight, diet intake, PA, QoL, cost effectiveness	Completed
Dr. Adam Bernstein FRESH Study The Cleveland Clinic	27	Diet instruction, PA, culinary education, and stress management for patients with prediabetes	Correlation between participation and health of participants	Completed

Abbreviations: BMI = body mass index; BP = blood pressure; CHD = coronary heart disease; CVD = cardiovascular disease; DBP = diastolic blood pressure; FBG = fasting blood glucose; HOMA-IR = homeostasis model assessment insulin resistance; HTN = hypertension; LDL = low-density lipoprotein; METS = metabolic syndrome; PA = physical activity; QALY = quality-adjusted life years; QOL = quality of life; SBP = systolic blood pressure; TC = total cholesterol.

Appendix C. Excluded Studies

This is a listing of studies excluded from the review by key question (KQ). If a study was included for one KQ, but excluded for others, it would still be listed here with the excluded KQs noted.

Exclusion Code

E1. Study relevance
  a. Does not focus on counseling intervention
  b. Primary aim is weight loss
  c. Not focused on cardiovascular disease

E2. Setting
  a. Human Development Index not >0.9
  b. Not generalizable to primary care

E3. Population
  a. Children, pregnant women, symptomatic patients, ≥50% with coronary heart disease or diabetes
  b. Biased recruitment or not generalizable to primary care
  c. Healthy Diet: specialized diet
  d. Physical Activity: specialized physical activity required
  e. The majority (≥50%) of participants do not meet high-risk criteria

E4: No relevant outcomes
E5: Not one of the specified interventions   **a.** Yoga or tai chi based intervention

E6: Study design
  a. Not a trial
  b. Less than 6 months followup
  c. Comparative effectiveness
  d. Physical Activity: CG told not to exercise

E7: Study quality
  a. Poor reporting
  b. Problematic baseline comparability
  c. Unblinded assessment
  d. High/differential attrition
  e. Other issues

E8: Precedes search (i.e., main outcomes published before 1990)
E9. Publication not in English

1. Aadahl M, von Huth SL, Pisinger C, et al. Five-year change in physical activity is associated with changes in cardiovascular disease risk factors: the Inter99 study. Prev Med 2009 Apr;48(4):326-31. PMID: 19463487. **KQ2E3e.**
2. Absetz P, Valve R, Oldenburg B, et al. Type 2 diabetes prevention in the "real world": one-year results of the GOAL Implementation Trial 1. Diabetes Care 2007 Oct;30(10):2465-70. PMID: 17586741. **KQ1E6a, KQ2E6a, KQ3E6a, KQ4E6a.**
3. Aggarwal B, Liao M, Allegrante JP, et al. Low social support level is associated with non-adherence to diet at 1 year in the Family Intervention Trial for Heart Health (FIT Heart). Journal of Nutrition Education & Behavior 2010 Nov;42(6):380-8. PMID: 20696617. **KQ1E3e, KQ2E3e, KQ3E3e, KQ4E3e.**
4. Aggarwal B, Liao M, Mosca L. Predictors of physical activity at 1 year in a randomized controlled trial of family members of patients with cardiovascular disease. Journal of Cardiovascular Nursing 2010 Nov;25(6):444-9. PMID: 20856131. **KQ1E3e, KQ2E3e, KQ3E3e, KQ4E3e.**
5. Aittasalo M, Miilunpalo S, Kukkonen HK, et al. A randomized intervention of physical activity promotion and patient self-monitoring in primary health care. Prev Med 2006;42(1):40-6. PMID: 16297442. **KQ3E3e.**
6. Aizawa K, Shoemaker JK, Overend TJ, et al. Effects of lifestyle modification on central artery stiffness in metabolic syndrome subjects with pre-hypertension and/or pre-diabetes. Diabetes Research & Clinical Practice 2009 Feb;83(2):249-56. PMID: 19097666. **KQ2E6a, KQ3E6a.**
7. Aizer A, Gaziano JM, Cook NR, et al. Relation of vigorous exercise to risk of atrial fibrillation. American Journal of Cardiology 2009 Jun 1;103(11):1572-7. PMID: 19463518. **KQ4E3e.**
8. Aldana SG, Greenlaw RL, Diehl HA, et al. Effects of an intensive diet and physical activity modification program on the health risks of adults. Journal of the American Dietetic Association 2005;105(3):371-81. PMID: 15746824. **KQ1E3e, KQ2E3e, KQ3E3e.**
9. Aldana SG, Greenlaw RL, Diehl HA, et al. The behavioral and clinical effects of therapeutic lifestyle change on middle-aged adults. Preventing

Appendix C. Excluded Studies

Chronic Disease 2006;3(1):A05. PMID: 16356358. **KQ2E3e, KQ3E3e.**

10. Alexander GL, McClure JB, Calvi JH, et al. A randomized clinical trial evaluating online interventions to improve fruit and vegetable consumption. American Journal of Public Health 2010 Feb;100(2):319-26. PMID: 20019315. **KQ3E3e.**

11. Alli C, Avanzini F, Bettelli G, et al. Feasibility of a long-term low-sodium diet in mild hypertension. J Hum Hypertens 1992 Aug;6(4):281-6. PMID: 1433163. **KQ1E7, KQ2E7, KQ3E7, KQ4E7.**

12. Almeida-Pittito B, Hirai AT, Sartorelli DS, et al. Impact of a 2-year intervention program on cardiometabolic profile according to the number of goals achieved. [References]. Brazilian Journal of Medical and Biological Research 2010 Nov;43(11):1088-94. PMID: 21088806. **KQ2E2a.**

13. Ammerman AS, Keyserling T, Atwood J, et al. High-quality nutrition counselling for hypercholesterolaemia by public health nurses in rural areas does not affect total blood cholesterol. Evidence Based Healthcare 2003;7(4):187-9. PMID: None. **KQ2E6a, KQ3E6a.**

14. Andersen LJ, Randers MB, Westh K, et al. Football as a treatment for hypertension in untrained 30-55-year-old men: a prospective randomized study. Scandinavian Journal of Medicine & Science in Sports 2010 Apr;20(Suppl 1):98-102. PMID: 20210907. **KQ2E5.**

15. Andersson EK, Moss TP. Imagery and implementation intention: A randomised controlled trial of interventions to increase exercise behaviour in the general population. Psychology of Sport and Exercise 2011;12(2):63-70. PMID: None. **KQ3E3e.**

16. Arciero PJ, Gentile CL, Martin PR, et al. Increased dietary protein and combined high intensity aerobic and resistance exercise improves body fat distribution and cardiovascular risk factors. International journal of sport nutrition and exercise metabolism 2006;16(4):373-92. PMID: 17136940. **KQ2E3e.**

17. Armit CM, Brown WJ, Marshall AL, et al. Randomized trial of three strategies to promote physical activity in general practice. Prev Med 2009 Feb;48(2):156-63. PMID: 19100282. **KQ2E3e, KQ3E3e.**

18. Armitage CJ, Arden MA. A volitional help sheet to increase physical activity in people with low socioeconomic status: A randomised exploratory trial. Psychology & Health 2010 Dec;25(10):1129-45. PMID: 20309777. **KQ3E6b.**

19. Ayres K, Conner M, Prestwich A, et al. Exploring the question-behaviour effect: randomized controlled trial of motivational and question-behaviour interventions. British Journal of Health Psychology 2013 Feb;18(1):31-44. PMID: 22519696. **KQ3E4.**

20. Bakx JC, Stafleu A, Van Staveren WA, et al. Long-term effect of nutritional counseling: a study in family medicine. Am J Clin Nutr 1997 Jun;65(6 Suppl):1946S-50S. PMID: 9174500. **KQ1E8, KQ2E8, KQ3E8, KQ4E8.**

21. Barclay C, Procter KL, Glendenning R, et al. Can type 2 diabetes be prevented in UK general practice? A lifestyle-change feasibility study (ISAIAH). The British journal of general practice : the journal of the Royal College of General Practitioners 2008;58(553):541-7. PMID: 18682012. **KQ2E6b, KQ3E6b, KQ4E6b.**

22. Beavers KM, Beavers DP, Nesbit BA, et al. Effect of an 18 month physical activity and weight loss intervention on body composition in overweight and obese older adults. Obesity (Silver Spring) 2013 Aug 20 PMID: 10.1002/oby.20607 [doi]. **KQ2E5.**

23. Bennett GG, Warner ET, Glasgow RE, et al. Obesity treatment for socioeconomically disadvantaged patients in primary care practice. Arch Intern Med 2012 Apr 9;172(7):565-74. PMID: 2412073. **KQ1E1b, KQ2E1b, KQ3E1b, KQ4E1b.**

24. Bennett JA, Perrin NA, Hanson G, et al. Healthy aging demonstration project: nurse coaching for behavior change in older adults 1. Res Nurs Health 2005 Jun;28(3):187-97. PMID: 15884026. **KQ1E3e, KQ2E3e, KQ3E3e, KQ4E3e.**

25. Bennett JA, Young HM, Nail LM, et al. A telephone-only motivational intervention to increase physical activity in rural adults: a randomized controlled trial. Nursing Research 2008;57(1):24-32. PMID: 18091289. **KQ3E3e.**

26. Berry SE, Mulla UZ, Chowienczyk PJ, et al. Increased potassium intake from fruit and vegetables or supplements does not lower blood pressure or improve vascular function in UK men and women with early hypertension: a randomised controlled trial. British Journal of Nutrition 2010 Dec;104(12):1839-47. PMID: 20673378. **KQ2E6b.**

27. Bickmore TW, Silliman RA, Nelson K, et al. A Randomized Controlled Trial of an Automated Exercise Coach for Older Adults. J Am Geriatr Soc 2013 Sep 3 PMID: 24001030. **KQ3E3e.**

28. Blaufox MD, Lee HB, Davis B, et al. Renin predicts diastolic blood pressure response to nonpharmacologic and pharmacologic therapy. JAMA 1992 Mar 4;267(9):1221-5. PMID: 1538559. **KQ1E1, KQ2E1, KQ3E1, KQ4E1.**

Appendix C. Excluded Studies

29. Blumenthal JA, Sherwood A, Gullette EC, et al. Exercise and weight loss reduce blood pressure in men and women with mild hypertension: effects on cardiovascular, metabolic, and hemodynamic functioning. Arch Intern Med 2000 Jul 10;160(13):1947-58. PMID: 10888969. **KQ1E4, KQ2E5, KQ3E4, KQ4E4.**

30. Blumenthal JA, Babyak MA, Hinderliter A, et al. Effects of the DASH diet alone and in combination with exercise and weight loss on blood pressure and cardiovascular biomarkers in men and women with high blood pressure: the ENCORE study. Arch Intern Med 2010 Jan 25;170(2):126-35. PMID: 20101007. **KQ2E5.**

31. Borschmann K, Moore K, Russell M, et al. Overcoming barriers to physical activity among culturally and linguistically diverse older adults: a randomised controlled trial. Australasian Journal on Ageing 2010 Jun;29(2):77-80. PMID: 20553538. **KQ3E3a.**

32. Bosak KA, Yates B, Pozehl B. Effects of an Internet physical activity intervention in adults with metabolic syndrome. Western Journal of Nursing Research 2010 Feb;32(1):5-22. PMID: 19357421. **KQ2E6b, KQ3E6b.**

33. Bouchonville M, Armamento-Villareal R, Shah K, et al. Weight loss, exercise or both and cardiometabolic risk factors in obese older adults: results of a randomized controlled trial. Int J Obes (Lond) 2013 Jul 4. PMID: 23823329. **KQ2E1c.**

34. Bray GA, Jablonski KA, Fujimoto WY, et al. Relation of central adiposity and body mass index to the development of diabetes in the Diabetes Prevention Program. Am J Clin Nutr 2008 May;87(5):1212-8. PMID: 18469241. **KQ2E4.**

35. Brekke HK, Jansson PA, Månsson JE, et al. Lifestyle changes can be achieved through counseling and follow-up in first-degree relatives of patients with type 2 diabetes. Journal of the American Dietetic Association 2003;103(7):835-43. PMID: 12830021. **KQ2E3e, KQ3E3e.**

36. Brekke HK, Jansson PA, Lenner RA. Long-term (1- and 2-year) effects of lifestyle intervention in type 2 diabetes relatives. Diabetes Research and Clinical Practice 2005;70(3):225-34. PMID: 15885845. **KQ1E3e, KQ2E3e, KQ3E3e, KQ4E3e.**

37. Bridgewater LE, Lodge MA, Reid RD. Description of a behavioural counselling strategy for risk factor modification in a Family Heart Health randomized controlled trial: preliminary results. Journal of Cardiopulmonary Rehabilitation and Prevention 2009;29(5):335. PMID: None. **KQ1E4, KQ2E4, KQ3E4, KQ4E4.**

38. Broekhuizen K, Poppel MN, Koppes LL, et al. A tailored lifestyle intervention to reduce the cardiovascular disease risk of individuals with Familial Hypercholesterolemia (FH): design of the PRO-FIT randomised controlled trial. BMC Public Health 2010;10:69. PMID: 20156339. **KQ1E4, KQ2E4, KQ3E4, KQ4E4.**

39. Buman MP, Giacobbi PR, Jr., Dzierzewski JM, et al. Peer volunteers improve long-term maintenance of physical activity with older adults: a randomized controlled trial. Journal of Physical Activity & Health 2011 Sep;8(Suppl 2):S257-S266. PMID: 21918240. **KQ3E3e.**

40. Burke L, Jancey J, Howat P, et al. Physical activity and nutrition program for seniors (PANS): protocol of a randomized controlled trial. BMC Public Health 2010;10:751. PMID: 21129226. **KQ1E4, KQ2E4, KQ3E4, KQ4E4.**

41. Burke L, Lee AH, Jancey J, et al. Physical activity and nutrition behavioural outcomes of a home-based intervention program for seniors: a randomized controlled trial. International Journal of Behavioral Nutrition & Physical Activity 2013;10:14. PMID: 23363616. **KQ3E3e.**

42. Burke LE, Dunbar-Jacob J, Orchard TJ, et al. Improving adherence to a cholesterol-lowering diet: a behavioral intervention study. Patient Education & Counseling 2005 Apr;57(1):134-42. PMID: 15797163. **KQ1E4, KQ2E6b, KQ3E6b, KQ4E4.**

43. Burke V, Giangiulio N, Gillam HF, et al. Physical activity and nutrition programs for couples: a randomized controlled trial. Journal of Clinical Epidemiology 2003;56(5):421-32. PMID: 12812815. **KQ2E3e, KQ3E3e.**

44. Burke V, Beilin LJ, Cutt HE, et al. Moderators and mediators of behaviour change in a lifestyle program for treated hypertensives: a randomized controlled trial (ADAPT). Health Education Research 2007;23(4):583-91. PMID: 17890759. **KQ2E4.**

45. Busnello FM, Bodanese LC, Pellanda LC, et al. Nutritional intervention and the impact on adherence to treatment in patients with metabolic syndrome. Arquivos Brasileiros de Cardiologia 2011 Sep;97(3):217-24. PMID: 21739068. **KQ2E2a.**

46. Byfield CL. Development and evaluation of a lifestyle physical activity intervention for obese sedentary women. Colorado State University PhD Thesis 2001 **KQ1E1b, KQ2E1b, KQ3E1b, KQ4E1b.**

47. Caggiula AW, Christakis G, Farrand M, et al. The multiple risk intervention trial (MRFIT). IV. Intervention on blood lipids. Prev Med 1981 Jul;10(4):443-75. PMID: 7027238. **KQ1E8, KQ2E8, KQ3E8, KQ4E8.**

Appendix C. Excluded Studies

48. Calfas KJ, Sallis JF, Zabinski MF, et al. Preliminary evaluation of a multicomponent program for nutrition and physical activity change in primary care: PACE+ for adults. Prev Med 2002;34(2):153-61. PMID: 11817910. **KQ3E6b.**

49. Camhi SM, Stefanick ML, Katzmarzyk PT, et al. Metabolic syndrome and changes in body fat from a low-fat diet and/or exercise randomized controlled trial. Obesity 2010 Mar;18(3):548-54. PMID: 19798074. **KQ2E3e.**

50. Campbell K, Foster-Schubert K, Xiao L, et al. Injuries in sedentary individuals enrolled in a 12-month, randomized, controlled, exercise trial. Journal of Physical Activity & Health 2012 Feb;9(2):198-207. PMID: 22368219. **KQ4E3e.**

51. Capewell S, O'Flaherty M. Can dietary changes rapidly decrease cardiovascular mortality rates? European Heart Journal 2011 May;32(10):1187-9. PMID: 21367835. **KQ1E6a, KQ2E6a, KQ3E6a.**

52. Carr LJ, Bartee RT, Dorozynski CM, et al. Eight-month follow-up of physical activity and central adiposity: results from an Internet-delivered randomized control trial intervention. Journal of Physical Activity & Health 2009 Jul;6(4):444-55. PMID: 19842458. **KQ1E7d, KQ2E7d, KQ3E7d, KQ4E7d.**

53. Carroll JK, Lewis BA, Marcus BH, et al. Computerized tailored physical activity reports. A randomized controlled trial. Am J Prev Med 2010;39:148-56. PMID: 2062162. **KQ3E3e.**

54. Carroll JK, Lewis BA, Marcus BH, et al. Eight-month follow-up of physical activity and central adiposity: results from an Internet-delivered randomized control trial intervention. Am J Prev Med 2010 Aug;39(2):148-56. PMID: 20621262. **KQ3E3a.**

55. Carroll S, Borkoles E, Polman R. Short-term effects of a non-dieting lifestyle intervention program on weight management, fitness, metabolic risk, and psychological well-being in obese premenopausal females with the metabolic syndrome. Applied physiology, nutrition, and metabolism = Physiologie appliquée, nutrition et métabolisme 2007;32(1):125-42. PMID: 17332789. **KQ1E4, KQ2E5, KQ1E4.**

56. Castro CM, Pruitt LA, Buman MP, et al. Physical activity program delivery by professionals versus volunteers: the TEAM randomized trial. Health Psychology 2011 May;30(3):285-94. PMID: 21553972. **KQ3E3e.**

57. Chandratilleke MG, Carson KV, Picot J, et al. Physical training for asthma. [Review]. Cochrane Database of Systematic Reviews 2012(5):CD001116. PMID: 22592674. **KQ4E3e.**

58. Chang AK, Fritschi C, Kim MJ. Nurse-led empowerment strategies for hypertensive patients with metabolic syndrome. Contemporary Nurse 2012 Aug;42(1):118-28. PMID: 23050578. **KQE5, KQ2E5, KQ3E5, KQ4E5.**

59. Chapman J, Armitage CJ. Do techniques that increase fruit intake also increase vegetable intake? Evidence from a comparison of two implementation intention interventions. [References]. Appetite 2012 Feb;58(1):28-33. PMID: 22001024. **KQ1E3e, KQ2E3e, KQ3E3e, KQ4E3e.**

60. Chellini E, Gorini G, Carreras G, et al. The Pap smear screening as an occasion for smoking cessation and physical activity counselling: baseline characteristics of women involved in the SPRINT randomized controlled trial. BMC Public Health 2011;11:906. PMID: 22151834. **KQ1E5, KQ2E5, KQ3E5, KQ4E5.**

61. Chiang CY, Sun FK. The effects of a walking program on older Chinese American immigrants with hypertension: a pretest and posttest quasi-experimental design. Public Health Nursing 2009 May;26(3):240-8. PMID: 19386059. **KQ2E6b, KQ3E6b.**

62. Claes N, Jacobs N. The PreCardio-study protocol-- a randomized clinical trial of a multidisciplinary electronic cardiovascular prevention programme. BMC Cardiovascular Disorders 2007;7:27. PMID: 17784946. **KQ1E2b, KQ2E2b, KQ3E2b.**

63. Coghill N, Cooper AR. The effect of a home-based walking program on risk factors for coronary heart disease in hypercholesterolaemic men. A randomized controlled trial. Prev Med 2008 Jun;46(6):545-51. PMID: 18316115. **KQ2E6b, KQ3E6b, KQ4E6b.**

64. Coghill N, Cooper AR. Motivators and de-motivators for adherence to a program of sustained walking. Prev Med 2009 Aug;49(1):24-7. PMID: 19426757. **KQ2E6b, KQ3E6b, KQ4E6b.**

65. Coleman KJ, Ngor E, Reynolds K, et al. Initial validation of an exercise "vital sign" in electronic medical records 4. Med Sci Sports Exerc 2012 Nov;44(11):2071-6. PMID: 22688832. **KQ1E1a, KQ2E1a, KQ3E1a, KQ4E1a.**

66. Colle B, Brusaferro S. [Cardiovascular risk reduction: impact of an international project]. Annali di igiene : medicina preventiva e di comunità 2008;20(3 Suppl 1):43-8. PMID: 18773604. **KQ2E9, KQ3E9.**

67. Cook NR, Cutler JA, Obarzanek E, et al. Long term effects of dietary sodium reduction on cardiovascular disease outcomes: Observational follow-up of the trials of hypertension prevention (TOHP). British Medical Journal 2007;334(7599):885-8. PMID: 17449506. **KQ1E3e.**

Appendix C. Excluded Studies

68. Cooper JN, Columbus ML, Shields KJ, et al. Effects of an intensive behavioral weight loss intervention consisting of caloric restriction with or without physical activity on common carotid artery remodeling in severely obese adults. Metabolism: Clinical & Experimental 2012 Nov;61(11):1589-97. PMID: 22579053. **KQ1E6c, KQ2E6c, KQ3E6c, KQ4E6c.**

69. Costa B, Barrio F, Cabre JJ, et al. Delaying progression to type 2 diabetes among high-risk Spanish individuals is feasible in real-life primary healthcare settings using intensive lifestyle intervention. Diabetologia 2012 May;55(5):1319-28. PMID: 22322921. **KQ1E6a, KQ2E6a, KQ3E6a, KQ4E6a.**

70. Couper MP, Alexander GL, Zhang N, et al. Engagement and retention: measuring breadth and depth of participant use of an online intervention. Journal of Medical Internet Research 2010;12(4):e52. PMID: 21087922. **KQ3E3e.**

71. Craigie AM, Barton KL, Macleod M, et al. A feasibility study of a personalised lifestyle programme (HealthForce) for individuals who have participated in cardiovascular risk screening. Preventive Medicine: An International Journal Devoted to Practice and Theory 2011;52(5):387-9. PMID: 21419792. **KQ2E6b, KQ3E6b.**

72. Critchley CR, Hardie EA, Moore SM. Examining the psychological pathways to behavior change in a group-based lifestyle program to prevent type 2 diabetes. Diabetes Care 2012 Apr;35(4):699-705. PMID: 22338102. **KQ1E4.**

73. Crowe FL, Key TJ, Appleby PN, et al. Dietary fibre intake and ischaemic heart disease mortality: the European Prospective Investigation into Cancer and Nutrition-Heart study. European Journal of Clinical Nutrition 2012 Aug;66(8):950-6. PMID: 22617277. **KQ1E6a, KQ2E6a, KQ3E6a, KQ4E6a.**

74. Curtis PJ, Adamson AJ, Mathers JC. Effects on nutrient intake of a family-based intervention to promote increased consumption of low-fat starchy foods through education, cooking skills and personalised goal setting: the Family Food and Health Project. British Journal of Nutrition 2012 Jun;107(12):1833-44. PMID: 22017999. **KQ1E3e, KQ2E3e, KQ3E3e, KQ4E3e.**

75. Dale KS, Mann JI, McAuley KA, et al. Sustainability of lifestyle changes following an intensive lifestyle intervention in insulin resistant adults: Follow-up at 2-years. Asia Pacific Journal of Clinical Nutrition 2009;18(1):114-20. PMID: 19329404. **KQ2E5, KQ3E5.**

76. Dansinger ML, Gleason JA, Griffith JL, et al. Comparison of the Atkins, Ornish, Weight Watchers, and Zone diets for weight loss and heart disease risk reduction: a randomized trial. JAMA 2005 Jan 5;293(1):43-53. PMID: 293/1/43 [pii];10.1001/jama.293.1.43 [doi]. **KQ1E6c, KQ2E6c, KQ3E6c, KQ4E6c.**

77. Dapp U, Anders JAM, von Renteln-Kruse W, et al. A randomized trial of effects of health risk appraisal combined with group sessions or home visits on preventive behaviors in older adults. The Journals of Gerontology: Series A: Biological Sciences and Medical Sciences 2011;66A(5):591-8. PMID: 21350242. **KQ3E3e.**

78. Darker CD, French DP, Eves FF, et al. An intervention to promote walking amongst the general population based on an 'extended' theory of planned behaviour: a waiting list randomised controlled trial. Psychology & Health 2010 Jan;25(1):71-88. PMID: 20391208. **KQ3E3e.**

79. Davey SG, Bracha Y, Svendsen KH, et al. Incidence of type 2 diabetes in the randomized multiple risk factor intervention trial. Ann Intern Med 2005 Mar 1;142(5):313-22. PMID: 15738450. **KQ1E8, KQ2E8, KQ3E8, KQ4E8.**

80. Davis BR, Oberman A, Blaufox MD, et al. Lack of effectiveness of a low-sodium/high-potassium diet in reducing antihypertensive medication requirements in overweight persons with mild hypertension. TAIM Research Group. Trial of Antihypertensive Interventions and Management. Am J Hypertens 1994 Oct;7(10 Pt 1):926-32. PMID: 7826557. **KQ1E1, KQ2E1, KQ3E1, KQ4E1.**

81. De CK, Spittaels H, Cardon G, et al. Web-based, computer-tailored, pedometer-based physical activity advice: development, dissemination through general practice, acceptability, and preliminary efficacy in a randomized controlled trial. Journal of Medical Internet Research 2012;14(2):e53. PMID: 22532102. **KQ1E3e, KQ2E3e, KQ3E3e, KQ4E3e.**

82. Delgadillo AT, Grossman M, Santoyo-Olsson J, et al. Description of an academic community partnership lifestyle program for lower income minority adults at risk for diabetes. Diabetes Educator 2010 Jul;36(4):640-50. PMID: 20576836. **KQ1E4, KQ2E4, KQ3E4, KQ4E4.**

83. Delichatsios HK, Friedman RH, Glanz K, et al. Randomized trial of a "talking computer" to improve adults' eating habits. American journal of health promotion : AJHP 2001;15(4):215-24. PMID: 11349340. **KQ1E3e, KQ2E3e, KQ3E3e, KQ4E3e.**

84. Dennison CR, Post WS, Kim MT, et al. Underserved urban african american men: hypertension trial outcomes and mortality during 5 years
1. Am J Hypertens 2007 Feb;20(2):164-71. PMID:

Appendix C. Excluded Studies

17261462. **KQ1E1a, KQ2E1a, KQ3E1a, KQ4E1a.**

85. Diaz-Lopez A, Bullo M, Martinez-Gonzalez MA, et al. Effects of Mediterranean diets on kidney function: a report from the PREDIMED trial. American Journal of Kidney Diseases 2012 Sep;60(3):380-9. PMID: 22541738. **KQ1E3a, KQ2E3a, KQ3E3a, KQ4E3a.**

86. Djuric Z, Vanloon G, Radakovich K, et al. Design of a Mediterranean exchange list diet implemented by telephone counseling. Journal of the American Dietetic Association 2008;108(12):2059-65. PMID: 19027409. **KQ1E3e, KQ2E3e, KQ3E3e, KQ4E3e.**

87. Djuric Z, Ellsworth JS, Ren J, et al. A randomized feasibility trial of brief telephone counseling to increase fruit and vegetable intakes. Prev Med 2010 May;50(5-6):265-71. PMID: 20226809. **KQ2E6b, kQ3E6b.**

88. Dubbert PM, Cushman WC, Meydrech EF, et al. Effects of dietary instruction and sodium excretion feedback in hypertension clinic patients. Behav Ther 1995;26(4):721-32. PMID: None. **KQ1E6b, KQ2E6b, KQ3E6b, KQ4E6b.**

89. Dubbert PM, Cooper KM, Kirchner KA, et al. Effects of nurse counseling on walking for exercise in elderly primary care patients. The journals of gerontology Series A, Biological sciences and medical sciences 2002;57(11):M733-M740. PMID: 12403802. **KQ2E4, KQ3E6c.**

90. Duncan MJ, Vandelanotte C, Rosenkranz RR, et al. Effectiveness of a website and mobile phone based physical activity and nutrition intervention for middle-aged males: trial protocol and baseline findings of the ManUp Study. BMC Public Health 2012;12:656. PMID: 22894747. **KQ1E4, KQ2E4, KQ3E4, KQ4E4.**

91. Dutton GR, Napolitano MA, Whiteley JA, et al. Is physical activity a gateway behavior for diet? Findings from a physical activity trial. Prev Med 2008;46(3):216-21. PMID: 18234327. **KQ1E3e, KQ2E3e, KQ3E3e, KQ4E3e.**

92. Eakin EG, Bull SS, Riley KM, et al. Resources for health: a primary-care-based diet and physical activity intervention targeting urban Latinos with multiple chronic conditions. Health psychology : official journal of the Division of Health Psychology, American Psychological Association 2007;26(4):392-400. PMID: 17605558. **KQ1E3e, KQ2E3e, KQ3E3e, KQ4E3e.**

93. Elley CR, Garrett S, Rose SB, et al. Cost-effectiveness of exercise on prescription with telephone support among women in general practice over 2 years. British Journal of Sports Medicine 2011 Dec;45(15):1223-9. PMID: 21081641. **KQ1E3e, KQ2E3e, KQ3E3e, KQ4E3e.**

94. Ellingsen I, Hjermann I, Abdelnoor M, et al. Dietary and antismoking advice and ischemic heart disease mortality in men with normal or high fasting triacylglycerol concentrations: a 23-y follow-up study. The American journal of clinical nutrition 2003;78(5):935-40. PMID: 14594779. **KQ1E8, KQ2E8, KQ3E8.**

95. Ellingsen I, Hjerkinn EM, Arnesen H, et al. Follow-up of diet and cardiovascular risk factors 20 years after cessation of intervention in the Oslo Diet and Antismoking Study. European Journal of Clinical Nutrition 2006 Mar;60(3):378-85. PMID: 16306931. **KQ1E8, KQ2E8, KQ3E8, KQ4E8.**

96. Endevelt R, Lemberger J, Bregman J, et al. Intensive dietary intervention by a dietitian as a case manager among community dwelling older adults: the EDIT study. Journal of Nutrition, Health & Aging 2011 Aug;15(8):624-30. PMID: 21968856. **KQ1E3e, KQ2E3e, KQ3E3e.**

97. Engberg S, Vistisen D, Lau C, et al. Progression to impaired glucose regulation and diabetes in the population-based Inter99 study. Diabetes Care 2009 Apr;32(4):606-11. PMID: 19114617. **KQ2E3e.**

98. Engberg S, Glumer C, Witte DR, et al. Differential relationship between physical activity and progression to diabetes by glucose tolerance status: the Inter99 Study. Diabetologia 2010 Jan;53(1):70-8. PMID: 19898830. **KQ2E4, KQ3E4.**

99. Eriksson MK, Franks PW, Eliasson M. A 3-year randomized trial of lifestyle intervention for cardiovascular risk reduction in the primary care setting: the Swedish Bjorknas study. PLoS ONE [Electronic Resource] 2009;4(4):e5195. PMID: 19365563. **KQ2E5, KQ3E5, KQ4E5.**

100. Estabrooks PA, Smith-Ray RL, Almeida FA, et al. Move More: Translating an efficacious group dynamics physical activity intervention into effective clinical practice. International Journal of Sport and Exercise Psychology 2011;9(1):4-18. PMID: None. **KQ4E3e.**

101. Evans AT, Rogers LQ, Peden JG, Jr., et al. Teaching dietary counseling skills to residents: patient and physician outcomes. The CADRE Study Group. Am J Prev Med 1996 Jul;12(4):259-65. PMID: 8874689. **KQ1E3a, KQ2E3a, KQ3E3a, KQ4E3a.**

102. Fahrenwald NL, Atwood JR, Walker SN, et al. A randomized pilot test of "Moms on the Move": a physical activity intervention for WIC mothers. Annals of behavioral medicine : a publication of the Society of Behavioral Medicine 2004;27(2):82-90. PMID: 15026292. **KQ3E3e.**

Appendix C. Excluded Studies

103. Fappa E, Yannakoulia M, Ioannidou M, et al. Telephone counseling intervention improves dietary habits and metabolic parameters of patients with the metabolic syndrome: a randomized controlled trial. The Review of Diabetic Studies 2012;9(1):36-45. PMID: 22972443. **KQ1E4, KQ2E7d, KQ3E7d, KQ4E4.**

104. Fappa E, Yannakoulia M, Skoumas Y, et al. Promoting only the consumption of healthy foods may be an alternative stategy for treating patients with the metabolic syndrome. Metabolism: Clinical & Experimental 2012 Oct;61(10):1361-9. PMID: 22503163. **KQ1E4, K12E7d, KQ3E7d, KQ4E4.**

105. Ferrara AL, Pacioni D, Di F, V, et al. Lifestyle educational program strongly increases compliance to nonpharmacologic intervention in hypertensive patients: a 2-year follow-up study. Journal of Clinical Hypertension 2012 Nov;14(11):767-72. PMID: 23126348. **KQ2E6c, KQ3E6c.**

106. Ferrer RL, Mody-Bailey P, Jaen CR, et al. A medical assistant-based program to promote healthy behaviors in primary care. Annals of Family Medicine 2009 Nov;7(6):504-12. PMID: 19901309. **KQ2E3e, KQ3E3e.**

107. Fitzsimons CF, Baker G, Gray SR, et al. Does physical activity counselling enhance the effects of a pedometer-based intervention over the long-term: 12-month findings from the Walking for Wellbeing in the west study. BMC Public Health 2012;12:206. PMID: 22429600. **KQ1E3e, KQ2E3e, KQ3E3e, KQ4E3e.**

108. Foy CG, Vitolins MZ, Case LD, et al. Incorporating prosocial behavior to promote physical activity in older adults: Rationale and design of the Program for Active Aging and Community Engagement (PACE). Contemporary Clinical Trials 2013 Sep;36(1):284-97. PMID: 23876672. **KQ3E3e.**

109. Francis SL, Taylor ML. A social marketing theory-based diet-education program for women ages 54 to 83 years improved dietary status. Journal of the American Dietetic Association 2009 Dec;109(12):2052-6. PMID: 19942023. **KQ3E3e.**

110. Francis SL, Taylor ML, Haldeman LM. Nutrition education improves morale and self-efficacy for middle-aged and older women. [References]. Journal of Nutrition for the Elderly 2009 Jul;28(3):272-86. PMID: 21184370. **KQ2E3e, KQ3E3e.**

111. Gabriel KK, Conroy MB, Schmid KK, et al. The impact of weight and fat mass loss and increased physical activity on physical function in overweight, postmenopausal women: results from the Women on the Move Through Activity and Nutrition study. Menopause 2011 Jul;18(7):759-65. PMID: 21705864. **KQ1E3e, KQ2E3e, KQ3E3e, KQ4E3e.**

112. Garcia-Ortiz L, Grandes G, Sanchez-Perez A, et al. Effect on cardiovascular risk of an intervention by family physicians to promote physical exercise among sedentary individuals. Revista Espanola de Cardiologia 2010 Nov;63(11):1244-52. PMID: 21070720. **KQ2E3e.**

113. García OL, Grandes G, Sánchez PA, et al. Effect on cardiovascular risk of an intervention by family physicians to promote physical exercise among sedentary individuals. Revista española de cardiología 2010;63:1244-52. PMID: None. **KQ2E3e.**

114. Geleijnse JM, Witteman JC, Bak AA, et al. Long-term moderate sodium restriction does not adversely affect the serum HDL/total cholesterol ratio. J Hum Hypertens 1995 Dec;9(12):975-9. PMID: 8746642. **KQ1E1a, KQ2E1a, KQ3E1a, KQ4E1a.**

115. Geller KS, Mendoza ID, Timbobolan J, et al. The decisional balance sheet to promote healthy behavior among ethnically diverse older adults. Public Health Nursing 2012 May;29(3):241-6. PMID: 22512425. **KQ1E6b, KQ2E6b, KQ3E6b, KQ4E6b.**

116. Gerber JB, Bloom PA, Ross JS. The physical activity contract--tailored to promote physical activity in a geriatric outpatient setting: a pilot study. Journal of the American Geriatrics Society 2010 Mar;58(3):604-6. PMID: 20398129. **KQ3E6b.**

117. Getchell WS, Svetkey LP, Appel LJ, et al. Summary of the Dietary Approaches to Stop Hypertension (DASH) Randomized Clinical Trial. Curr Treat Options Cardiovasc Med 1999 Dec;1(4):295-300. PMID: 11096495. **KQ1E4, KQ2E4, KQ3E4, KQ4E4.**

118. Gidlow CJ, Cochrane T, Davey R, et al. One-year cardiovascular risk and quality of life changes in participants of a health trainer service. Perspect Public Health 2013 May 8 PMID: 23656746. **KQ1E6a, KQ2E6a, KQ3E6a, KQ4E6a.**

119. Gillison F, Greaves C, Stathi A, et al. 'Waste the waist': The development of an intervention to promote changes in diet and physical activity for people with high cardiovascular risk. [References]. British Journal of Health Psychology 2012 May;17(2):327-45. PMID: 22107451. **KQ1E6a, KQ2E6a, KQ3E6a.**

120. Gine-Garriga M, Martin C, Martin C, et al. Referral from primary care to a physical activity programme: establishing long-term adherence? A randomized controlled trial. Rationale and study design. BMC Public Health 2009(9):31. PMID: 19161605. **KQ1E4, KQ2E4, KQ3E4, KQ4E4.**

Appendix C. Excluded Studies

121. Godin G, Belanger-Gravel A, Amireault S, et al. The effect of mere-measurement of cognitions on physical activity behavior: a randomized controlled trial among overweight and obese individuals. International Journal of Behavioral Nutrition & Physical Activity 2011;8:2. PMID: 21223565. **KQ3E3e.**

122. Goodrich DE, Larkin AR, Lowery JC, et al. Adverse events among high-risk participants in a home-based walking study: a descriptive study. International Journal of Behavioral Nutrition & Physical Activity 2007;4:20. PMID: 17521443. **KQ4E6c.**

123. Gorbach SL, Morrill-LaBrode A, Woods MN, et al. Changes in food patterns during a low-fat dietary intervention in women. J Am Diet Assoc 1990 Jun;90(6):802-9. PMID: 23455252. **KQ1E5, KQ2E5, KQ3E5, KQ4E5.**

124. Gorini G, Carreras G, Giordano L, et al. The Pap smear screening as an occasion for smoking cessation and physical activity counselling: effectiveness of the SPRINT randomized controlled trial. BMC Public Health 2012;12:740. PMID: 22950883. **KQ1E1a, KQ2E1a, KQ3E1a, KQ4E1a.**

125. Grandes G, Sanchez A, Sanchez-Pinilla RO, et al. Effectiveness of physical activity advice and prescription by physicians in routine primary care: a cluster randomized trial. Arch Intern Med 2009 Apr 13;169(7):694-701. PMID: 19364999. **KQ3E3e.**

126. Grandes G, Sanchez A, Montoya I, et al. Two-year longitudinal analysis of a cluster randomized trial of physical activity promotion by general practitioners. PLoS ONE [Electronic Resource] 2011;6(3):e18363. PMID: 21479243. **KQ3E3e.**

127. Granner ML, Liguori G, Kirkner GJ, et al. Health care provider counseling for physical activity among black and white South Carolinians. Journal of the South Carolina Medical Association 2001;97:338-41. PMID: 11534474. **KQ1E6a, KQ2E6a, KQ3E6a, KQ4E6a.**

128. Greaves CJ, Middlebrooke A, O'Loughlin L, et al. Motivational interviewing for modifying diabetes risk: a randomised controlled trial. The British journal of general practice : the journal of the Royal College of General Practitioners 2008;58(553):535-40. PMID: 18682011. **KQ3E3e.**

129. Green BB, McAfee T, Hindmarsh M, et al. Effectiveness of telephone support in increasing physical activity levels in primary care patients. Am J Prev Med 2002;22(3):177-83. PMID: 11897462. **KQ3E3e.**

130. Greenberger HM. Modifiers of the effectiveness of a diet intervention in family members of cardiovascular disease patients. Dissertation Abstracts International: Section B: The Sciences and Engineering 2011(9-B) PMID: None. **KQ1E3e, KQ2E3e, KQ3E3e.**

131. Guillaumie L, Godin G, Manderscheid JC, et al. The impact of self-efficacy and implementation intentions-based interventions on fruit and vegetable intake among adults. Psychology & Health 2012;27(1):30-50. PMID: 21678169. **KQ1E6b, KQ2E6b, KQ3E6b, KQ4E6b.**

132. Hansen AW, Gronbaek M, Helge JW, et al. Effect of a Web-based intervention to promote physical activity and improve health among physically inactive adults: a population-based randomized controlled trial. Journal of Medical Internet Research 2012;14(5):e145. PMID: 23111127. **KQ1E3e, KQ2E3e, KQ3E3e, KQ4E3e.**

133. Hardcastle S, Taylor A, Bailey M, et al. A randomised controlled trial on the effectiveness of a primary health care based counselling intervention on physical activity, diet and CHD risk factors. Patient Education and Counseling 2008;70(1):31-9. PMID: 17997263. **KQ1E4, KQ4E4.**

134. Hardeman W, Kinmonth AL, Michie S, et al. Impact of a physical activity intervention program on cognitive predictors of behaviour among adults at risk of Type 2 diabetes (ProActive randomised controlled trial). International Journal of Behavioral Nutrition & Physical Activity 2009;6:16. PMID: 19292926. **KQ3E3e.**

135. Hardeman W, Kinmonth AL, Michie S, et al. Theory of planned behaviour cognitions do not predict self-reported or objective physical activity levels or change in the ProActive trial. British Journal of Health Psychology 2011 Feb;16(Pt:1):1-50. PMID: 21226788. **KQ3E3e.**

136. Harrison RA, Roberts C, Elton PJ. Does primary care referral to an exercise programme increase physical activity one year later? A randomized controlled trial. Journal of Public Health 2005 Mar;27(1):25-32. PMID: 15564275. **KQ3E3a.**

137. Hatzitolios AI, Athyros VG, Karagiannis A, et al. Implementation of strategy for the management of overt dyslipidemia: the IMPROVE-dyslipidemia study. International Journal of Cardiology 2009 May 29;134(3):322-9. PMID: 19268376. **KQ2E6a.**

138. Helland-Kigen KM, Raberg Kjollesdal MK, Hjellset VT, et al. Maintenance of changes in food intake and motivation for healthy eating among Norwegian-Pakistani women participating in a culturally adapted intervention. Public Health Nutrition 2013 Jan;16(1):113-22. PMID: 22781507. **KQ3E3e.**

139. Hellenius ML, de FU, Berglund B, et al. Diet and exercise are equally effective in reducing risk for cardiovascular disease. Results of a randomized

Appendix C. Excluded Studies

controlled study in men with slightly to moderately raised cardiovascular risk factors. Atherosclerosis 1993 Oct;103(1):81-91. PMID: 8280188. **KQ1E3e, KQ2E3e, KQ3E3e, KQ4E3e.**

140. Henkin Y, Shai I, Zuk R, et al. Dietary treatment of hypercholesterolemia: do dietitians do it better? A randomized, controlled trial. Am J Med 2000 Nov;109(7):549-55. PMID: 11063956. **KQ2E6c.**

141. Herman C, Thompson J, Wolfe V, et al. Six-month results from a healthy lifestyles diabetes primary prevention program among urban Native American women. American Public Health Association 134th.Annual Meeting & Exposition; Nov 4 2006; Boston,MA. 2006. PMID: None. **KQ2E3e.**

142. Hertogh EM, Vergouwe Y, Schuit AJ, et al. Behavioral changes after a 1-yr exercise program and predictors of maintenance. Medicine & Science in Sports & Exercise 2010 May;42(5):886-92. PMID: 19996989. **KQ1E5, KQ2E5, KQ3E5, KQ4E5.**

143. Hillier FC, Batterham AM, Nixon CA, et al. A community-based health promotion intervention using brief negotiation techniques and a pledge on dietary intake, physical activity levels and weight outcomes: lessons learnt from an exploratory trial. Public Health Nutrition 2012 Aug;15(8):1446-55. PMID: 22122753. **KQ1E3e, KQ2E3e, KQ3E3e, KQ4E3e.**

144. Hillsdon M, Thorogood M, White I, et al. Advising people to take more exercise is ineffective: a randomized controlled trial of physical activity promotion in primary care. International Journal of Epidemiology 2002;31(4):808-15. PMID: 12177026. **KQ2E4, KQ3E4.**

145. Hind D, Scott EJ, Copeland R, et al. A randomised controlled trial and cost-effectiveness evaluation of "booster" interventions to sustain increases in physical activity in middle-aged adults in deprived urban neighbourhoods. BMC Public Health 2010;10:3. PMID: 20047672. **KQ1E3e, KQ2E3e, KQ3E3e, KQ4E3e.**

146. Hirvensalo M, Heikkinen E, Lintunen T, et al. The effect of advice by health care professionals on increasing physical activity of older people. Scandinavian Journal of Medicine Science & Sports 2003;13:231-6. PMID: 12859605. **KQ1E6a, KQ2E6a, KQ3E6a, KQ4E4.**

147. Holme I, Hostmark AT, Anderssen SA. ApoB but not LDL-cholesterol is reduced by exercise training in overweight healthy men. Results from the 1-year randomized Oslo Diet and Exercise Study. Journal of Internal Medicine 2007 Aug;262(2):235-43. PMID: 17645591. **KQ1E4, KQ2E4, KQ3E4, KQ4E4.**

148. Horner-Johnson W, Drum CE, Abdullah N. A randomized trial of a health promotion intervention for adults withdisabilities. Disability & Health Journal 2011 Oct;4(4):254-61. PMID: 22014673. **KQ3E3e.**

149. Hosper K, Deutekom M, Stronks K. The effectiveness of "Exercise on Prescription" in stimulating physical activity among women in ethnic minority groups in the Netherlands: protocol for a randomized controlled trial. BMC Public Health 2008;8:406. PMID: 19077190. **KQ1E4, KQ2E4, KQ3E4, KQ4E4.**

150. Howard BV, Van HL, Hsia J, et al. Low-fat dietary pattern and risk of cardiovascular disease: the Women's Health Initiative Randomized Controlled Dietary Modification Trial. JAMA 2006 Feb 8;295(6):655-66. PMID: 16467234. **KQ1E3e, KQ2E3e, KQ3E3e.**

151. Howard BV, Curb JD, Eaton CB, et al. Low-fat dietary pattern and lipoprotein risk factors: the Women's Health Initiative Dietary Modification Trial
1. Am J Clin Nutr 2010 Apr;91(4):860-74. PMID: 20164311. **KQ1E3e, KQ2E3e, KQ3E3e.**

152. Hughes SL, Seymour RB, Campbell RT, et al. Best-practice physical activity programs for older adults: findings from the national impact study. American Journal of Public Health 2009 Feb;99(2):362-8. PMID: 19059858. **KQ1E5, KQ2E5, KQ3E5, KQ4E5.**

153. Hyman DJ, Herd JA, Ho KS, et al. Maintenance of cholesterol reduction using automated telephone calls. Am J Prev Med 1996 Mar;12(2):129-33. PMID: 8777066. **KQ1E6c, KQ2E6c, KQ3E6c, KQ4E6c.**

154. Hypertension Prevention Trial Research Group. The Hypertension Prevention Trial: three-year effects of dietary changes on blood pressure. Arch Intern Med 1990 Jan;150(1):153-62. PMID: 2404477. **KQ1E3e, KQ2E3e, KQ3E3e, KQ4E3e.**

155. Inoue S, Odagiri Y, Wakui S, et al. Randomized controlled trial to evaluate the effect of a physical activity intervention program based on behavioral medicine. Zasshi/Tokyo Ika Daigaku 2003;61(2):154-65. PMID: 15479705. **KQ3E5.**

156. Irvine AB, Gelatt VA, Seeley JR, et al. Web-based intervention to promote physical activity by sedentary older adults: randomized controlled trial. Journal of Medical Internet Research 2013;15(2):e19. PMID: 23470322. **KQ2E3e, KQ3E3e.**

157. Jackson J, Mandel D, Blanchard J, et al. Confronting challenges in intervention research with ethnically diverse older adults: The USC Well Elderly II Trial. Clinical Trials 2009;6(1):90-101. PMID: 19254939. **KQ1E4, KQ2E4, KQ3E4, KQ4E4.**

Appendix C. Excluded Studies

158. Jacobs AD, Ammerman AS, Ennett ST, et al. Effects of a tailored follow-up intervention on health behaviors, beliefs, and attitudes. Journal of Women's Health 2004 Jun;13(5):557-68. PMID: 15257847. **KQ1E7e, KQ2E7e, KQ3E7e.**

159. Jacobs N, Evers S, Ament A, et al. Cost-utility of a cardiovascular prevention program in highly educated adults: intermediate results of a randomized controlled trial. International Journal of Technology Assessment in Health Care 2010 Jan;26(1):11-9. PMID: 20059776. **KQ1E3e, KQ2E3e, KQ3E3e, KQ4E3e.**

160. Jacobs N, De B, I, Thijs H, et al. Effect of a cardiovascular prevention program on health behavior and BMI in highly educated adults: a randomized controlled trial. Patient Education & Counseling 2011 Oct;85(1):122-6. PMID: 20888728. **KQ2E3e, KQ3E3e.**

161. Jacobs N, Clays E, De BD, et al. Effect of a tailored behavior change program on a composite lifestyle change score: a randomized controlled trial. Health Education Research 2011 Oct;26(5):886-95. PMID: 21712501. **KQ2E3e, KQ3E3e.**

162. Jantchou P, Morois S, Clavel-Chapelon F, et al. Animal protein intake and risk of inflammatory bowel disease: The E3N prospective study. American Journal of Gastroenterology 2010 Oct;105(10):2195-201. PMID: 20461067. **KQ4E3e.**

163. Jehn ML, Patt MR, Appel LJ, et al. One year follow-up of overweight and obese hypertensive adults following intensive lifestyle therapy. J Hum Nutr Diet 2006 Oct;19(5):349-54. PMID: 16961681. **KQ1E1b, KQ2E1b, KQ3E1b, KQ4E1b.**

164. Jiang Y, Maddison R, McRobbie H, et al. Can exercise enhance smoking cessation outcomes? A pragmatic randomized controlled trial (fit2quit Study). Clinical Trials 2012;9(4):484-5. PMID: None. **KQ3E5.**

165. Jimmy G, Martin BW. Implementation and effectiveness of a primary care based physical activity counselling scheme. Patient Education and Counseling 2005;56(3):323-31. PMID: 15721975. **KQ1E3e, KQ2E3e, KQ3E3e.**

166. Johansen KS, Bjorge B, Hjellset VT, et al. Changes in food habits and motivation for healthy eating among Pakistani women living in Norway: results from the InnvaDiab-DEPLAN study. Public Health Nutrition 2010 Jun;13(6):858-67. PMID: 19941691. **KQ3E3e.**

167. Jolly K, Duda JL, Daley A, et al. Evaluation of a standard provision versus an autonomy promotive exercise referral programme: rationale and study design. BMC Public Health 2009;9:176. PMID: 19505293. **KQ1E4, KQ2E4, KQ3E4, KQ4E4.**

168. Jula A, Ronnemaa T, Rastas M, et al. Long-term nopharmacological treatment for mild to moderate hypertension. J Intern Med 1990 Jun;227(6):413-21. PMID: 2191071. **KQ1E2b, KQ2E2b, KQ3E2b, KQ4E2b.**

169. Jula AM, Karanko HM. Effects on left ventricular hypertrophy of long-term nonpharmacological treatment with sodium restriction in mild-to-moderate essential hypertension. Circulation 1994 Mar;89(3):1023-31. PMID: 8124787. **KQ1E7a, KQ2E7a, KQ3E7a, KQ4E7a.**

170. Kallings LV. Physical activity on prescription: studies on physical activity level, adherence, and cardiovascular risk factors. Stockholm, Sweden: Karolinska Institutet; 2008. PMID: None. **KQ1E3e, KQ2E3e, KQ3E3e, KQ4E3e.**

171. Kawano M, Shono N, Yoshimura T, et al. Improved cardio-respiratory fitness correlates with changes in the number and size of small dense LDL: randomized controlled trial with exercise training and dietary instruction. Internal Medicine 2009;48(1):25-32. PMID: 19122353. **KQ2E5.**

172. Kegler MC, Alcantara I, Veluswamy JK, et al. Results from an intervention to improve rural home food and physical activity environments. Progress in Community Health Partnerships 2012;6(3):265-77. PMID: 22982840. **KQ2E3e, KQ3E3e.**

173. Kelders SM, Van Gemert-Pijnen JE, Werkman A, et al. Effectiveness of a Web-based intervention aimed at healthy dietary and physical activity behavior: a randomized controlled trial about users and usage. Journal of Medical Internet Research 2011;13(2):e32. PMID: 21493191. **KQ3E3e.**

174. Kemmler W, von SS, Engelke K, et al. Exercise decreases the risk of metabolic syndrome in elderly females. Medicine & Science in Sports & Exercise 2009 Feb;41(2):297-305. PMID: 19127197. **KQ2E5.**

175. Kennedy MF, Meeuwisse WH. Exercise counselling by family physicians in Canada. Prev Med 2003;37:226-32. PMID: 12914828. **KQ1E6a, KQ2E6a, KQ3E6a.**

176. Kerr DA, Pollard CM, Howat P, et al. Connecting Health and Technology (CHAT): protocol of a randomized controlled trial to improve nutrition behaviours using mobile devices and tailored text messaging in young adults. BMC Public Health 2012;12:477. PMID: 22726532. **KQ1E4, KQ2E4, KQ3E4, KQ4E4.**

177. Ketola E, Makela M, Klockars M. Individualised multifactorial lifestyle intervention trial for high-risk cardiovascular patients in primary care. Br J Gen Pract 2001 Apr;51(465):291-4. PMID: 11458482. **KQ2E3a, KQ3E3a.**

Appendix C. Excluded Studies

178. Khare MM, Huber R, Carpenter RA, et al. A lifestyle approach to reducing cardiovascular risk factors in underserved women: design and methods of the Illinois WISEWOMAN Program. Journal of Women's Health 2009;18(3):409-19. PMID: 19821324. **KQ1E3e, KQ2E3e, KQ3E3e.**

179. Khare MM, Carpenter RA, Huber R, et al. Lifestyle intervention and cardiovascular risk reduction in the Illinois WISEWOMAN Program. Journal of Women's Health 2012;21(3):294-301. PMID: 22136298. **KQ1E3e, KQ2E3e, KQ3E3e.**

180. Kim BH, Newton RA, Sachs ML, et al. The effect of guided relaxation and exercise imagery on self-reported leisure-time exercise behaviors in older adults. Journal of Aging & Physical Activity 2011 Apr;19(2):137-46. PMID: 21558568. **KQ3E6b.**

181. Kim C, Draska M, Hess ML, et al. A web-based pedometer programme in women with a recent history of gestational diabetes. Diabetic Medicine 2012 Feb;29(2):278-83. PMID: 21838764. **KQ1E3e, KQ2E3e, KQ3E3e, KQ4E3e.**

182. Kim J, Bea W, Lee K, et al. Effect of the telephone-delivered nutrition education on dietary intake and biochemical parameters in subjects with metabolic syndrome. Clinical Nutrition Research 2013 Jul;2(2):115-24. PMID: 23908978. **KQ2E6b, KQ3E6b.**

183. Kim Y, Pike J, Adams H, et al. Telephone intervention promoting weight-related health behaviors. Prev Med 2010 Mar;50(3):112-7. PMID: 20006642. **KQ3E3e.**

184. King AC, Castro CM, Buman MP, et al. Behavioral Impacts of Sequentially versus Simultaneously Delivered Dietary Plus Physical Activity Interventions: the CALM Trial. Annals of Behavioral Medicine 2013 Oct;46(2):157-68. **KQ3E3e.**

185. Kinmonth AL, Wareham NJ, Hardeman W, et al. Efficacy of a theory-based behavioural intervention to increase physical activity in an at-risk group in primary care (ProActive UK): a randomised trial. Lancet 2008;371(9606):41-8. PMID: 18177774. **KQ3E3e.**

186. Kirwan M, Duncan MJ, Vandelanotte C, et al. Using smartphone technology to monitor physical activity in the 10,000 Steps program: a matched case-control trial. Journal of Medical Internet Research 2012;14(2):e55. PMID: 22522112. **KQ3E6a.**

187. Kitaoka K, Nagaoka J, Matsuoka T, et al. Dietary intervention with cooking instructions and self-monitoring of the diet in free-living hypertensive men. Clinical & Experimental Hypertension (New York) 2013;35(2):120-7. PMID: 22799766. **KQ2E6b, KQ3E6b.**

188. Kjelsberg MO, Cutler JA, Dolecek TA. Brief description of the Multiple Risk Factor Intervention Trial. Am J Clin Nutr 1997 Jan;65(1 Suppl):191S-5S. PMID: 8988937. **KQ1E8, KQ2E8, KQ3E8, KQ4E8.**

189. Knutsen SF, Knutsen R. The Tromso Survey: the Family Intervention study--the effect of intervention on some coronary risk factors and dietary habits, a 6-year follow-up. Prev Med 1991 Mar;20(2):197-212. PMID: 2057468. **KQ1E8, KQ2E8, KQ3E8, KQ4E8.**

190. Ko LK, Campbell MK, Lewis MA, et al. Information processes mediate the effect of a health communication intervention on fruit and vegetable consumption. Journal of Health Communication 2011 Mar;16(3):282-99. PMID: 21132593. **KQ3E3e.**

191. Koelewijn-van-Loon MS, Weijden T, Ronda G, et al. Improving lifestyle and risk perception through patient involvement in nurse-led cardiovascular risk management: a cluster-randomized controlled trial in primary care. Prev Med 2010;50(1-2):35-44. PMID: 19944713. **KQ2E6b, KQ3E6b.**

192. Koelewijn-van Loon MS, Eurlings JW, Winkens B, et al. Small but important errors in cardiovascular risk calculation by practice nurses: a cross-sectional study in randomised trial setting. Int J Nurs Stud 2011 Mar;48(3):285-91. PMID: 20439105. **KQ2E4, KQ3E4.**

193. Koizumi D, Rogers NL, Rogers ME, et al. Efficacy of an accelerometer-guided physical activity intervention in community-dwelling older women. Journal of Physical Activity & Health 2009 Jul;6(4):467-74. PMID: 19842461. **KQ1E6b, KQ2E6b, KQ3E6b, KQ4E6b.**

194. Kolt GS, Schofield GM, Kerse N, et al. Effect of telephone counseling on physical activity for low-active older people in primary care: a randomized, controlled trial. Journal of the American Geriatrics Society 2007;55(7):986-92. PMID: 17608869. **KQ3E3e.**

195. Koopman H, Spreeuwenberg C, Westerman RF, et al. Dietary treatment of patients with mild to moderate hypertension in a general practice: a pilot intervention study (2). Beyond three months. J Hum Hypertens 1990 Aug;4(4):372-4. PMID: 2258877. **KQ1E6b, KQ2E6b, KQ3E6b, KQ4E6b.**

196. Korhonen M, Kastarinen M, Uusitupa M, et al. Advice from primary care physicians and nurses may improve diet in people with hypertension. Evidence based Cardiovascular Medicine {EVID BASED CARDIOVASC MED} 2003;7:94-6. PMID: None. **KQ1E6a, KQ2E6a, KQ3E6a, KQ4E6a.**

Appendix C. Excluded Studies

197. Korhonen MH, Litmanen H, Rauramaa R, et al. Adherence to the salt restriction diet among people with mildly elevated blood pressure. Eur J Clin Nutr 1999 Nov;53(11):880-5. PMID: 10557001. **KQ1E1, KQ2E1, KQ3E1, KQ4E1.**

198. Kovelis D, Zabatiero J, Furlanetto KC, et al. Short-term effects of using pedometers to increase daily physical activity in smokers: a randomized trial. Respiratory Care 2012 Jul;57(7):1089-97. PMID: 22272985. **KQ3E6b.**

199. Kreausukon P, Gellert P, Lippke S, et al. Planning and self-efficacy can increase fruit and vegetable consumption: a randomized controlled trial. Journal of Behavioral Medicine 2012 Aug;35(4):443-51. PMID: 21822980. **KQ3E6b.**

200. Kuller LH, Simkin-Silverman LR, Wing RR, et al. Women's Healthy Lifestyle Project: A randomized clinical trial: results at 54 months. Circulation 2001;103(1):32-7. PMID: 11136682. **KQ3E3e.**

201. Kuller LH, Pettee Gabriel KK, Kinzel LS, et al. The Women on the Move Through Activity and Nutrition (WOMAN) study: final 48-month results. Obesity 2012 Mar;20(3):636-43. PMID: 21494228. **KQ2E3e, KQ3E3e.**

202. Kupka-Schutt L, Mitchell ME. Positive effect of a nutrition instruction model on the dietary behavior of a selected group of elderly. J Nutr Elder 1992;12(2):29-53. PMID: 1296987. **KQ3E3e.**

203. Laan EK, Kraaijenhagen RA, Peek N, et al. Effectiveness of a web-based health risk assessment with individually-tailored feedback on lifestyle behaviour: study protocol. BMC Public Health 2012;12:200. PMID: 22429308. **KQ1E4, KQ2E4, KQ3E4, KQ4E4.**

204. Lamb SE, Bartlett HP, Ashley A, et al. Can lay-led walking programmes increase physical activity in middle aged adults? A randomised controlled trial. Journal of Epidemiology and Community Health 2002;56(4):246-52. PMID: 11896130. **KQ2E3e, KQ3E3e.**

205. Lammes E, Rydwik E, Akner G. Effects of nutritional intervention and physical training on energy intake, resting metabolic rate and body composition in frail elderly. a randomised, controlled pilot study. Journal of Nutrition, Health & Aging 2012 Feb;16(2):162-7. PMID: 22323352. **KQ3E5.**

206. Langford HG, Davis BR, Blaufox D, et al. Effect of drug and diet treatment of mild hypertension on diastolic blood pressure. The TAIM Research Group. Hypertension 1991 Feb;17(2):210-7. PMID: 1671380. **KQ1E1, KQ2E1, KQ3E1, KQ4E1.**

207. Lee RE, Medina AV, Mama SK, et al. Health is Power: an ecological, theory-based health intervention for women of color. [Review]. Contemporary Clinical Trials 2011 Nov;32(6):916-23. PMID: 21782975. **KQ3E4.**

208. Leijon ME, Bendtsen P, Stahle A, et al. Factors associated with patients self-reported adherence to prescribed physical activity in routine primary health care. BMC Family Practice 2010;11:38. PMID: 20482851. **KQ1E3e, KQ2E3e, KQ3E3e, KQ4E3e.**

209. Lesley ML. Social problem solving training for African Americans: effects on dietary problem solving skill and DASH diet-related behavior change. Patient Education and Counseling 2007;65(1):137-46. PMID: 16950591. **KQ3E4.**

210. Lewis BA, Williams DM, Martinson BC, et al. Healthy for life: A randomized trial examining physical activity outcomes and psychosocial mediators. [References]. Annals of Behavioral Medicine 2013 Apr;Vol.45(2):203-12. PMID: 23229158. **KQ3E3e.**

211. Liao D, Asberry PJ, Shofer JB, et al. Improvement of BMI, body composition, and body fat distribution with lifestyle modification in Japanese Americans with impaired glucose tolerance. Diabetes Care 2002 Sep;25(9):1504-10. PMID: 12196418. **KQ2E5, KQ3E5.**

212. Lien LF, Brown AJ, Ard JD, et al. Effects of PREMIER lifestyle modifications on participants with and without the metabolic syndrome. Hypertension 2007;50(4):609-16. PMID: 17698724. **KQ1E4.**

213. Lim HJ, Choi YM, Choue R. Dietary intervention with emphasis on folate intake reduces serum lipids but not plasma homocysteine levels in hyperlipidemic patients. Nutrition Research 2008;28(11):767-74. PMID: 19083486. **KQ2E6b, KQ3E6b.**

214. Lindahl B, Nilsson TK, Borch-Johnsen K, et al. A randomized lifestyle intervention with 5-year follow-up in subjects with impaired glucose tolerance: pronounced short-term impact but long-term adherence problems.[Erratum appears in Scand J Public Health. 2009 Jun;37(4):443]. Scandinavian Journal of Public Health 2009 Jun;37(4):434-42. PMID: 19181821. **KQ2E5a, KQ3E5a, KQ4E5a.**

215. Lindholm LH, Ekbom T, Dash C, et al. The impact of health care advice given in primary care on cardiovascular risk. CELL Study Group. BMJ 1995 Apr 29;310(6987):1105-9. PMID: 7742677. **KQ1E4, KQ2E6c, KQ3E6c, KQ4E4.**

216. Lindholm LH, Ekbom T, Dash C, et al. Changes in cardiovascular risk factors by combined pharmacological and nonpharmacological strategies: the main results of the CELL Study. J Intern Med 1996 Jul;240(1):13-22. PMID: 8708586. **KQ1E4, KQ2E6c, KQ3E6c, KQ4E4.**

Appendix C. Excluded Studies

217. Lindström J, Peltonen M, Eriksson JG, et al. High-fibre, low-fat diet predicts long-term weight loss and decreased type 2 diabetes risk: the Finnish Diabetes Prevention Study. Diabetologia 2006;49(5):912-20. PMID: 16541277. **KQ2E6a, KQ3E6a.**
218. Lippke S, Schwarzer R, Ziegelmann JP, et al. Testing stage-specific effects of a stage-matched intervention: a randomized controlled trial targeting physical exercise and its predictors. Health Education & Behavior 2010 Aug;37(4):533-46. PMID: 20547760. **KQ1E6b, KQ2E6b, KQ3E6b, KQ4E6b.**
219. Little P, Dorward M, Gralton S, et al. A randomised controlled trial of three pragmatic approaches to initiate increased physical activity in sedentary patients with risk factors for cardiovascular disease. Br J Gen Pract 2004 Mar;54(500):189-95. PMID: 15006124. **KQ2E6b, KQ3E6b, KQ4E6b.**
220. Luszczynska A, Schwarzer R, Lippke S, et al. Self-efficacy as a moderator of the planning-behaviour relationship in interventions designed to promote physical activity. Psychology & Health 2011 Feb;26(2):151-66. PMID: 21318927. **KQ3E3a.**
221. Ma J, King AC, Wilson SR, et al. Evaluation of lifestyle interventions to treat elevated cardiometabolic risk in primary care (E-LITE): a randomized controlled trial. BMC Family Practice 2009;10:71. PMID: 19909549. **KQ2E4, KQ3E4.**
222. Macmillan F, Fitzsimons C, Black K, et al. Evaluation of lifestyle interventions to treat elevated cardiometabolic risk in primary care (E-LITE): a randomized controlled trial. BMC Public Health 2011;11:120. PMID: 21333020. **KQ1E4, KQ2E4, KQ3E4, KQ4E4.**
223. Maindal HT, Toft U, Lauritzen T, et al. Three-year effects on dietary quality of health education: a randomized controlled trial of people with screen-detected dysglycaemia (The ADDITION study, Denmark). Eur J Public Health 2012 Jun 13;23(3):393-8. PMID: 23132875. **KQ1E3a, KQ2E3a, KQ3E3a, KQ4E3a.**
224. Malin SK, Gerber R, Chipkin SR, et al. Independent and combined effects of exercise training and metformin on insulin sensitivity in individuals with prediabetes. Diabetes Care 2012 Jan;35(1):131-6. PMID: 22040838. **KQ2E5.**
225. Mancuso CA, Choi TN, Westermann H, et al. Increasing physical activity in patients with asthma through positive affect and self-affirmation: a randomized trial. Arch Intern Med 2012 Feb 27;172(4):337-43. PMID: 22269593. **KQ4E3e.**
226. Martinson BC, Sherwood NE, Crain AL, et al. Maintaining physical activity among older adults: 24-month outcomes of the Keep Active Minnesota randomized controlled trial. Prev Med 2010 Jul;51(1):37-44. PMID: 20382179. **KQ3E3e.**
227. Mascola AJ, Yiaslas TA, Meir RL, et al. Framing physical activity as a distinct and uniquely valuable behavior independent of weight management: A pilot randomized controlled trial from overweight and obese sedentary persons. [References]. Eating and Weight Disorders 2009 Jun;14(2-3):e148-e152. PMID: 19934630. **KQ3E6b.**
228. Mason C, Foster-Schubert KE, Imayama I, et al. Dietary weight loss and exercise effects on insulin resistance in postmenopausal women. Am J Prev Med 2011 Oct;41(4):366-75. PMID: 21961463. **KQ2E5.**
229. Mayer JA, Jermanovich A, Wright BL, et al. Changes in health behaviors of older adults: the San Diego Medicare Preventive Health Project. Prev Med 1994 Mar;23(2):127-33. PMID: 8047517. **KQ1E3e, KQ2E3e, KQ3E3e, KQ4E3e.**
230. Márquez-Celedonio FG, Téxon FO, Chávez NA, et al. [Clinical effect of lifestyle modification on cardiovascular risk in prehypertensives: PREHIPER I study]. Revista española de cardiología 2009;62(1):86-90. PMID: 19150019. **KQ2E2a.**
231. McAuley KA, Williams SM, Mann JI, et al. Intensive lifestyle changes are necessary to improve insulin sensitivity: a randomized controlled trial. Diabetes Care 2002 Mar;25(3):445-52. PMID: 11874928. **KQ2E5, KQ3E5, KQ4E5.**
232. McClure JB, Catz SL, Ludman EJ, et al. Feasibility and acceptability of a multiple risk factor intervention: the Step Up randomized pilot trial. BMC Public Health 2011;11:167. PMID: 21414216. **KQ3E6b.**
233. McGuire HL, Svetkey LP, Harsha DW, et al. Comprehensive lifestyle modification and blood pressure control: a review of the PREMIER trial. Journal of Clinical Hypertension 2004;6(7):383-90. PMID: 15249794. **KQ1E4, KQ2E4, KQ3E4, KQ4E4.**
234. McMurdo ME, Sugden J, Argo I, et al. Do pedometers increase physical activity in sedentary older women? A randomized controlled trial. Journal of the American Geriatrics Society 2010 Nov;58(11):2099-106. PMID: 21054290. **KQ3E3e.**
235. Meland E, Laerum E, Ulvik RJ. Effectiveness of two preventive interventions for coronary heart disease in primary care. Scand J Prim Health Care 1997 Mar;15(1):57-64. PMID: 9101627. **KQ1E6c, KQ2E6c, KQ3E6c, KQ4E6c.**
236. Merom D, Bauman A, Phongsavan P, et al. Can a motivational intervention overcome an unsupportive environment for walking--findings

Appendix C. Excluded Studies

from the Step-by-Step Study. Annals of Behavioral Medicine 2009 Oct;38(2):137-46. PMID: 19806414. **KQ1E4, KQ2E4, KQ3E4, KQ4E4.**

237. Merriam PA, Persuitte G, Olendzki BC, et al. Dietary intervention targeting increased fiber consumption for metabolic syndrome. Journal of the Academy of Nutrition & Dietetics 2012 May;112(5):621-3. PMID: 22709766. **KQ2E4, KQ3E4.**

238. Miettinen TA, Huttunen JK, Naukkarinen V, et al. Multifactorial primary prevention of cardiovascular diseases in middle-aged men. Risk factor changes, incidence, and mortality. JAMA 1985 Oct 18;254(15):2097-102. PMID: 4046137. **KQ1E8, KQ2E8, KQ3E8, KQ4E8.**

239. Milkereit J, Graves JS. Follow-up dietary counseling benefits attainment of intake goals for total fat, saturated fat, and fiber. J Am Diet Assoc 1992 May;92(5):603-5. PMID: 1315350. **KQ1E7e, KQ2E7e, KQ3E7e, KQ4E7e.**

240. Miner JT. Enabling exercise prescription: Developing a comprehensive intervention strategy for exercise counseling and prescription in Family Medicine. Dissertation Abstracts International Section A: Humanities and Social Sciences 2012;72(12-A):4438. PMID: None. **KQ1E4, KQ2E4, KQ3E4, KQ4E4.**

241. Miura S, Yamaguchi Y, Urata H, et al. Efficacy of a multicomponent program (patient-centered assessment and counseling for exercise plus nutrition [PACE+ Japan]) for lifestyle modification in patients with essential hypertension. Hypertension research : official journal of the Japanese Society of Hypertension 2004;27(11):859-64. PMID: 15824468. **KQ2E7e, KQ3E7e.**

242. Mochari-Greenberger H, Terry MB, Mosca L. Does stage of change modify the effectiveness of an educational intervention to improve diet among family members of hospitalized cardiovascular disease patients? Journal of the American Dietetic Association 2010 Jul;110(7):1027-35. PMID: 20630159. **KQ1E3e, KQ2E3e, KQ3E3e, KQ4E3e.**

243. Mochari-Greenberger H, Terry MB, Mosca L. Sex, age, and race/ethnicity do not modify the effectiveness of a diet intervention among family members of hospitalized cardiovascular disease patients. Journal of Nutrition Education & Behavior 2011 Sep;43(5):366-73. PMID: 21906549. **KQ3E3e.**

244. Mok Y, Won S, Kimm H, et al. Physical activity level and risk of death: the severance cohort study. Journal of Epidemiology 2012;22(6):494-500. PMID: 22850543. **KQ4E6a.**

245. Morey MC, Peterson MJ, Pieper CF, et al. The Veterans Learning to Improve Fitness and Function in Elders Study: a randomized trial of primary care-based physical activity counseling for older men. Journal of the American Geriatrics Society 2009 Jul;57(7):1166-74. PMID: 19467149. **KQ1E3e, KQ2E3e, KQ3E3e, KQ4E3e.**

246. Mosca L, Mochari H, Liao M, et al. A novel family-based intervention trial to improve heart health: FIT Heart: results of a randomized controlled trial. Circ Cardiovasc Qual Outcomes. 2008;1:98-106. PMID: None. **KQ1E3e, KQ2E3e, KQ3E3e, KQ4E3e.**

247. Mouttapa M, Robertson TP, McEligot AJ, et al. The Personal Nutrition Planner: a 5-week, computer-tailored intervention for women. Journal of Nutrition Education & Behavior 2011 May;43(3):165-72. PMID: 21550532. **KQ2E6b, KQ3E6b.**

248. MR FIT Research Team. Multiple risk factor intervention trial. Risk factor changes and mortality results. Multiple Risk Factor Intervention Trial Research Group. JAMA 1982 Sep 24;248(12):1465-77. PMID: 7050440. **KQ1E8, KQ2E8, KQ3E8, KQ4E8.**

249. Mulholland Y, Nicokavoura E, Broom J, et al. Very-low-energy diets and morbidity: a systematic review of longer-term evidence. British Journal of Nutrition 2012;108(5):832-51. PMID: 22800763. **KQ1E1b, KQ2E1b.**

250. Mutrie N, Doolin O, Fitzsimons CF, et al. Increasing older adults' walking through primary care: Results of a pilot randomized controlled trial. Family Practice 2012;29(6):633-42. PMID: 22843637. **KQ3E3e.**

251. Nanri A, Tomita K, Matsushita Y, et al. Effect of six months lifestyle intervention in Japanese men with metabolic syndrome: randomized controlled trial. Journal of Occupational Health 2012;54(3):215-22. PMID: 22790524. **KQ2E2b, KQ3E2b.**

252. Neaton JD, Broste S, Cohen L, et al. The multiple risk factor intervention trial (MRFIT). VII. A comparison of risk factor changes between the two study groups. Prev Med 1981 Jul;10(4):519-43. PMID: 7027241. **KQ1E8, KQ2E8, KQ3E8, KQ4E8.**

253. Nelson MR, Alkhateeb AN, Ryan P, et al. Physical activity, alcohol and tobacco use and associated cardiovascular morbidity and mortality in the Second Australian National Blood Pressure study cohort. Age & Ageing 2010 Jan;39(1):112-6. PMID: 19903774. **KQ1E1a.**

254. Newton RL, Perri MG. A randomized pilot trial of exercise promotion in sedentary African-American

Appendix C. Excluded Studies

adults. Ethnicity & Disease 2004;14(4):548-57. PMID: 15724775. **KQ3E3e.**

255. No ai. Development of an intervention to "Waste the waist". Journal of Sport & Exercise Psychology 2012;34(6):844-5. PMID: None. **KQ1E6a, KQ2E6a, KQ3E6a.**

256. Nolan RP, Upshur RE, Lynn H, et al. Therapeutic benefit of preventive telehealth counseling in the Community Outreach Heart Health and Risk Reduction Trial. The American journal of cardiology 2011;107(5):690-6. PMID: 21215382. **KQ2E3a, KQ3E3a.**

257. Noordman J, van der Weijden T, van DS. Communication-related behavior change techniques used in face-to-face lifestyle interventions in primary care: a systematic review of the literature. Patient Education and Counseling 2012;89(2):227-44. PMID: 22878028. **KQ1E1a, KQ2E1a, KQ3E1a, KQ4E1a.**

258. Norton LH, Norton KI, Lewis N, et al. Communication-related behavior change techniques used in face-to-face lifestyle interventions in primary care: a systematic review of the literature. The International Journal of Behavioral Nutrition and Physical Activity 2011;8:133. PMID: 22136578. **KQ3E3e.**

259. Norton LH, Norton KI, Lewis N, et al. A comparison of two short-term intensive physical activity interventions: Methodological considerations. [References]. The International Journal of Behavioral Nutrition and Physical Activity 2011;Vol.8. PMID: 22136578. **KQ3E3e.**

260. Oberman A, Wassertheil-Smoller S, Langford HG, et al. Pharmacologic and nutritional treatment of mild hypertension: changes in cardiovascular risk status. Ann Intern Med 1990 Jan 15;112(2):89-95. PMID: 1967210. **KQ1E1, KQ2E1, KQ3E1, KQ4E1.**

261. Ockene IS, Hebert JR, Ockene JK, et al. Effect of training and a structured office practice on physician-delivered nutrition counseling: the Worcester-Area Trial for Counseling in Hyperlipidemia (WATCH). Am J Prev Med 1996 Jul;12(4):252-8. PMID: 8874688. **KQ1E4, KQ2E4, KQ3E4, KQ4E4.**

262. Oh EG, Bang SY, Hyun SS, et al. Effects of a 6-month lifestyle modification intervention on the cardiometabolic risk factors and health-related qualities of life in women with metabolic syndrome. Metabolism: Clinical & Experimental 2010 Jul;59(7):1035-43. PMID: 20045151. **KQ2E8.**

263. Okayama A, Chiba N, Ueshima H. Non-pharmacological intervention study of hypercholesterolemia among middle-aged people. Environmental Health and Preventive Medicine {ENVIRON HEALTH PREV MED} 2004;9(4):165-9. PMID: 21432327. **KQ2E2b.**

264. Panagiotakos D, Pitsavos C, Chrysohoou C, et al. Dietary patterns and 5-year incidence of cardiovascular disease: a multivariate analysis of the ATTICA study. Nutrition Metabolism & Cardiovascular Diseases 2009 May;19(4):253-63. PMID: 18722096. **KQ1E4, KQ2E4, KQ3E4, KQ4E4.**

265. Panunzio MF, Caporizzi R, Antoniciello A, et al. Randomized, controlled nutrition education trial promotes a Mediterranean diet and improves anthropometric, dietary, and metabolic parameters in adults. Annali di Igiene 2011 Jan;23(1):13-25. PMID: 21736003. **KQ2E3e, KQ3E3e.**

266. Park YH, Song M, Cho BL, et al. The effects of an integrated health education and exercise program in community-dwelling older adults with hypertension: a randomized controlled trial. Patient Education & Counseling 2011 Jan;82(1):133-7. PMID: 20434864. **KQ2E6b.**

267. Parra-Medina D, Wilcox S, Wilson DK, et al. Heart Healthy and Ethnically Relevant (HHER) Lifestyle trial for improving diet and physical activity in underserved African American women. Contemporary Clinical Trials 2010 Jan;31(1):92-104. PMID: 19781665. **KQ3E3a.**

268. Parra-Medina D, Wilcox S, Salinas J, et al. Results of the Heart Healthy and Ethnically Relevant Lifestyle trial: a cardiovascular risk reduction intervention for African American women attending community health centers. American Journal of Public Health 2011 Oct;101(10):1914-21. PMID: 21852629. **KQ3E3a.**

269. Peels DA, van Stralen MM, Bolman C, et al. Results of the Heart Healthy and Ethnically Relevant Lifestyle trial: a cardiovascular risk reduction intervention for African American women attending community health centers. Journal of Medical Internet Research 2012;14(2):e39. PMID: 22390878. **KQ1E4, KQ2E4, KQ3E4, KQ4E4.**

270. Pekmezi D, Dunsiger S, Gans K, et al. Rationale, design, and baseline findings from Seamos Saludables: a randomized controlled trial testing the efficacy of a culturally and linguistically adapted, computer-tailored physical activity intervention for Latinas. Contemporary Clinical Trials 2012 Nov;33(6):1261-71. PMID: 22789455. **KQ1E4, KQ2E4, KQ3E4, KQ4E4.**

271. Pekmezi DW, Neighbors CJ, Lee CS, et al. A culturally adapted physical activity intervention for Latinas: a randomized controlled trial. Am J Prev Med 2009 Dec;37(6):495-500. PMID: 19944914. **KQ3E3e.**

Appendix C. Excluded Studies

272. Pekmezi DW, Williams DM, Dunsiger S, et al. Feasibility of using computer-tailored and internet-based interventions to promote physical activity in underserved populations. Telemedicine Journal & E-Health 2010 May;16(4):498-503. PMID: 20507203. **KQ3E3e.**

273. Petersen CB, Severin M, Hansen AW, et al. A population-based randomized controlled trial of the effect of combining a pedometer with an intervention toolkit on physical activity among individuals with low levels of physical activity or fitness. Preventive Medicine: An International Journal Devoted to Practice and Theory 2012;54(2):125-30. PMID: 22200586. **KQ3E3e.**

274. Peterson JA, Ward-Smith P. Choose to Move for Positive Living: physical activity program for obese women. Holistic Nursing Practice 2012 May;26(3):120-8. PMID: 22517347. **KQ3E6a.**

275. Petrella RJ, Lattanzio CN, Shapiro S, et al. Improving aerobic fitness in older adults: effects of a physician-based exercise counseling and prescription program. Canadian Family Physician 2010 May;56(5):e191-e200. PMID: 20463260. **KQ2E3e, KQ3E3e.**

276. Petrogianni M, Kanellakis S, Kallianioti K, et al. A multicomponent lifestyle intervention produces favourable changes in diet quality and cardiometabolic risk indices in hypercholesterolaemic adults. J Hum Nutr Diet 2013 Mar 20 PMID: 10.1111/jhn.12041 [doi]. **KQ2E6b, KQ3E6b.**

277. Pettman TL, Misan GMH, Owen K, et al. Self-management for obesity and cardio-metabolic fitness: description and evaluation of the lifestyle modification program of a randomised controlled trial. International Journal of Behavioral Nutrition and Physical Activity 2008;5:53. PMID: 18954466. **KQ1E4, KQ2E5, KQ3E5.**

278. Pignol AM. Self-management for obesity and cardio-metabolic fitness: description and evaluation of the lifestyle modification program of a randomised controlled trial. University of North Dakota: University of North Dakota; 2008. PMID: None. **KQ3E3e.**

279. Pignol AM. Effects of motivational interviewing on levels of physical activity in older adults. Dissertation Abstracts International: Section B: The Sciences and Engineering 2009(4-B) PMID: None. **KQ3E3e.**

280. Pinto BM, Goldstein MG, Ashba J, et al. Randomized controlled trial of physical activity counseling for older primary care patients. Am J Prev Med 2005;29(4):247-55. PMID: 16242586. **KQ3E3a.**

281. Pisinger C, Ladelund S, Glumer C, et al. Five years of lifestyle intervention improved self-reported mental and physical health in a general population: the Inter99 study. Prev Med 2009 Nov;49(5):424-8. PMID: 19664653. **KQ2E4, KQ3E4.**

282. Poston WS, Haddock CK, Olvera NE, et al. Evaluation of a culturally appropriate intervention to increase physical activity. American Journal of Health Behavior 2001;25(4):396-406. PMID: 11488550. **KQ3E3e.**

283. Prestwich A, Perugini M, Hurling R. Can implementation intentions and text messages promote brisk walking? A randomized trial. Health Psychology 2010 Jan;29(1):40-9. PMID: 20063934. **KQ2E6b. KQ3E6b.**

284. Prestwich A, Conner MT, Lawton RJ, et al. Randomized controlled trial of collaborative implementation intentions targeting working adults' physical activity. Health Psychology 2012 Jul;31(4):486-95. PMID: 22468716. **KQ3E3e.**

285. Price HC, Griffin SJ, Holman RR. Impact of personalized cardiovascular disease risk estimates on physical activity-a randomized controlled trial. Diabetic Medicine 2011 Mar;28(3):363-72. PMID: 21309847. **KQ1E6b, KQ2E6b, KQ3E6b, KQ4E6b.**

286. Prochaska JO, Velicer WF, Rossi JS, et al. Multiple risk expert systems interventions: impact of simultaneous stage-matched expert system interventions for smoking, high-fat diet, and sun exposure in a population of parents. Health psychology : official journal of the Division of Health Psychology, American Psychological Association 2004;23(5):503-16. PMID: 15367070. **KQ3E3e.**

287. Qian J, Wang B, Dawkins N, et al. Reduction of risk factors for cardiovascular diseases in African Americans with a 12-week nutrition education program. Nutrition Research 2007;27(5):252-7. PMID: None. **KQ2E6b, KQ3E6b.**

288. Rasinaho M, Hirvensalo M, Tormakangas T, et al. Effect of physical activity counseling on physical activity of older people in Finland (ISRCTN 07330512). Health Promotion International 2012 Dec;27(4):463-74. PMID: 21911336. **KQ3E3e.**

289. Ratner RE, Christophi CA, Metzger BE, et al. Prevention of diabetes in women with a history of gestational diabetes: effects of metformin and lifestyle interventions. J Clin Endocrinol Metab 2008 Dec;93(12):4774-9. PMID: 18826999. **KQ2E3e, KQ3E3e.**

290. Råberg-Kjøllesdal MK, Hjellset VT, Bjørge B, et al. Intention to change dietary habits, and weight loss among Norwegian-Pakistani women participating in a culturally adapted intervention. Journal of immigrant and minority health / Center for Minority Public Health 2011;13:1150-8. PMID: 21082252. **KQ3E3e.**

Appendix C. Excluded Studies

291. Reed J, Malvern L, Muthukrishnan S, et al. An ecological approach with primary-care counseling to promote physical activity. Journal of Physical Activity & Health 2008;5:169-83. PMID: 18209262. **KQ1E3e, KQ2E3e, KQ3E3e, KQ4E3e.**

292. Reinhardt JA, van der Ploeg HP, Grzegrzulka R, et al. Implementing lifestyle change through phone-based motivational interviewing in rural-based women with previous gestational diabetes mellitus. Health Promotion Journal of Australia 2012 Apr;23(1):5-9. PMID: 22730940. **KQ2E3e, KQ3E3e.**

293. Rejeski WJ, Mihalko SL, Ambrosius WT, et al. Weight loss and self-regulatory eating efficacy in older adults: the cooperative lifestyle intervention program. Journals of Gerontology Series B-Psychological Sciences & Social Sciences 2011 May;66(3):279-86. PMID: 21292809. **KQ2E5, KQ3E5.**

294. Rejeski WJ, Brubaker PH, Goff DC, Jr., et al. Translating weight loss and physical activity programs into the community to preserve mobility in older, obese adults in poor cardiovascular health. Arch Intern Med 2011 May 23;171(10):880-6. PMID: 21263080. **KQ2E5, KQ3E5.**

295. Reseland JE, Anderssen SA, Solvoll K, et al. Effect of long-term changes in diet and exercise on plasma leptin concentrations. Am J Clin Nutr 2001 Feb;73(2):240-5. PMID: 11157319. **KQ1E4, KQ4E4.**

296. Rikkonen T, Salovaara K, Sirola J, et al. Physical activity slows femoral bone loss but promotes wrist fractures in postmenopausal women: a 15-year follow-up of the OSTPRE study. Journal of Bone & Mineral Research 2010 Nov;25(11):2332-40. PMID: 20533310. **KQ4E3e.**

297. Robare JF, Milas NC, Bayles CM, et al. The key to life nutrition program: results from a community-based dietary sodium reduction trial. Public Health Nutrition 2010 May;13(5):606-14. PMID: 19781124. **KQ3E6a.**

298. Robare JF, Bayles CM, Newman AB, et al. The "10 keys" to healthy aging: 24-month follow-up results from an innovative community-based prevention program. Health Education & Behavior 2011 Aug;38(4):379-88. PMID: 21652780. **KQ2E5, KQ3E5.**

299. Roca-Cusachs A, Sort D, Altimira J, et al. The impact of a patient education programme in the control of hypertension. J Hum Hypertens 1991 Oct;5(5):437-41. PMID: 1770472. **KQ1E7, KQ2E7, KQ3E7, KQ4E7.**

300. Rodriguez Cristobal JJ, Panisello Royo JM, Alonso-Villaverde GC, et al. Group motivational intervention in overweight/obese patients in primary prevention of cardiovascular disease in the primary healthcare area. BMC Family Practice 2010;11:23. PMID: 20298557. **KQ1E4, KQ2E4, KQ3E4, KQ4E4.**

301. Rodríguez S, I, Escortell ME, Rico BM, et al. EDUCORE project: a clinical trial, randomised by clusters, to assess the effect of a visual learning method on blood pressure control in the primary healthcare setting. BMC Public Health 2010;10:449. PMID: 20673325. **KQ1E4, KQ2E4, KQ3E4, KQ4E4.**

302. Romé A, Persson U, Ekdahl C, et al. Physical activity on prescription (PAP): costs and consequences of a randomized, controlled trial in primary healthcare. Scandinavian Journal of Primary Health Care 2009;27:216-22. **KQ2E6b, KQ3E6b.**

303. Rosamond WD, Ammerman AS, Holliday JL, et al. Cardiovascular disease risk factor intervention in low-income women: the North Carolina WISEWOMAN project. Prev Med 2000;2000(4):370-9. PMID: 11006062. **KQ1E7e, KQ2E7e, KQ3E7e, KQ4E7e.**

304. Rose SB, Lawton BA, Elley CR, et al. The 'Women's Lifestyle Study', 2-year randomized controlled trial of physical activity counselling in primary health care: rationale and study design. BMC Public Health 2007;7:166. PMID: 17645805. **KQ2E3e, KQ3E3e, KQ4E3e.**

305. Ruffin MT, Nease DE, Jr., Sen A, et al. Effect of preventive messages tailored to family history on health behaviors: the Family Healthware Impact Trial. Annals of Family Medicine 2011 Jan;9(1):3-11. PMID: 21242555. **KQ3E3e.**

306. Saaristo T, Peltonen M, Keinanen-Kiukaanniemi S, et al. National type 2 diabetes prevention programme in Finland: FIN-D2D. Int J Circumpolar Health 2007 Apr;66(2):101-12. PMID: 17515250. **KQ1E5, KQ2E5, KQ3E5, KQ4E5.**

307. Sabti Z, Handschin M, Joss MK, et al. Evaluation of a physical activity promotion program in primary care. Family Practice 2010 Jun;27(3):279-84. PMID: 20332179. **KQ3E3e.**

308. Salkeld G, Phongsavan P, Oldenburg B, et al. The cost-effectiveness of a cardiovascular risk reduction program in general practice. Health Policy 1997 Aug;41(2):105-19. PMID: 10169297. **KQ1E4, KQ2E4, KQ3E4, KQ4E4.**

309. Schneider JK, Cook JH, Luke DA. Unexpected effects of cognitive-behavioural therapy on self-reported exercise behaviour and functional outcomes in older adults. Age & Ageing 2011 Mar;40(2):163-8. PMID: 21059615. **KQ3E1a.**

310. Serwe KM, Swartz AM, Hart TL, et al. Effectiveness of long and short bout walking on

Appendix C. Excluded Studies

310. increasing physical activity in women. Journal of Women's Health 2011;20(2):247-53. PMID: 21314449. **KQ3E6b.**
311. Shahnazari M, Ceresa C, Foley S, et al. Nutrition-focused wellness coaching promotes a reduction in body weight in overweight US veterans. Journal of the Academy of Nutrition & Dietetics 2013 Jul;113(7):928-35. PMID: 23706353. **KQ2E1b, KQ3E1b.**
312. Simmons RK, van Sluijs EM, Hardeman W, et al. Who will increase their physical activity? Predictors of change in objectively measured physical activity over 12 months in the ProActive cohort. BMC Public Health 2010;10:226. PMID: 20433700. **KQ3E3e.**
313. Smeets T, Kremers SP, Brug J, et al. Effects of tailored feedback on multiple health behaviors. Annals of behavioral medicine : a publication of the Society of Behavioral Medicine 2007;33(2):117-23. PMID: 17447863. **KQ3E6b.**
314. Sohn AJ, Hasnain M, Sinacore JM. Impact of exercise (walking) on blood pressure levels in African American adults with newly diagnosed hypertension. Ethnicity & Disease 2007;17(3):503-7. PMID: 17985505. **KQ2E6c, KQ3E6c, KQ4E6c.**
315. Soureti A, Murray P, Cobain M, et al. Web-based risk communication and planning in an obese population: exploratory study. Journal of Medical Internet Research 2011;13(4):e100. PMID: 22126827. **KQ3E6b.**
316. Soureti A, Murray P, Cobain M, et al. Exploratory study of web-based planning and mobile text reminders in an overweight population. [References]. Journal of Medical Internet Research 2011 Oct;13(4):232-42. PMID: 22182483. **KQ3E3e.**
317. Spink KS, Wilson KS. Physician counseling and longer term physical activity. Journal of Primary Care & Community Health 2010 Oct 1;1(3):173-7. **KQ3E3e.**
318. St George A, Bauman A, Johnston A, et al. Effect of a lifestyle intervention in patients with abnormal liver enzymes and metabolic risk factors. Journal of Gastroenterology & Hepatology 2009 Mar;24(3):399-407. PMID: 19444870. **KQ2E6b, KQ3E6b.**
319. Stadler G, Oettingen G, Gollwitzer PM. Intervention effects of information and self-regulation on eating fruits and vegetables over two years. Health Psychology 2010 May;29(3):274-83. PMID: 20496981. **KQ3E3e.**
320. Staffileno BA, Braun LT, Rosenson RS. The accumulative effects of physical activity in hypertensive post-menopausal women. Journal of cardiovascular risk 2001;8(5):283-90. PMID: 11702034. **KQ2E6b, KQ3E6b.**
321. Staffileno BA, Minnick A, Coke LA, et al. Blood pressure responses to lifestyle physical activity among young, hypertension-prone African-American women. The Journal of cardiovascular nursing 2007;22(2):107-17. PMID: 17318036. **KQ2E6b, KQ3E6b.**
322. Stamler J, Briefel RR, Milas C, et al. Relation of changes in dietary lipids and weight, trial years 1-6, to changes in blood lipids in the special intervention and usual care groups in the Multiple Risk Factor Intervention Trial. Am J Clin Nutr 1997 Jan;65(1 Suppl):272S-88S. PMID: 8988942. **KQ1E8, KQ2E8, KQ3E8, KQ4E8.**
323. Staudter M, Dramiga S, Webb L, et al. Effectiveness of pedometer use in motivating active duty and other military healthcare beneficiaries to walk more. US Army Medical Department Journal 2011 Jul:108-19. PMID: 21805462. **KQ2E3e, KQ3E3e.**
324. Steptoe A, Perkins PL, McKay C, et al. Behavioural counselling to increase consumption of fruit and vegetables in low income adults: randomised trial. BMJ 2003;326(7394):855. PMID: 12702620. **KQ3E3e.**
325. Stevens VJ, Obarzanek E, Cook NR, et al. Long-term weight loss and changes in blood pressure: results of the Trials of Hypertension Prevention, phase II. Ann Intern Med 2001;134(1):1-11. PMID: 11187414. **KQ1E3e, KQ2E3e, KQ3E3e.**
326. Stewart AL, Verboncoeur CJ, McLellan BY, et al. Physical activity outcomes of CHAMPS II: a physical activity promotion program for older adults. The journals of gerontology Series A, Biological sciences and medical sciences 2001;56(8):M465-M470. PMID: 11487597. **KQ3E3e.**
327. Stralen MM, Vries H, Mudde AN, et al. The long-term efficacy of two computer-tailored physical activity interventions for older adults: main effects and mediators. Health psychology : official journal of the Division of Health Psychology, American Psychological Association 2011;30:442-52. PMID: 21639638. **KQ3E3e.**
328. Strandberg TE, Salomaa VV, Naukkarinen VA, et al. Long-term mortality after 5-year multifactorial primary prevention of cardiovascular diseases in middle-aged men. JAMA 1991 Sep 4;266(9):1225-9. PMID: 1870247. **KQ1E8, KQ2E8, KQ3E8, KQ4E8.**
329. Strandberg TE, Salomaa VV, Vanhanen HT, et al. Mortality in participants and non-participants of a multifactorial prevention study of cardiovascular diseases: a 28 year follow up of the Helsinki Businessmen Study. Br Heart J 1995

Appendix C. Excluded Studies

Oct;74(4):449-54. PMID: 7488463. **KQ1E8, KQ2E8, KQ3E8, KQ4E8.**

330. Strath SJ, Swartz AM, Parker SJ, et al. A pilot randomized controlled trial evaluating motivationally matched pedometer feedback to increase physical activity behavior in older adults. Journal of Physical Activity & Health 2011 Sep;8(Suppl 2):S267-S274. PMID: 21918241. **KQ3E6b.**

331. Suurkula M, Agewall S, Fagerberg B, et al. Multiple risk intervention in high-risk hypertensive patients. A 3-year ultrasound study of intima-media thickness and plaques in the carotid artery. Risk Intervention Study (RIS) Group. Arterioscler Thromb Vasc Biol 1996 Mar;16(3):462-70. PMID: 8630674. **KQ1E8, KQ2E8, KQ3E8, KQ4E8.**

332. Svetkey LP, Stevens VJ, Brantley PJ, et al. Comparison of strategies for sustaining weight loss: the weight loss maintenance randomized controlled trial. JAMA 2008 Mar 12;299(10):1139-48. PMID: 18334689. **KQ1E1b, KQ2E1b, KQ3E1b, KQ4E1b.**

333. Swanson CM, Bersoux S, Larson MH, et al. An outpatient-based clinical program for diabetes prevention: an update. Endocrine Practice 2012 Mar;18(2):200-8. PMID: 22068253. **KQ2E6a.**

334. Swearingin B. The comparison of the effects of lifestyle activity and structured cardiovascular exercise on obesity-related risk factors of African-American women ages 22--55. Dissertation Abstracts International: Section B: The Sciences and Engineering 2009(12-B) PMID: None. **KQ2E6b, KQ3E6b.**

335. Teri L, McCurry SM, Logsdon RG, et al. A randomized controlled clinical trial of the Seattle Protocol for Activity in older adults. Journal of the American Geriatrics Society 2011 Jul;59(7):1188-96. PMID: 21718259. **KQ3E5.**

336. Tessaro I, Rye S, Parker L, et al. Effectiveness of a nutrition intervention with rural low-income women. American Journal of Health Behavior 2007;31(1):35-43. PMID: 17181460. **KQ3E6b.**

337. The Trials of Hypertension Prevention Collaborative Research Group. The effects of nonpharmacologic interventions on blood pressure of persons with high normal levels. Results of the Trials of Hypertension Prevention, Phase I. JAMA 1992 Mar 4;267(9):1213-20. PMID: 1586398. **KQ1E3e, KQ2E3e, KQ3E3e, KQ4E3e.**

338. The Trials of Hypertension Prevention Collaborative Research Group. Effects of weight loss and sodium reduction intervention on blood pressure and hypertension incidence in overweight people with high-normal blood pressure. The Trials of Hypertension Prevention, phase II. Arch Intern Med 1997 Mar 24;157(6):657-67. PMID: 9080920. **KQ1E3e, KQ2E3e, KQ3E3e, KQ4E3e.**

339. Thomas GN, Macfarlane DJ, Guo B, et al. Health promotion in older Chinese: a 12-month cluster randomized controlled trial of pedometry and "peer support". Medicine & Science in Sports & Exercise 2012 Jun;44(6):1157-66. PMID: 22143109. **KQ2E6d, KQ3E6d.**

340. Thompson JL, Allen P, Helitzer DL, et al. Reducing diabetes risk in American Indian women. Am J Prev Med 2008;34(3):192-201. PMID: 18312806. **KQ2E3e.**

341. Toft U, Jakobsen M, Aadahl M, et al. Does a population-based multi-factorial lifestyle intervention increase social inequality in dietary habits? The Inter99 study. Prev Med 2012 Jan;54(1):88-93. PMID: 22036837. **KQ4E4.**

342. Toft UN, Kristoffersen LH, Aadahl M, et al. Diet and exercise intervention in a general population--mediators of participation and adherence: the Inter99 study. Eur J Public Health 2006;17(5):455-63. PMID: 17170019. **KQ3E4.**

343. Trovato GM, Pirri C, Martines GF, et al. Lifestyle interventions, insulin resistance, and renal artery stiffness in essential hypertension. Clinical and experimental hypertension 2009;32:262-9. **KQ2E6a, KQ3E6a.**

344. Trovato GM, Pirri C, Martines GF, et al. Lifestyle interventions, insulin resistance, and renal artery stiffness in essential hypertension. Clinical & Experimental Hypertension (New York) 2010;32(5):262-9. PMID: 20662726. **KQ2E6a.**

345. Trøseid M, Arnesen H, Hjerkinn EM, et al. Serum levels of interleukin-18 are reduced by diet and n-3 fatty acid intervention in elderly high-risk men. Metabolism: clinical and experimental 2009;58:1543-9. PMID: 19595382. **KQ2E1a.**

346. Tsai AC, Tsai HJ. The association of age, gender, body fatness and lifestyle factors with plasma C-reactive protein concentrations in older Taiwanese. Journal of Nutrition, Health & Aging 2010 Jun;14(6):412-6. PMID: 20617281. **KQ2E6b.**

347. Tudor-Locke C. Promoting Lifestyle Physical Activity: Experiences with the First Step Program. Am J Lifestyle Med 2009 Jul 1;3(1 Suppl):508-48. PMID: 20161372. **KQ1E4, KQ2E4, KQ3E4, KQ4E4.**

348. Turner JE, Markovitch D, Betts JA, et al. Nonprescribed physical activity energy expenditure is maintained with structured exercise and implicates a compensatory increase in energy intake. The American journal of clinical nutrition 2010;92(5):1009-16. PMID: 20826629. **KQ4E3e.**

349. van Stralen MM, de VH, Mudde AN, et al. Efficacy of two tailored interventions promoting physical activity in older adults. Am J Prev Med

Appendix C. Excluded Studies

2009 Nov;37(5):405-17. PMID: 19840695. **KQ3E3e.**

350. van Stralen MM, de VH, Bolman C, et al. Exploring the efficacy and moderators of two computer-tailored physical activity interventions for older adults: a randomized controlled trial. Annals of Behavioral Medicine 2010 May;39(2):139-50. PMID: 20182833. **KQ3E3e.**

351. van Stralen MM, de VH, Mudde AN, et al. The long-term efficacy of two computer-tailored physical activity interventions for older adults: main effects and mediators. Health Psychology 2011 Jul;30(4):442-52. PMID: 21639638. **KQ3E3e.**

352. van Teeffelen WM, de Beus MF, Mosterd A, et al. Risk factors for exercise-related acute cardiac events. A case-control study. British Journal of Sports Medicine 2009 Sep;43(9):722-5. PMID: 19734508. **KQ1E3e, KQ2E3e, KQ3E3e, KQ4E3e.**

353. Vandelanotte C, Bourdeaudhuij I, Sallis JF, et al. Efficacy of sequential or simultaneous interactive computer-tailored interventions for increasing physical activity and decreasing fat intake. Annals of behavioral medicine : a publication of the Society of Behavioral Medicine 2005;29(2):138-46. PMID: 15823787. **KQ1E3e, KQ2E3e, KQ3E3e, KQ4E3e.**

354. Verheijden M, Bakx JC, Akkermans R, et al. Web-based targeted nutrition counselling and social support for patients at increased cardiovascular risk in general practice: randomized controlled trial. J Med Internet Res 2004 Dec 16;6(4):e44. PMID: 15631968. **KQ1E4, KQ2E4, KQ3E4, KQ4E4.**

355. Vrdoljak D, Markovic BB, Puljak L, et al. Lifestyle intervention in general practice for physical activity, smoking, alcohol consumption and diet in elderly: A randomized controlled trial. Arch Gerontol Geriatr 2013 Aug 24 PMID: 24012131. **KQ3E3e.**

356. Walden CE, Retzlaff BM, Buck BL, et al. Lipoprotein lipid response to the National Cholesterol Education Program step II diet by hypercholesterolemic and combined hyperlipidemic women and men. Arterioscler Thromb Vasc Biol 1997 Feb;17(2):375-82. PMID: 9081694. **KQ1E7d, KQ2E7d, KQ3E7d, KQ4E7d.**

357. Walker SN, Pullen CH, Hageman PA, et al. Maintenance of activity and eating change after a clinical trial of tailored newsletters with older rural women. Nursing Research 2010 Sep;59(5):311-21. PMID: 20697307. **KQ3E3e.**

358. Wang X, Hsu FC, Isom S, et al. Effects of a 12-month physical activity intervention on prevalence of metabolic syndrome in elderly men and women. Journals of Gerontology Series A-Biological Sciences & Medical Sciences 2012 Apr;67(4):417-24. PMID: 22054949. **KQ2E5.**

359. Wang YF, Yancy WS, Yu D, et al. The relationship between dietary protein intake and blood pressure: results from the PREMIER study. Journal of Human Hypertension 2008;22(11):745-54. PMID: 18580887. **KQ1E4, KQ2E4, KQ3E4, KQ4E4.**

360. Wassertheil-Smoller S, Oberman A, Blaufox MD, et al. The Trial of Antihypertensive Interventions and Management (TAIM) Study. Final results with regard to blood pressure, cardiovascular risk, and quality of life. Am J Hypertens 1992 Jan;5(1):37-44. PMID: 1736933. **KQ1E1, KQ2E1, KQ3E1, KQ4E1.**

361. Watson A, Bickmore T, Cange A, et al. An Internet-based virtual coach to promote physical activity adherence in overweight adults: Randomized controlled trial. [References]. Journal of Medical Internet Research 2012 Jan;14(1):e1. PMID: 22281837. **KQ2E3e, KQ3E3e.**

362. Wenrich TR, Brown JL, Wilson RT, et al. Impact of a community-based intervention on serving and intake of vegetables among low-income, rural Appalachian families. Journal of Nutrition Education & Behavior 2012 Jan;44(1):36-45. PMID: 22023910. **KQE3e.**

363. Werkman A, Hulshof PJ, Stafleu A, et al. Effect of an individually tailored one-year energy balance programme on body weight, body composition and lifestyle in recent retirees: a cluster randomised controlled trial. BMC Public Health 2010;10:110. PMID: 20205704. **KQ3E3e.**

364. Will JC, Massoudi B, Mokdad A, et al. Reducing risk for cardiovascular disease in uninsured women: combined results from two WISEWOMAN projects. Journal of the American Medical Women's Association 2001;56(4):161-5. PMID: 11759784. **KQE7e, KQ2E7e, KQ3E7e.**

365. Williams DM, Papandonatos GD, Jennings EG, et al. Does tailoring on additional theoretical constructs enhance the efficacy of a print-based physical activity promotion intervention? Health Psychology 2011 Jul;30(4):432-41. PMID: 21574710. **KQ3E3e.**

366. Wilson DK, Trumpeter NN, St George SM, et al. An overview of the "Positive Action for Today's Health" (PATH) trial for increasing walking in low income, ethnic minority communities. Contemporary Clinical Trials 2010 Nov;31(6):624-33. PMID: 20801233. **KQ1E4, KQ2E4, KQ3E4, KQ4E4.**

367. Witmer JM, Hensel MR, Holck PS, et al. Heart disease prevention for Alaska Native women: a review of pilot study findings. Journal of Women's

Appendix C. Excluded Studies

Health 2004;13(5):569-78. PMID: 15257848. **KQ2E3e, KQ3E3e.**

368. Wolf RL, Lepore SJ, Vandergrift JL, et al. Tailored telephone education to promote awareness and adoption of fruit and vegetable recommendations among urban and mostly immigrant black men: a randomized controlled trial. Prev Med 2009 Jan;48(1):32-8. PMID: 19010349. **KQ3E3e.**

369. Woodall WG, Buller DB, Saba L, et al. Effect of emailed messages on return use of a nutrition education website and subsequent changes in dietary behavior. Journal of Medical Internet Research 2007;9(3):e27. PMID: 17942389. **KQ3E6b.**

370. Woollard J, Burke V, Beilin LJ, et al. Effects of a general practice-based intervention on diet, body mass index and blood lipids in patients at cardiovascular risk. Journal of cardiovascular risk 2003;10(1):31-40. PMID: 12569235. **KQ2E7, KQ3E7.**

371. Wright JL, Sherriff JL, Dhaliwal SS, et al. Tailored, iterative, printed dietary feedback is as effective as group education in improving dietary behaviours: results from a randomised control trial in middle-aged adults with cardiovascular risk factors. International Journal of Behavioral Nutrition & Physical Activity 2011;8:43. PMID: 21595978. **KQ3E6b.**

372. Yancy WS, Jr., Westman EC, McDuffie JR, et al. A randomized trial of a low-carbohydrate diet vs orlistat plus a low-fat diet for weight loss. Arch Intern Med 2010 Jan 25;170(2):136-45. PMID: 20101008. **KQ1E6c, KQ2E6c, KQ3E6c, KQ4E6c.**

373. Yates BC, Pullen CH, Santo JB, et al. The influence of cognitive-perceptual variables on patterns of change over time in rural midlife and older women's healthy eating. Social Science & Medicine 2012 Aug;75(4):659-67. PMID: 22365936. **KQ3E3e.**

374. Yen WJ, Lewis NM. MyPyramid-omega-3 fatty acid nutrition education intervention may improve food groups and omega-3 fatty acid consumption in university middle-aged women. Nutrition Research 2013 Feb;33(2):103-8. PMID: 23399660. **KQ1E3e, KQ2E3e, KQ3E3e, KQ4E3e.**

375. Zoellner JM, Connell CC, Madson MB, et al. H.U.B city steps: methods and early findings from a community-based participatory research trial to reduce blood pressure among African Americans. International Journal of Behavioral Nutrition & Physical Activity 2011;8:59. PMID: 21663652. **KQ2E3e.**

Appendix D Table 1. Results of Included Studies for Systolic Blood Pressure

Study	FU (mo)	IG N	CG N	BL Mean IG	BL SD IG	BL Mean CG	BL SD CG	FU Mean IG	FU SD IG	FU Mean CG	FU SD CG	Change Mean IG	Change SD IG	Change Mean CG	Change SD CG	Mean Difference of Change Between Groups	SE Difference of Change
ADAPT, 2006[138]	36	123	118	128.00	11.32	125.00	11.08	127.00	11.32	126.00	11.08						
Applegate, 1992[127]	6	21	26	142.60	11.70	144.50	9.70	133.90		140.00		-8.70		-4.50			
Arroll, 1995[128]	6	48	43	145.00		145.30		139.80		139.10							
Bo, 2007[146]	12	169	166	142.60	14.10	141.50	15.20	140.70	17.70	146.30	18.20	-1.99	18.77	4.79	16.99		
CA WISEWOMAN, 2010[108]	12	433	436	125.10		124.70		119.20		121.00		-5.90		-3.70			
DEER, 1998[71]	12	95	91									-2.60	7.90	-1.00	7.80		
DPP, 2002[89]	24	1079	1082	123.70	14.80	123.50	14.40					-3.40	13.14	-0.52	13.16		
DPP, 2002[89]	36	1079	1082	123.70	14.80	123.50	14.40					-3.27	16.42	-0.57	16.45		
EDIPS, 2001[90]	6	35	32	137.20	19.90	132.80	16.40	129.30	19.50	132.60	14.40	-7.90	16.70	-0.27	14.30	-7.60	3.88
EUROACTION, 2008[106]	12	1019	332									-7.60		-2.80		-4.80	2.76
FDPS, 2001[118]	24	256	250	140.00	18.00	136.00	17.00					-5.00	14.00	0.00	15.00		
GOAL, 2009[139]	12	201	215	146.00	18.50	145.00	15.50					-6.86	18.59	-3.66	14.88		
Green Prescription Program, 2003[123]	12	451	427	135.10	19.60	135.40	17.90					-2.58	15.66	-1.21	14.34	-1.31	1.12
Hardcastle, 2008[167]	6	203	131	134.05	19.38	133.29	18.77					-2.90	10.83	-0.60	10.64		
Hardcastle, 2008[167]	18	203	131	133.12	16.53	132.41	17.33	128.98	14.43	129.96	17.75						
HIP, 2009[136]	6	132	132	133.80	16.30	131.60	14.60					-9.70	12.70	-6.70	12.80		
HIP, 2009[136]	18	128	122	133.80	16.30	131.60	14.60					-8.60		-7.50			
HTTP, 1993[134]	18	86	74	162.00	14.00	161.00	13.00	154.00	16.00	158.00	18.00	-8.00	17.00	-3.00	18.00	-5.00	2.55
Hyman, 2007[135]	6	188	93	139.75	18.64	137.20	17.20	133.03	19.94	133.90	19.10						
Hyman, 2007[135]	18	188	93	139.75	18.64	137.20	17.20	132.53	19.26	134.30	18.40						
IMPALA, 2009[133]	12	286	261	144.00	19.00	150.00	19.00	138.00	16.00	142.00	16.00						
Kallings, 2009[141]	6	41	50	137.60	2.20	142.30	2.60					0.20	14.70	-4.10	12.45		
LIFE, 2010[130]	11	60	66	148.60	17.82	142.90	17.87					-9.30		-4.10			
LIHEF, 2002[137]	24	360	355	149.00	16.00	148.00	16.00					-6.20		-4.20		-2.00	1.17
Migneault, 2012[126]	8	169	168	130.60	19.80	131.80	18.60					-2.06		0.25		-2.31	
Moreau, 2001[104]	6	15	9	142.00	11.62	142.00	9.00	131.00		143.00	9.00	-11.00	4.94	-0.80	4.29		
NC WISEWOMAN, 2008[110]	6	107	110	126.00	18.62	129.00	20.98	125.00	15.52	125.00	15.73					0.50	2.1
NC WISEWOMAN, 2008[110]	12	105	105	126.00	18.62	129.00	20.98	126.00	15.37	125.00	15.37					0.50	2.1
Nilsson, 1992[119]	12	30	29	147.50	15.50	151.80	19.50	139.80	19.40	148.00	19.10						
ODES, 1995[80]	12	52	43	132.80	15.14	128.70	9.84					-6.40	10.10	-0.50	11.15		
PEGASE, 2008[120]	6	274	199									-0.63		0.34			
PHPP, 2007[121]	12	46	41	127.60	15.70	132.00	17.80	122.40	16.30	123.30	15.20						
PREDIAS, 2009[95]	12	91	91	141.80	18.60	139.10	15.90	137.20	17.10	139.10	15.30	-4.60	19.10	-1.00	16.70		

Appendix D Table 1. Results of Included Studies for Systolic Blood Pressure

Study	FU (mo)	IG N	CG N	BL Mean IG	BL SD IG	BL Mean CG	BL SD CG	FU Mean IG	FU SD IG	FU Mean CG	FU SD CG	Change Mean IG	Change SD IG	Change Mean CG	Change SD CG	Mean Difference of Change Between Groups	SE Difference of Change
PREMIER, 2003[116]	6	97	97	144.10	7.10	143.50	8.20					-14.20	10.10	-7.80	10.30	-6.30	1.3
PREMIER, 2003[116]	18	96	97	139.00	15.00	141.00	15.00					-11.00	13.00	-9.90	13.20	-1.00	1.51
PREPARE, 2009[99]	6	29	29	139.00	15.00	141.00	15.00					-3.30	18.27	-2.60	11.13	0.20	3.49
PREPARE, 2009[99]	12	29	29	139.00	15.00	141.00	15.00					-0.4	13.33	-3.5	14.01	2.70	3.34
RIS, 1998[112]	12	239	238	155.00	18.00	155.00	20.00					-3.00	16.00	-2.00	20.00	-2.00	1.79
RIS, 1998[112]	79.2	248	252	155.00	18.00	155.00	20.00					-1.00	15.27	1.00	17.01	-2.00	1.43
Rodriguez, 2012	6	154	168	135.96	13.78	137.15	17.52	131.19	14.58	131.65	16.82						
Rodriguez, 2012	12	151	158	135.96	13.78	137.15	17.52	130.58	14.39	130.90	20.98						
Rodriguez-Cristobal, 2012[172]	24	146	154	133.80	17.40	134.70	18.00	129.60	15.10	136.90	14.80					-6.80	2.02
SLIM, 2011[149]	24	56	58	141.60	16.70	145.00	14.60	137.20	14.70	139.90	13.50						
SLIM, 2011[149]	49.2	57	58	141.60	16.70	145.00	14.60	138.60	14.30	141.20	13.90						
TONE, 1998[117]	36	147	341	127.60	12.10	127.70	12.10										
Wister, 2007[140]	12	157	158	139.00	15.20	136.10	14.30					-7.49	15.85	-3.58	16.03		
SPRING, 2012[100]	12	89	90	158.00	17.10	158.00	16.30					-6.80	17.09	-5.60	14.28	1.20	2.35
MDPS, 2012[85]	12	38	41	135.90	18.61	132.10	14.04					-6.55	14.73	-0.45	18.31	-6.10	3.75
Live Well, Be Well, 2012[86]	6	113	117	126.90	18.07	127.60	21.63					0.70	14.88	-1.20	14.06		
Live Well, Be Well, 2012[86]	12	113	117	126.90	18.07	127.60	21.63					0.30	14.88	0.30	17.31		
Cochrane, 2012[102]	12	236	365	144.40	16.20	146.00	17.00					-5.64	14.85	-6.65	16.67		
HIPS, 2012[103]	12	355	300														
E-LITE, 2013[87]	15	81	81	118.20	11.50	118.40	11.20					-0.40	13.50	0.10	14.40		
PRO-FIT, 2012[68]	12	169	143	123.00	14.40	126.30	15.70	123.00	14.10	125.20	14.40						
Bosworth, 2009[84]	24	110	128	126.00	20.00	124.00	18.00									-3.90	1.5

Abbreviations: BL = baseline; CG = CG; FU = followup; IG = intervention group; mo = months; SD = standard deviation; SE = standard error.

Appendix D Table 2. Results of Included Studies for Diastolic Blood Pressure

Study	FU (mo)	IG N	CG N	BL Mean IG	BL SD IG	BL Mean CG	BL SD CG	FU Mean IG	FU SD IG	FU Mean CG	FU SD CG	Change Mean IG	Change SD IG	Change Mean CG	Change SD CG	Mean Difference of Change Between Groups	SE Difference of Change
Hardcastle, 2008[167]	6	203	131	83.52	10.26	82.41	10.42	82.40	9.03	82.81	8.13	-1.98	7.27	0.49	7.21		
Hardcastle, 2008[167]	18	203	131	83.42	9.63	81.92	9.27										
HIP, 2009[136]	6	132	132	75.30	11.10	73.30	10.50					-5.40		-3.60			
HIP, 2009[136]	18	128	122	75.30	11.10	73.30	10.50					-5.30		-4.90			
HTTP, 1993[134]	18	86	74	100.00	7.00	98.00	7.00	95.00	9.00	96.00	11.00	-6.00	11.00	-2.00	10.00	-4.00	1.53
Hyman, 2007[135]	6	188	93	85.59	9.46	84.80	8.90	82.37	10.82	81.70	9.40						
Hyman, 2007[135]	18	188	93	85.59	9.46	84.80	8.90	82.81	10.53	81.70	9.60						
Kallings, 2009[141]	6	41	50	79.90	1.50	81.60	1.30					-1.00	8.33	-1.70	9.56		
LIFE, 2010[130]	11	60	66	87.90	10.07	84.60	9.75					-6.40		-5.80			
LIHEF, 2002[137]	24	360	355	91.00	9.00	91.00	8.00					-4.30		-3.20		-1.10	0.66
Migneault, 2012[126]	8	169	168	80.90	12.50	80.30	11.80					-1.28		-0.10		-1.18	
Moreau, 2001[104]	6	15	9	84.00	3.87	86.00	6.00	81.00	3.87	87.00	9.00					0.90	1.2
NC WISEWOMAN, 2008[110]	6	107	110	77.00	10.34	80.00	12.59	81.00	8.28	80.00	9.44						
NC WISEWOMAN, 2008[110]	12	105	106	77.00	10.34	80.00	12.59	79.00	8.20	79.00	9.27					0.00	1.2
Nilsson, 1992[119]	12	30	29	86.00	6.20	85.80	7.50	79.90	7.20	81.80	8.80						
ODES, 1995[80]	12	52	43	87.50	8.65	87.00	7.21					-3.40	7.21	-0.70	8.52		
PHPP, 2007[121]	12	46	41	78.20	9.00	79.30	11.80	74.50	10.20	75.00	10.20						
PREDIAS, 2009[95]	12	91	91	88.50	10.50	87.30	9.70	84.10	10.40	85.20	12.30	-4.40	11.70	-2.10	12.60		
PREMIER, 2003[116]	6	97	97									-7.40	7.10	-3.80	7.10	-3.60	0.89
PREMIER, 2003[116]	18	96	97	87.20	4.00	87.80	4.50					-7.40	8.80	-6.50	9.60	-1.00	1.02
RIS, 1998[112]	12	239	238	91.00	8.00	91.00	9.00					-2.50	8.00	-0.80	9.20	-1.60	0.79
RIS, 1998[112]	79.2	248	252	91.00	8.00	91.00	9.00					-4.00	6.43	-3.00	7.69	-1.00	0.66
Rodriguez-Cristobal, 2012[72]	24	146	154	80.70	9.80	81.70	9.40	75.50	9.70	80.40	8.70					-4.40	1.22
SLIM, 2011[149]	24	56	58	89.00	9.40	89.10	7.80	87.60	7.30	85.40	8.00						
SLIM, 2011[149]	49.2	57	58	89.00	9.40	89.10	7.80	83.80	7.90	84.90	7.60						
TONE, 1998[117]	36	147	341	71.30	8.90	71.50	8.50										
SPRING, 2012[100]	12	89	90	92.00	9.50	91.00	8.50					-4.40	9.39	-3.30	7.26	1.10	1.25
MDPS, 2012[85]	12	38	41	80.10	7.85	78.40	7.84					0.70	9.55	1.43	11.21	-0.73	2.35
Cochrane, 2012[102]	12	236	365	85.30	9.60	84.90	9.50					-3.31	8.35	-3.56	9.31		
E-LITE, 2013[87]	15	81	81	73.90	7.20	72.50	9.20					-1.10	9.90	-0.30	9.90		

Abbreviations: BL = baseline; CG = CG; FU = followup; IG = intervention group; mo = months; SD = standard deviation; SE = standard error.

Appendix D Table 3. Results of Included Studies for Total Cholesterol

Study	FU (mo)	IG N	CG N	BL Mean IG	BL SD IG	BL Mean CG	BL SD CG	FU Mean IG	FU SD IG	FU Mean CG	FU SD CG	Change Mean IG	Change SD IG	Change Mean CG	Change SD CG	Mean Difference of Change Between Groups	SE Difference of Change
Hardcastle, 2008[167]	6	203	131	5.48	1.14	5.42	1.03	5.36	1.03	5.52	1.03	-0.14	0.71	0.00	0.69		
Hardcastle, 2008[167]	18	203	131	5.51	1.01	5.39	0.93										
Hyman, 1998[76]	6	65	58	273.20	40.30	272.40	42.30	265.00		267.60		-8.20		-4.80		-3.40	
Hyman, 2007[135]	6	188	93	197.71	35.50	192.80	46.70	192.86	40.93	194.10	41.90						
Hyman, 2007[135]	18	188	93	197.71	35.50	192.80	46.70	191.16	38.97	188.60	42.40						
Johnston, 1995[77]	6	80	39	6.17		6.10											
Kallings, 2009[141]	6	41	50	5.60	0.10	5.50	0.10					-0.30	0.98	0.10	0.36		
LIFE, 2010[130]	11	60	66	240.70	42.60	237.80	43.06					-4.10		-7.80			
LIHEF, 2002[137]	24	360	355	5.66	0.91	5.59	0.93					-0.03		0.07		-0.11	0.05
NC WISEWOMAN, 2008[110]	6	106	110	205.00	41.18	215.00	36.71	203.00	30.89	205.00	31.46					-2.00	4.2
NC WISEWOMAN, 2008[110]	12	106	106	205.00	41.18	215.00	36.71	199.00	29.86	199.00	30.89					-0.30	4.2
Neil, 1995[78]	6	207	102	7.08	0.63	7.23	0.63	6.94	0.73	7.10	0.63						
NFPMP, 2002[79]	12	67	63									-2.30		-6.20			
Nilsson, 1992[119]	12	30	29	5.74	0.72	5.64	0.81	5.78	0.77	5.87	0.84						
ODES, 1995[80]	12	52	43	6.37	0.94	6.58	0.85					-0.23	0.65	-0.16	0.59		
PAC, 2011[122]	6.25	20	15	4.90	0.90	5.00	1.20	4.90	0.90	4.70	1.20						
PEGASE, 2008[120]	6	274	199									-7.64		-3.40			
PHPP, 2007[121]	12	46	41	204.30	31.80	207.00	30.20	201.90	32.20	209.60	32.40	-10.30	35.90	-2.00	35.10		
PREDIAS, 2009[95]	12	91	91	212.20	43.80	209.90	36.60	201.90	35.60	207.90	36.80						
PREPARE, 2009[99]	6	29	29	4.70	1.10	4.70	0.90					-0.26	0.56	0.04	0.80	-0.31	0.18
PREPARE, 2009[99]	12	29	29	4.70	1.10	4.70	0.90					-0.04	0.81	0.11	0.84	-0.17	0.19
RHPP, 1993[69]	36	643	258	267.80		264.70											
RIS, 1998[112]	12	239	238	6.70	1.20	6.60	1.20					-0.50	1.00	-0.10	0.70	-0.40	0.08
RIS, 1998[112]	79.2	248	252	6.70	1.20	6.60	1.20					-0.70	0.80	-0.20	0.81	-0.50	0.08
Rodriguez-Cristobal, 2012[172]	24	146	154	211.10	26.70	210.20	25.50	204.40	30.50	224.40	32.00					-19.20	3.29
SLIM, 2011[149]	24	56	58	5.17	0.83	5.27	0.85	5.40	0.85	5.55	0.89						
SLIM, 2011[149]	49.2	57	58	5.17	0.83	5.27	0.85	5.51	0.82	5.48	0.97						
SE Cholesterol Project, 1997[81]	7	143	150	6.64		6.53						-0.33	0.72	-0.20	0.73	-0.13	0.0714
SE Cholesterol Project, 1997[81]	12	165	176	6.64		6.53						-0.25	0.64	-0.21	0.66	-0.04	0.0663
Stevens, 2003[82]	12	277	271	230.81	23.17	232.08	25.18	223.42	26.79	225.89	29.24	-7.39		-6.19		-2.47	
Tomson, 1995[83]	12	41	35	7.28	0.24	7.30	0.24	7.01	0.86	7.06	0.85						
Wister, 2007[140]	12	157	158	5.80	1.30	5.60	1.20					-0.41	1.15	-0.14	1.15		0.14
SPRING, 2012[100]	12	89	90	5.60	0.85	5.60	0.94					-0.32	0.99	-0.14	0.82	0.17	0.14

Appendix D Table 3. Results of Included Studies for Total Cholesterol

Study	FU (mo)	IG N	CG N	BL Mean IG	BL SD IG	BL Mean CG	BL SD CG	FU Mean IG	FU SD IG	FU Mean CG	FU SD CG	Change Mean IG	Change SD IG	Change Mean CG	Change SD CG	Mean Difference of Change Between Groups	SE Difference of Change
MDPS, 2012[85]	12	37	39	4.97	1.15	5.05	0.88					-0.09	0.73	0.06	0.94	-0.15	0.19
Cochrane, 2012[102]	12	236	365	5.70	0.90	5.70	0.90					-0.56	0.94	-0.54	0.93		
E-LITE, 2013[87]	15	81	81	185.70	31.10	188.40	31.80					4.40	50.40	10.60	49.50		
PRO-FIT, 2012[68]	12	169	146	5.30	1.40	5.20	1.20	5.20	1.20	5.10	1.20						

Abbreviations: BL = baseline; CG = CG; FU = followup; IG = intervention group; mo = months; SD = standard deviation; SE = standard error.

Appendix D Table 4. Results of Included Studies for Low-Density Lipoprotein Cholesterol

Study	FU (mo)	IG N	CG N	BL Mean IG	BL SD IG	BL Mean CG	BL SD CG	FU Mean IG	FU SD IG	FU Mean CG	FU SD CG	Change Mean IG	Change SD IG	Change Mean CG	Change SD CG	Mean Difference of Change Between Groups	SE Difference of Change
Hardcastle, 2008[167]	6	203	131	1.46	0.43	1.53	0.46	1.33	0.35	1.39	0.41	-0.05	0.14	-0.07	0.34		
Hardcastle, 2008[167]	18	203	131	1.46	0.38	1.52	0.43										
HLC, 2011[92]	6	114	65	1.37	0.39	1.45	0.37	1.37	0.41	1.38	0.30						
Johnston, 1995[77]	6	80	39	1.35		1.50											
Kallings, 2009[141]	6	41	50	1.70	0.07	1.70	0.05					0.00	0.33	0.00	0.36		
LIFE, 2010[130]	11	60	66	53.50	12.39	54.10	12.19					0.40		-0.10			
LIHEF, 2002[137]	24	360	355	1.32	0.33	1.36	0.38					0.10		0.07		0.03	0.02
Moy, 2001[73]	24	117	118									0.044	0.300	0.008	0.200		
NC WISEWOMAN, 2008[110]	6	106	110	57.00	14.41	56.00	14.68	59.00	8.24	58.00	8.39					0.60	1.1
NC WISEWOMAN, 2008[110]	12	106	106	57.00	14.41	56.00	14.68	57.00	8.24	58.00	8.24					-0.05	1.1
Neil, 1995[78]	6	207	102	1.21	0.27	1.23	0.28	1.23	0.29	1.25	0.30						
NFPMP, 2002[176]	12	67	63									3.90		2.70			
Nilsson, 1992[119]	12	30	29	0.88	0.22	0.88	0.23	0.97	0.27	0.98	0.24						
ODES, 1995[80]	12	52	43	1.010	0.220	1.040	0.200					0.050	0.115	0.015	0.098		
PAC, 2001[122]	6.25	20	15	1.30	0.40	1.50	0.50	1.30	0.40	1.40	0.50						
PEGASE, 2008[120]	6	274	199									0.87		0.38			
PHPP, 2007[121]	12	46	41	54.50	13.40	55.70	12.90	56.70	14.20	56.50	15.60	-1.30	6.90	-2.20	9.40		
PREDIAS, 2009[95]	12	91	91	55.90	14.10	53.50	13.20	54.60	14.90	51.30	14.50						
PREPARE, 2009[99]	6	29	29	1.20		1.30						-0.08	0.16	-0.04	0.16	-0.04	0.05
PREPARE, 2009[99]	12	29	29	1.20		1.30						-0.03	0.21	0.02	0.16	0.00	0.05
RIS, 1998[112]	12	239	238	1.30	0.40	1.20	0.40					-0.06	0.27	-0.08	0.30	0.02	0.03
RIS, 1998[112]	79.2	248	252	1.30	0.40	1.20	0.40					-0.06	0.24	-0.08	0.24	0.02	0.02
Rodriguez-Cristobal, 2012[172]	24	146	154	54.20	12.00	55.20	13.10	61.70	15.10	60.30	14.60					2.10	1.53
SLIM, 2011[149]	24	56	58	1.14	0.30	1.11	0.28	1.21	0.33	1.16	0.30						
SLIM, 2011[149]	49.2	57	58	1.14	0.30	1.11	0.28	1.25	0.37	1.18	0.31						
Tomson, 1995[83]	12	41	35					1.29	0.28	1.44	0.43						
Wister, 2007[140]	12	157	158	1.30	0.30	1.30	0.30					0.04	0.19	0.03	0.19		
SPRING, 2012[100]	12	89	90	1.30	0.29	1.30	0.34					0.07	0.19	0.10	0.22	0.02	0.03
MDPS, 2012[85]	12	37	39	1.43	0.35	1.59	0.48					0.07	0.18	-0.05	0.25	0.12	0.05
Live Well, Be Well, 2012[86]	6	113	117	53.00	17.01	54.70	17.31					1.80	7.44	0.60	7.57		
Live Well, Be Well, 2012[86]	12	113	117	53.00	17.01	54.70	17.31					3.20	9.57	1.70	8.65		
Cochrane, 2012[102]	12	236	365	1.20	0.30	1.20	0.30					0.01	0.16	0.01	0.15		
HIPS, 2012[103]	12	355	300														

Appendix D Table 4. Results of Included Studies for Low-Density Lipoprotein Cholesterol

Study	FU (mo)	IG N	CG N	BL Mean IG	BL SD IG	BL Mean CG	BL SD CG	FU Mean IG	FU SD IG	FU Mean CG	FU SD CG	Change Mean IG	Change SD IG	Change Mean CG	Change SD CG	Mean Difference of Change Between Groups	SE Difference of Change
E-LITE, 2013[87]	15	81	81	46.20	13.10	46.70	10.70					2.60	11.70	2.90	12.60		
PRO-FIT, 2012[68]	12	169	143	1.20	0.40	1.20	0.40	1.20	0.40	1.20	0.40						

Abbreviations: BL = baseline; CG = CG; FU = followup; IG = intervention group; mo = months; SD = standard deviation; SE = standard error.

Appendix D Table 5. Results of Included Studies for High-Density Lipoprotein Cholesterol

Study	FU (mo)	IG N	CG N	BL Mean IG	BL SD IG	BL Mean CG	BL SD CG	FU Mean IG	FU SD IG	FU Mean CG	FU SD CG	Change Mean IG	Change SD IG	Change Mean CG	Change SD CG	Mean Difference of Change Between Groups	SE Difference of Change
Hardcastle, 2008[167]	6	203	131	2.94	1.28	3.03	1.14	3.28	1.05	3.48	0.94	0.09	1.00	0.25	0.92		
Hardcastle, 2008[167]	18	203	131	2.96	1.14	3.01	1.08	2.71	0.82	2.96	0.90						
HLC, 2011[92]	6	114	64	2.86	0.86	2.94	0.83										
Johnston, 1995[77]	6	67	30	4.12		4.00											
Kallings, 2009[141]	6	41	50	3.40	0.12	3.20	0.09					-0.10	0.49	0.10	0.72		
LIFE, 2010[130]	11	60	66	149.40	31.76	147.70	32.50					-2.80		-6.00			
LIFEF, 2002[137]	24	360	355	3.64	0.81	3.56	0.79					-0.11		0.04		-0.15	0.05
Moy, 2001[73]	24	117	118	4.70	1.40	4.30	1.20					-0.69	1.10	-0.40	0.80		
NC WISEWOMAN, 2008[110]	6	102	103	121.00	33.33	130.00	33.49	119.00	25.25	121.00	27.40					-2.00	3.7
NC WISEWOMAN, 2008[110]	12	103	101	121.00	33.33	130.00	33.49	114.00	25.37	115.00	27.13					-1.10	3.7
Neil, 1995[78]	6	207	102	5.14	0.64	5.25	0.65	4.99	0.69	5.06	0.62						
NFPMP, 2002[176]	12	67	63									-6.20		-7.70			
Nilsson, 1992[119]	12	30	29	4.02	0.80	3.97	0.72	3.95	0.81	4.00	0.73						
ODES, 1995[80]	12	52	43	4.27	0.87	4.57	0.85					-0.18	0.72	-0.22	0.59		
PAC, 2001[122]	6.25	20	15	2.90	0.80	2.90	1.10	2.90	0.90	2.70	1.10						
PEGASE, 2008[120]	6	274	199									2.00		10.00		8.00	
PHPP, 2007[121]	12	46	41	121.00	29.20	123.80	28.20	119.60	28.00	123.90	26.60						
RIS, 1998[112]	12	239	238	4.60	1.00	4.50	1.10	3.59	0.81	3.66	0.81	-0.30	0.80	-0.10	0.80	-0.30	0.08
RIS, 1998[112]	79.2	248	252	4.60	1.00	4.50	1.10	3.57	0.86	3.57	0.72	-0.70	0.80	-0.20	0.81	-0.40	0.08
Rodriguez-Cristobal, 2012[172]	24	146	154	134.60	26.90	134.30	28.60	131.10	28.00	129.60	31.40					1.90	4.06
SLIM, 2011[149]	24	56	58	3.39	0.81	3.51	0.75										
SLIM, 2011[149]	49.2	57	58	3.39	0.81	3.51	0.75										
SE Cholesterol Project, 1997	7	135	145	4.71		4.62						-0.32	0.70	-0.19	0.72	-0.13	0.071
SE Cholesterol Project, 1997	12	153	164	4.71		4.62						-0.24	0.74	-0.19	0.64	-0.04	0.07
SPRING, 2012[100]	12	89	90	3.60	0.78	3.60	0.81					-0.34	0.87	-0.18	0.77	0.16	0.12
MDPS, 2012[85]	12	37	39	2.89	1.01	2.79	0.84					-0.12	0.67	0.11	0.75	-0.23	0.17
Live Well, Be Well, 2012[86]	6	113	117	112.00	31.89	114.80	32.45					-6.60	19.13	-2.40	22.71		
Live Well, Be Well, 2012[86]	12	113	117	112.00	31.89	114.80	32.45					-5.80	24.45	-3.60	23.80		
HIPS, 2012[103]	12	355	300														
E-LITE, 2013[87]	15	81	81	104.60	27.40	108.90	27.00					5.20	44.10	10.60	45.00		
PRO-FIT, 2012[68]	12	128	105	3.60	1.30	3.70	1.20	3.50	1.10	3.60	1.20						

Abbreviations: BL = baseline; CG = CG; FU = followup; IG = intervention group; mo = months; SD = standard deviation; SE = standard error.

Appendix D Table 6. Results of Included Studies for Triglycerides

Study	FU (mo)	IG N	CG N	BL Mean IG	BL SD IG	BL Mean CG	BL SD CG	FU Mean IG	FU SD IG	FU Mean CG	FU SD CG	Change Mean IG	Change SD IG	Change Mean CG	Change SD CG	Mean Difference of Change Between Groups	SE Difference of Change
Hardcastle, 2008[167]	6	203	131	1.96	1.28	1.73	1.03	1.65	1.01	1.55	0.78	-0.17	1.14	-0.15	0.92		
Hardcastle, 2008[167]	18	203	131	1.96	0.79	1.77	1.02										
HLC, 2011[92]	6	118	69	1.71	1.05	1.74	1.04	1.52	0.86	1.55	0.87						
Johnston, 1995[77]	6	80	39	1.10		1.20											
Kallings, 2009[141]	6	41	50	1.40	0.10	1.30	0.10					-0.20	0.49	0.00	0.36		
LIFE, 2010[130]	11	60	66	134.40	63.52	122.20	64.99					-2.60		8.70			
LIHEF, 2002[137]	24	360	355	1.56	1.01	1.49	1.00					-0.06		-0.06		0.00	0.05
Moy, 2001[73]	24	117	118									-0.40	2.00	-0.06	1.90		
Neil, 1995[78]	6	207	102	1.52		1.54											
NFPMP, 2002[79]	12	67	63									-0.80		-3.10			
Nilsson, 1992[119]	12	30	29	1.86	0.68	1.84	0.90	1.93	0.73	1.98	0.90						
ODES, 1995[80]	12	52	43	2.38	1.30	2.18	0.85					-0.23	1.01	0.17	0.92		
PAC, 2001[122]	6.25	20	15	1.70	0.60	1.40	0.70	1.50	0.80	1.40	0.50						
PHPP, 2007[121]	12	46	41	174.80	103.50	166.00	87.70	146.90	70.90	167.40	91.10	-35.60	136.80	-2.50	100.30		
PREDIAS, 2009[95]	12	91	91	156.20	151.00	144.10	102.10	120.60	65.50	141.60	99.50						
PREPARE, 2009[99]	6	29	29	1.40		1.20						-0.02	0.47	0.11	0.52	-0.17	0.15
PREPARE, 2009[99]	12	29	29	1.40		1.20						0.03	0.56	0.04	0.47	0.03	0.14
RIS, 1998[112]	12	239	238	1.90	1.10	1.90	1.00					0.01	0.84	0.17	1.43	-0.18	0.11
RIS, 1998[112]	79.2	248	252	1.90	1.10	1.90	1.00					0.02	0.76	0.24	0.89	-0.22	0.07
Rodriguez-Cristobal, 2012	24	146	154	116.50	54.30	116.60	59.60	115.10	56.50	119.20	55.40					-5.60	6.63
SLIM, 2011[149]	24	56	58	1.52	1.18	1.44	0.79	1.24	0.56	1.45	1.60						
SLIM, 2011[149]	49.2	57	58	1.52	1.18	1.44	0.79	1.74	1.87	1.53	1.06						
Tomson, 1995[83]	12	41	35					1.97	1.01	1.79	0.81						
MDPS, 2012[85]	12	37	39	1.41	0.50	1.44	0.64					-0.09	0.49	0.01	0.50	-0.10	0.11
Live Well, Be Well, 2012[86]	6	113	117	148.30	113.74	128.10	93.02					-8.80	81.85	14.40	69.23		
Live Well, Be Well, 2012[86]	12	113	117	148.30	113.74	128.10	93.02					-1.60	72.28	4.90	54.08		
HIPS, 2012[103]	12	355	300														
E-LITE, 2013[87]	15	81	81	174.50	71.20	164.00	65.80					-28.80	97.20	-18.80	99.00		
PRO-FIT, 2012[68]	12	128	110	1.20	0.60	1.30	0.70	1.30	0.70	1.20	0.60						

Abbreviations: BL = baseline; CG = CG; FU = followup; IG = intervention group; mo = months; SD = standard deviation; SE = standard error.

Appendix D Table 7. Results of Included Studies for Fasting Plasma Glucose

Study	FU (mo)	IG N	CG N	BL Mean IG	BL SD IG	BL Mean CG	BL SD CG	FU Mean IG	FU SD IG	FU Mean CG	FU SD CG	Change Mean IG	Change SD IG	Change Mean CG	Change SD CG	Mean Difference of Change Between Groups	SE Difference of Change
HLC, 2011[92]	6	142	83	5.87	0.58	5.91	0.58	5.66	0.82	5.89	0.86	-0.20	0.33	-0.10	0.36		
Kallings, 2009[141]	6	41	50	5.50	0.10	5.40	0.10					0.30		0.70			
LIFE, 2010[130]	11	60	66	95.60	11.62	93.50	12.19										
LLDP, 2012[94]	12	147	142	104.41	11.90	105.61	12.30					0.50	11.82	-1.50	15.81		
Moreau, 2001[104]	6	15	9	5.60	1.16	5.70	1.20	5.50	0.77	5.70	0.90						
Nilsson, 1992[119]	12	30	29	5.14	0.59	5.17	0.52	5.17	0.41	5.28	0.70						
ODES, 1995[80]	12	52	43	5.65	0.81	5.41	0.52					-0.20	0.10	0.00	0.10		
PAC, 2001[92]	6.25	20	15	5.30	1.10	6.30	3.20	5.70	1.00	6.40	2.40						
PHPP, 2007[121]	12	46	41	5.50	0.60	5.40	0.40	5.50	0.40	5.40	0.40						
PREDIAS, 2009[95]	12	91	91	105.70	12.40	105.50	12.40	101.40	11.30	107.30	14.30	-4.30	11.30	1.80	13.10	-0.30	0.14
PREPARE, 2009[99]	6	28	29	5.60	0.50	5.70	0.50					-0.35	0.60	-0.08	0.62	-0.30	0.18
PREPARE, 2009[99]	24	22	29	5.60	0.50	5.70	0.50	5.40	0.70	5.70	1.00						
RIS, 1998[112]	12	239	238	5.80	2.40	5.80	2.00					-0.40	4.50	0.20	1.40	-0.60	0.31
RIS, 1998[112]	79.2	248	252	5.80	2.40	5.80	2.00					-0.20	1.45	0.00	1.17	-0.20	0.12
SLIM, 2011[149]	24	56	58	6.01	0.84	5.92	0.70	6.05	1.09	6.31	0.84						
SLIM, 2011[149]	49.2	57	58	6.01	0.84	5.92	0.70	6.30	1.07	6.48	0.86						
Watanabe, 2003[97]	12	79	77	6.10	0.55	5.50	0.55					-0.37	3.07	0.01	2.69		
Wister, 2007[140]	12	157	158	8.30	2.60	8.10	2.30					0.17	0.55	0.28	0.63	0.11	0.07
SPRING, 2012[100]	12	89	90	5.40	0.50	5.40	0.68					-0.03	0.36	0.05	0.44	-0.08	0.1
MDPS, 2012[85]	12	37	39	5.17	0.44	5.17	0.44					-0.70	9.57	0.40	10.82		
Live Well, Be Well, 2012[86]	6	113	117	93.80	11.69	93.50	11.90										
Live Well, Be Well, 2012[86]	12	113	117	93.80	11.69	93.50	11.90					-0.90	10.63	-1.40	10.82		
E-LITE, 2013[87]	15	81	81	100.10	9.70	99.30	9.00					-2.70	14.40	0.20	15.30		
PRO-FIT, 2012[68]	12	169	145	4.90	0.80	4.90	1.00	4.70	0.70	4.80	0.80						

Abbreviations: BL = baseline; CG = CG; FU = followup; IG = intervention group; mo = months; SD = standard deviation; SE = standard error.

Appendix D Table 8. Results of Included Studies for Adiposity

Study	FU (mo)	IG N	CG N	BL Mean IG	BL SD IG	BL Mean CG	BL SD CG	FU Mean IG	FU SD IG	FU Mean CG	FU SD CG	Change Mean IG	Change SD IG	Change Mean CG	Change SD CG	Mean Difference of Change Between Groups	SE Difference of Change
ADAPT, 2006[138]	12	123	118	86.50	12.73	84.40	6.10	85.00	12.73	83.70	11.92	-3.52	2.72	-0.96	1.88		
ADAPT, 2006[138]	36	123	118	86.50	12.73	84.40	6.10										
Ammerman, 2003[74]	6	154	189	79.50	29.39	80.00	30.16					-1.41	6.37	-0.45	4.17	-0.95	0.46
Ammerman, 2003[74]	12	189	196	79.50	29.39	80.00	30.16					-0.73	4.91	0.00		0.73	0.487
Anderson, 1992[70]	12	95	51	71.55	10.86	71.44	9.91										
APHRODITE, 2011[88]	6	350	318	29.00	4.40	28.50	4.10					-0.30	1.10	-0.20	1.00		
APHRODITE, 2011[88]	18	330	305	29.00	4.40	28.50	4.10					-0.20	1.70	-0.10	1.60		
Applegate, 1992[127]	6	21	26	88.70		79.70		86.60		79.40		-2.10		0.30			
Beckman, 1995[111]	6	32	32	87.20	12.45	83.60	13.01	84.80	11.31	84.40	14.14	-2.70	2.83	0.06	1.86		
Beckman, 1995[111]	12	32	32	87.20	12.45	83.60	13.01	84.50	11.88	83.90	13.58	-0.94	2.68	0.61	1.97		
Bloemberg, 1991[75]	6	39	41	80.80	9.90	83.30	8.60										
Bo, 2007[146]	12	169	166	29.70	4.10	29.80	4.60	29.40	4.40	30.40	4.80	-0.29	1.79	0.00			
CA WISEWOMAN, 2010[108]	12	433	436	31.60		32.00		31.40		32.00		-0.20					
DEER, 1998[71]	12	95	91									-2.80	3.50	0.60	3.50		
Delahanty, 2001[72]	6	44	44	79.60	15.40	83.20	15.00	77.70	15.40	83.20	15.00						
Delahanty, 2001[72]	12	43	44	79.60	15.40	83.20	15.00	78.20	15.40	83.20	15.00						
DPP, 2002[89]	24			94.10	20.80	94.30	20.20					-5.40		-0.20			
DPP, 2002[89]	36			94.10	20.80	94.30	20.20					-4.00		0.30			
Edelman, 2006[129]	10	77	77	33.30	7.80	34.10	7.70	32.10		33.50							
EDIPS, 2001[90]	6	35	32	83.30	16.10	85.50	14.20	81.90	16.60	86.10	13.80	-1.50	2.60	0.54	2.20	-2.00	0.61
EDIPS, 2001[90]	24	30	24	83.30	16.10	85.50	14.20					-1.80	5.90	1.50	2.60		
EDIPS-Newcastle, 2009[91]	12	39	43	93.40	16.00	90.60	12.50					-2.30		0.01		-2.50	1.25
Enhanced Fitness Trial, 2012[98]	12	180	122	31.35	3.75	30.97	3.45	30.74	3.88	30.64	3.62						
EUROACTION, 2008	12	1019	332									-0.47		0.13		-0.56	0.16
FDPS, 2001[118]	24	256	250	86.70	14.00	85.50	14.40					-3.50	5.50	-0.80	4.40		
FDPS, 2001[118]	36	231	203	86.70	14.00	85.50	14.40					-3.50	5.10	-0.90	5.40		
GOAL, 2009[139]	12	169	172	88.30	12.10	87.60	13.70					-1.90		-0.90			
GOAL, 2009[139]	36	148	165	88.30	12.10	87.60	13.70					-1.40	5.40	-1.00	5.20		
Green Prescription Program, 2003[123]	12	451	427	30.00	6.70	29.90	6.40					-0.11	1.46	-0.05	1.32	-0.06	0.09
Hardcastle, 2008[167]	6	203	131	33.67	5.41	34.28	6.98					-0.21	1.42	0.15	1.14		
Hardcastle, 2008[167]	18	203	131	33.66	5.12	33.37	4.47	33.68	4.77	34.04	4.88						
HIP, 2009[136]	6	132	132	202.50	37.50	202.10	39.60					-7.00	10.70	-0.30	6.30		
HIP, 2009[136]	18	128	122	202.50	37.50	202.10	39.60					-3.80	9.80	-2.10	12.00		
HLC, 2011[92]	6	179	70	29.66	5.33	29.79	4.94	28.72	5.00	29.50	5.24	-1.40					
Hyman, 1998[76]	6	65	58	86.64	19.53	87.37	20.25	85.60		86.55		-1.09		-0.77		-0.32	

Appendix D Table 8. Results of Included Studies for Adiposity

Study	FU (mo)	IG N	CG N	BL Mean IG	BL SD IG	BL Mean CG	BL SD CG	FU Mean IG	FU SD IG	FU Mean CG	FU SD CG	Change Mean IG	Change SD IG	Change Mean CG	Change SD CG	Mean Difference of Change Between Groups	SE Difference of Change
Hyman, 2007[135]	6	188	93	31.85	7.63	33.40	8.20	31.80	7.46	33.30	8.10						
Hyman, 2007[135]	18	188	93	31.85	7.63	33.40	8.20	32.05	8.17	32.80	8.00						
Johnston, 1995[77]	6	84	47	24.63		25.10											
Kallings, 2009[141]	6	41	50	29.70	3.40	30.40	2.90					-0.60	0.98	-0.20	0.72		
Kosaka, 2005[93]	24	102	356									-2.20	8.24	-0.45	12.51		
Kosaka, 2005[93]	48	102	356									-2.18	1.63	-0.39	1.42		
LIFE, 2010[130]	11	60	66	26.50	3.95	26.80	3.66					-0.20		0.00			
LIHEF, 2002[137]	24	360	355	81.10	15.70	80.00	14.80					-1.50		-0.30		-1.20	0.26
LLDP, 2012[94]	12	147	142	33.57	5.10	34.18	5.90					-0.40	1.58	0.11	1.82		
Moreau, 2001[104]	6	15	9	81.10	22.85	79.10	22.20	79.80	22.46	79.70	22.50						
Moy, 2001[73]	24	117	118	28.50	5.00	29.50	7.00					-0.10	1.00	0.21	2.00		
NC WISEWOMAN, 2008[110]	6	108	110	181.00	49.88	180.00	49.29	179.00	9.35	179.00	8.39					-0.70	1.2
NC WISEWOMAN, 2008[110]	12	106	106	181.00	49.88	180.00	49.29	180.00	9.27	180.00	8.24					0.40	1.2
Neil, 1995[78]	6	207	102	26.47	3.99	26.32	4.32	26.32	4.10	26.08	4.29						
NFPMP, 2002[79]	6	70	67	28.10	4.30	29.20	4.80					-0.50	0.60	-0.20	0.70		
NFPMP, 2002[79]	12	67	63	28.10	4.30	29.20	4.80					0.00	1.10	-0.20	1.00		
Nilsson, 1992[119]	12	30	29	87.00	11.01	84.40	12.80	84.80	11.20	84.30	13.20						
ODES, 1995[80]	12	52	43	93.40	12.98	89.30	13.77					-4.00	5.05	1.10	2.62		
PAC, 2001[122]	6.25	20	15	28.80	6.60	30.60	7.30	28.50	7.00	30.80	6.90						
PHPP, 2007[121]	12	46	41	23.60	3.20	24.00	2.50	23.10	3.20	23.90	2.40						
PREDIAS, 2009[95]	12	91	91	31.00	4.70	32.00	5.70	29.70	4.70	31.50	5.80						
PREMIER, 2003[116]	6	97	97	98.10	18.40	94.70	16.00					-1.30	1.70	-0.50	1.40		
PREPARE, 2009[99]	6	29	29	79.40	16.40	81.10	15.00					-5.90	5.90	-1.30	3.40		
PREPARE, 2009[99]	24	22	29	79.40	16.40	81.10	15.00	82.00	15.40	80.00	15.90	-0.61	3.37	-0.45	2.28	-0.15	0.76
RIS, 1998[112]	12	239	238	83.40	14.10	82.10	11.90					-1.90	3.60	-0.60	3.10	1.50	1.43
RIS, 1998[112]	79.2	248	252	83.40	14.10	82.10	11.90					-2.20	4.42	-0.60	3.64	-1.30	0.33
Rodriguez-Cristobal, 2012[172]	24	146	154	30.30	5.80	30.50	5.10	29.60	4.80	31.80	4.90					-1.50	0.36
SLIM, 2011[149]	24	56	58	29.89	4.16	29.65	3.42	29.16	3.84	29.19	3.14					-1.70	0.28
SLIM, 2011[149]	49.2	57	58	29.89	4.16	29.65	3.42	29.19	3.90	29.37	3.32						
Wister, 2007[140]	12	157	158	31.80	6.90	33.20	7.60					-0.47	1.95	-0.33	1.80		
SPRING, 2012[100]	12	89	90	28.00	3.30	29.00	4.00					-0.10	1.32	-0.10	1.67	0.04	0.23
MDPS, 2012[85]	12	38	41	31.40	4.82	30.10	4.19					-0.98	1.60	-0.21	0.77	-0.77	0.29
Live Well, Be Well, 2012[86]	6	113	117	177.90	39.33	176.50	40.02					-2.30	7.44	-0.40	6.49		
Live Well, Be Well, 2012[86]	12	113	117	177.90	39.33	176.50	40.02					-1.30	7.44	-0.40	8.65		

Appendix D Table 8. Results of Included Studies for Adiposity

Study	FU (mo)	IG N	CG N	BL Mean IG	BL SD IG	BL Mean CG	BL SD CG	FU Mean IG	FU SD IG	FU Mean CG	FU SD CG	Change Mean IG	Change SD IG	Change Mean CG	Change SD CG	Mean Difference of Change Between Groups	SE Difference of Change
Cochrane, 2012[102]	12	236	365	28.70	5.00	27.50	4.10					-0.22	1.96	-0.02	1.46		
HIPS, 2012[103]	12	355	300									-0.07	5.77	0.05	6.30		
E-LITE, 2013[87]	6	81	81	31.70	4.70	32.40	6.30					-1.50	2.70	-0.30	2.70		
E-LITE, 2013[87]	15	81	81	31.70	4.70	32.40	6.30					-1.60	2.70	-0.90	2.70		
PRO-FIT, 2012[68]	12	167	147	25.90	4.50	27.10	5.40	25.80	4.40	27.10	5.20						

Abbreviations: BL = baseline; CG = CG; FU = followup; IG = intervention group; mo = months; SD = standard deviation; SE = standard error.

Appendix D Table 9. Results of Included Studies for Diabetes Incidence

Study	Followup (mo)	N IG	N CG	DM Events IG	DM Events CG	Relative Risk	Lower 95% CI	Upper 95% CI
PHPP, 2007[121]	12	46	41	1	3			
LLDP, 2012[94]	12	147	142	2	5			
DPP, 2002[89]	36	1079	1082	155	313			
APHRODITE, 2011[88]	18	479	446	32	32			
EDIPS, 2001[90]	24	37	32	7	8			
EDIPS-Newcastle, 2009[91]	37.3	51	51	5	11	0.45	0.2	1.2
FDPS, 2001[118]	24	265	257	15	37			
FDPS, 2001[118]	84	238	237	75	110			
Kosaka, 2005[93]	48	102	356	3	32			
SLIM, 2011[149]	49.2	74	73			0.53	0.29	0.97
Enhanced Fitness Trial, 2012[98]	12	180	122	7	4			
PREPARE, 2009[99]	12	29	26	0	3			
Inter99, 2008[107]	60	2454	284	187	21			
Bo, 2007[146]	12	169	166	3	12			
HLC, 2011[92]	6	183	91	24	7			

Abbreviations: DM = diabetes mellitus; CG = CG; CI = confidence interval; IG = intervention group.

Appendix E. Intervention Descriptions of Included Studies by Intervention Focus and Intensity

Author, Year	Intervention	Description
Edelman, 2006[129]	Healthy diet & physical activity counseling	Multidimensional intervention on risk education and development/execution of personal health plan. Risk assessments using the "Know Your Number" tool and individual assessments with medical providers to interpret and understand their risk. Small group sessions: 1) first 7 week phase of the intervention, participants learned about integrative health, explored healthier behavior changes, and developed 1–3 personal health goals to prioritize during the remainder of the intervention; 2) next 21 sessions, participants learned about techniques for changing the behaviors identified in their personal goals. Group sessions included mind-body approaches to self-care, nutritional education, physical activity education, and strategies for behavior change. Individual telephone sessions to reinforce group session techniques, to clarify their priorities and set or update goals, and to enhance their motivation. Two opportunities to meet with a nutritionist for more information and development of an individualized eating plan.
	Usual care	The group received a mailed report including their health assessment and baseline blood test results.
PREMIER, 2003[116]	Healthy diet & physical activity counseling (IG 1)	Participant goals were: 1) weight loss ≥15 lb at 6 months for those with BMI ≥25 kg/m^2; 2) ≥180 minutes/week of moderate-intensity physical activity; 3) daily intake ≤100 mEq of dietary sodium; and 4) daily intake ≤1 oz alcohol (2 drinks) for men and ½ oz of alcohol (1 drink) for women. No goals for fruit, vegetable, or dairy intake; saturated fat goal ≤10% and total fat goal ≤30% of energy. To achieve weight loss, increased physical activity and reduced total energy intake was emphasized. Participants kept food diaries and recorded physical activity.
	Healthy diet & physical activity counseling (IG 2 [DASH diet])	Same goals as IG 1 plus instruction and counseling on the Dietary Approaches to Stop Hypertension (DASH) diet. Goals related to DASH diet were: increased consumption of fruits and vegetables (9–12 servings/day) and low-fat dairy products (2–3 servings/day) and reduced intake of saturated fat (≤7% of energy) and total fat (≤25% of energy). To achieve weight loss, increased physical activity and reduced total energy intake was emphasized (as in IG 1), but IG 2 also emphasized substitution of fruits and vegetables for high-fat, high-calorie foods. In addition to food diaries, recording physical activity, and monitoring calorie and sodium intake (as with IG 1), IG 2 participants also monitored intake of fruits, vegetables, dairy products, and fats.
	Usual care	Interventionist discussed nonpharmacological factors that affect blood pressure (weight, sodium intake, physical activity, and the DASH diet) and provided printed educational materials. Counseling on behavior change not provided.
Nilsson, 1992[119]	Healthy diet & physical activity counseling	Intensive nonpharmacological program for improving knowledge and lifestyle. Run-in period of 1 month with seminars, videotapes, and individual counseling; groups continued to meet monthly and encouraged to meet between sessions. Special physical activity given to all participants and relatives (outdoor walking for 2 hours) and every 2 weeks to the 8 most sedentary men; participation in other sports strongly recommended. Special guided tours to supermarkets as well as cooking instruction and distribution of free olive oil to provide adherence to healthier lifestyle. Goals: low-fat, high-fiber diet recommended; fat energy <30%, polyunsaturated fat/saturated fat ratio of 0.8/1.0; more mono and polyunsaturated fat; cholesterol <200 mg/day; fiber 30 g/day (mostly water soluble oat and beans); fruits and vegetable intake; cold water fish (fatty fish such as salmon, mackerel); dietary salt and caloric intake reduced in overweight (BMI ≥27 kg/m^2) or increased abdominal obesity distribution; stop smoking; increase physical activity; no overconsumption of alcohol.
	Usual care	No special intervention offered. Told of metabolic disturbances, risk of hyperinsulinaemia, and how to treat it with nonpharmacological methods; opportunity to know findings of 4-day diet recordings.
DPP, 2002[89]	Healthy diet & physical activity counseling	Goals were to achieve and maintain weight reduction ≥7% of initial body weight through a healthy low-calorie, low-fat diet and engage in moderate-intensity physical activity, such as brisk walking for ≥150 minutes/week. Intervention was designed to maximize success by: interactive training in diet, exercise, and behavior modification skills; frequent support for behavior change; interventions that are flexible, culturally sensitive, and acceptable in specific communities where they are implemented; combination of structured protocol and flexibility to tailor strategies individually; and emphasis on self-esteem, empowerment, and social support. Participants taught to record diet and exercise. Offered supervised exercise sessions twice per week for duration of intervention (not mandatory).
	Minimal intervention	Staff reviews written information addressing importance of healthy lifestyle to prevent diabetes with each participant. Encouraged to follow Food Pyramid guidelines and consume equivalent of National Cholesterol Education Program Step 1 diet, lose 5%–10% of initial weight through diet and exercise, increase physical activity gradually to 30 minutes of an activity, such as walking 5 days/week, and avoid excessive alcohol intake. Smokers encouraged to stop smoking. Placebo tablet taken twice daily. Recommendations reviewed annually.

Appendix E. Intervention Descriptions of Included Studies by Intervention Focus and Intensity

Author, Year	Intervention	Description
TONE, 1998[117]	Healthy diet counseling: sodium reduction (IG 1)	Participants advised on ways to change eating patterns. Interventionists provided information using both centrally and locally prepared materials, motivated participants to make and sustain long-term lifestyle changes, monitored individual and group progress at frequent intervals, and helped participants customize intervention to meet individual needs. Centrally prepared materials included food counters, scorekeepers, manuals, and audiovisual aids. Each active intervention consisted of 3 phases (intensive, extended, and maintenance). Primary goal during intensive phase was to provide core knowledge and behavior skills necessary to achieve and maintain reductions in sodium and body weight. During extended phase, focus was on problem solving and relapse prevention. During maintenance phase, continued attempts made to maintain or reengage participant interest in the intervention. Goal was 24-hour dietary sodium intake ≤1800 mg (as measured by 24-hour urine collection).
	Physical activity counseling: weight loss (IG 2)	Participants advised on ways to increase physical activity for weight loss. Goal was weight loss ≥4.5 kg (10 lb).
	Healthy diet & physical activity counseling: sodium reduction & weight loss (IG 3)	Combination of IG 1 & IG 2. Participants advised on ways to change eating patterns (all active interventions) and increase physical activity (weight loss interventions).
	Usual care (partial attention control)	Usual care groups received no study-related counseling in lifestyle change techniques, but were invited to meetings on topics unrelated to diet, physical activity, and cardiovascular disease.
HIP[136]	Healthy diet & physical activity counseling: patient only (IG 1)	Weekly small group sessions focusing on behavior change using the following strategies: frequent contact, group interaction and social support, goal setting and self-monitoring, identification of barriers and problem solving, and motivational interviewing. Participants kept records of dietary intake, physical activity, and medication use. Group sessions and the participant manual emphasized diet, physical activity, and changing behaviors. Community health advisors attended and helped to lead group sessions and also provided 1-on-1 telephone counseling during and after the group session period.
	Healthy diet & physical activity counseling: patient + physician (IG 2)	Same as above, plus physician-focused training. Physician: training modules (CME) aimed at JNC-7 guidelines and lifestyle modification for blood pressure control. An evaluation and treatment algorithm summarizing the major JNC-7 guidelines and formatted as a decision tree was provided to each physician. Assessment and quarterly feedback to physicians on their adherence to guidelines, including lifestyle counseling that assessed the proportion of patients with hypertension whose blood pressure was controlled, proportion not at goal, proportion that received lifestyle counseling, proportion with diabetes or chronic kidney disease who were at goal blood pressure and prescribed a thiazide diuretic or angiotensin-converting enzyme inhibitor/angiotensin receptor blocker, and comparisons of physicians with peers.
	Usual care	Patients: brief visit after randomization during which they received advice and brochures on lifestyle modification for blood pressure control consistent with JNC-7 guidelines.
PREDIAS, 2009[95]	Healthy diet & physical activity counseling	Group sessions (median size, 7 people) based on the self-management approach. PREDIAS goals were: weight loss (minimum 5%), change of unhealthy eating habits, and increase in physical activity to >150 minutes/week. First 8 weeks were comprised of weekly core lessons covering 8 topics: motivational challenge, weight reduction, healthy diet, analysis and modification of eating habits, physical activity, analysis and modification of physical activity, social support, and maintenance of lifestyle modification. Booster session topics included: dealing with failure, stress management, activating resources, and maintaining new lifestyle. Group leaders provided with curriculum and patients were given a book that contained information about diabetes prevention, resources, and worksheets for each lesson (i.e., eating diaries and physical activity logs).
	Minimal intervention	Controls received the PREDIAS written group information and written patient materials.

Appendix E. Intervention Descriptions of Included Studies by Intervention Focus and Intensity

Author, Year	Intervention	Description
FDPS, 2001[118]	Healthy diet & physical activity counseling	Goals of the intervention were: weight reduction ≥5%; fat intake <30% of energy; saturated fat intake <10% of energy (mono or polyunsaturated fats, 20% of energy, or ≤25% if surplus from monounsaturated fat); carbohydrate intake >50% of energy; increase fiber to ≥15 g/1,000 kcal; and moderate exercise for ≥30 minutes/day. Frequent ingestion of whole-grain products, vegetables, fruits, low-fat milk and meat products, soft margarines, and vegetable oils rich in monounsaturated fats recommended. Dietary advice tailored to each subject on the basis of 3-day food records completed 4 times/year. Subjects received individual guidance on increasing physical activity. Endurance exercise (e.g., walking, jogging, swimming, aerobic ball games) was recommended. Optional supervised, progressive, individually tailored, circuit-type resistance-training sessions offered up to twice per week (participation rates varied from 50%–85% at different centers).
	Usual care	General nontailored verbal and written advice (2-page leaflet) to adjust total energy intake in order to reduce BMI to <25 kg/m²; keep fat to <30% of daily energy; reduce alcohol intake; and stop smoking as appropriate. Verbal general information about health effects of recreational exercise provided, but no specific individual advice given.
LLDP, 2012[94]	Healthy diet & physical activity counseling	Increasing intake of whole grains and nonstarchy vegetables and reducing sodium, total and saturated fat, portion sizes, and refined carbohydrates and starches. The physical activity goal was to increase walking by 4,000 steps per day from baseline. Participants received a pedometer. Skill building included cooking classes, shopping skills, goal setting, self-monitoring, problem solving, and information on opportunities to engage in safe physical activity. The previous DPP intervention was tailored to be culturally and low-literacy sensitive by focusing on traditional Latino foods, using a video series featuring Latino actors, and illustrated, colorful workbooks and materials.
	Usual care	No description provided.
Inter99, 2008[107]	Healthy diet & physical activity counseling	Three kinds of group counseling offered: a smoking cessation course, a diet and physical activity course, and a course on diet and physical activity. Choice of group depended on risk factors and the preference of the individual. Those who were not ready to decide if they wanted to participate in group counseling were encouraged to consider the invitation and were contacted by mail after 3 months and offered participation in a group. Relatives of participants were offered to participate in 1 of the meetings. After 1 and 3 years, individuals still fulfilling high-risk criteria were again offered group counseling. Group counseling included didactic and open-ended discussion and committing to specific diet and physical activity goals; dietary and physical activity advice mirrored advice in individual sessions. In group sessions, the physical activity aim was to achieve small positive changes in physical activity in everyday life.
	Minimal intervention	Based on a personal risk assessment, each participant received an individual "lifestyle counseling talk" focusing on smoking, physical activity, diet, and alcohol. Counseling addressed all individuals who smoked, had <30 minutes physical activity daily, had a high saturated fat diet, <300 g fruits/vegetables daily, or alcohol consumption >14 drinks/week for women and >21 for men. Written materials provided as appropriate. Overall goal was to achieve small but sustained dietary changes. Specifically, decreasing total saturated fat intake, substituting unsaturated for saturated fat, and increasing intake of fruits/vegetables and fish. Participants advised to aim for 4 hours/week of physical activity (some papers report 30 minutes/day); only minimal counseling time spent on physical activity. Participants reinvited after 1 and 3 years for risk assessment and counseling and at 5 years for a short final lifestyle counseling session.
PEGASE, 2008[120]	Healthy diet & physical activity counseling	Assessment and counseling for healthy diet and physical activity. Sessions focused on 3 stages: increasing awareness on CVD risks, start action, and maintain action. Group sessions included self-reflection on risks and threats to health, physical activity and healthy diet education, and information on cholesterol management, plus written materials. Educational messages were reinforced during individual sessions, along with focusing on translating individual goals into small, achievable steps and actions related to healthy behaviors.
	Usual care	Physicians received no training; patients received usual care.
Applegate 1992[127]	Healthy diet & physical activity counseling	Focused on calorie and sodium restriction and increase in moderate levels of physical activity. Weight loss goal was 4.5 kg and calorie restrictions were individualized (women advised to not eat <1200 calories per day and men not <1500). Daily sodium consumption was reduced to 1400 mg. Advised to increase physical activity to 120 minutes/week.
	No advice	Received no treatment; if diastolic blood pressure exceeded 105 mm Hg, participants were placed on medication and removed from trial.

Appendix E. Intervention Descriptions of Included Studies by Intervention Focus and Intensity

Author, Year	Intervention	Description
EDIPS-Newcastle, 2009[91]	Healthy diet & physical activity counseling	Counseling sessions included individually tailored plans for behavior change with the following goals: >50% energy from carbohydrates, <30% energy from fat, reduce saturated fat, increase fiber intake, and physical activity of 30 minutes of moderate aerobic activity each day. Weight goal was BMI <25 kg/m². Three-day food diaries, activity diaries, weight, and waist circumference used to track behaviors. Group sessions included healthy cooking demonstrations and tastings and healthy behavior education. Quarterly newsletters were mailed and included information on healthy recipes, nutrition labels, and opportunities for exercise in the community. Information packs with information about local exercise facilities and opportunities, along with a City Card (offering discounts on facilities), and the opportunity to meet with a trainer for an initial session were offered.
	Usual care	Standard advice plus widely available educational leaflets on healthy eating and physical activity.
APHRODITE, 2011[88]	Healthy diet & physical activity counseling	Stages of change-based intervention with the following goals: weight reduction ≥5% if overweight; moderate- to high-intensity physical activity ≥30 minutes, 5 days/week; fat <30% of energy; saturated fat <10% of energy; and dietary fiber intake ≥3.4 g/MJ. A 3-day food record informed a dietician consultation.
	Usual care	Received oral and written information about type 2 diabetes, risk for developing diabetes, and benefits of exercise and healthy diet.
WISEWOMAN NC, 2008[110]	Healthy Diet & physical activity counseling	Individual sessions consisted of education about barriers to behavior change and "tip sheets" were used to facilitate tailored messaging. An action plan with 2–3 specific goals related to healthy diet and physical activity was created in the first session and progress was monitored at each subsequent session. A motivational videotape was given to view at home. Group sessions focused on teaching problem solving skills, lifestyle behavior change strategies, and emphasized the importance of social support. Education regarding heart-healthy eating, portion sizes, meal planning, and how to read nutrition labels also included. Group sessions also included recipe taste testing and 15-minute physical activity sessions (chair exercises). Food and exercise diaries and pedometers were used to track activity and diet. Participants received monthly phone calls offering support, followup on goal setting, and linkages to community resources.
	Usual care	One-time mailing of two AHA pamphlets on healthy dietary and physical activity practices.
SLIM, 2011[149]	Healthy diet & physical activity counseling	Diet: dietary goals based on Dutch guidelines and included carbohydrate intake ≥55% of total energy; total fat intake <30%–35% of total energy, with <10% total energy intake of saturated fats; cholesterol intake <33 mg/MJ; protein intake 10%–15% total energy, and dietary fiber intake ≥3 g/MJ. Weight loss goal was 5% to 7%, depending on the degree of obesity. Initially, this was achieved by stimulating people to change their daily dietary intake and increase physical activity according to recommendations. If necessary, subjects received example of a mild energy-restricted diet during second year. Detailed dietary advice based on 3-day food record. At each meeting, new goals (including physical activity) were set for the next visit. Topics covered in sessions included fat, carbohydrates, label reading, artificial sweeteners, special occasions, vegetarian food, vitamins and minerals, and lifestyle and diabetes. Physical activity: physical activity goal was to increase low- to moderate-physical activity to ≥30 minutes/day, 5 days/week. Individual advice was given on how to increase daily physical activity. Participants were offered supervised training sessions as part of an exercise program designed for the study that emphasized aerobic exercise and resistance training. Subjects had free access to training sessions and were stimulated to participate for ≥1 hour/week.
	Usual care	Oral and written information on healthy diet, weight loss, and increased physical activity. No individualized advice or information provided.
Migneault, 2012[126]	Healthy diet & physical activity counseling	Telephone-linked care: automated system delivered 3 tailored behavior intervention modules using social cognitive theory, transtheoretical model of behavioral change, and motivational interviewing. The first 3 calls introduced targeted behaviors, how they help with blood pressure control, and oriented users to the system. Subsequent calls were modules on medication adherence (8 calls), physical activity (12 calls), and diet (9 calls). The physical activity module focused on increasing moderate- or greater-intensity physical activity. The diet module focused on fruits/vegetables, fiber, sodium, and fat and intended to promote the DASH diet. Participants and their providers received printouts of their tracked health behaviors. Before randomization, all eligible participants had an in-home visit for health education (and to collect baseline data).
	Minimal intervention	Pre-randomization, everyone had 1 visit for health education; a 75-page resource manual that described hypertension, dietary recommendations, food recipes, and local resources for exercise; and support for medication adherence; also received a pedometer and digital scale. Followed by usual primary care, details not reported.

Appendix E. Intervention Descriptions of Included Studies by Intervention Focus and Intensity

Author, Year	Intervention	Description
Kosaka, 2005[93]	Healthy diet & physical activity counseling	Individual advice was given to help patients lower their BMI if it was above the desirable range for Japanese men (≥22 kg/m²). Patients were instructed to weigh themselves at home weekly. Patients were giving instructions based on their current dietary habits to help them achieve a BMI of 22 kg/m². Patients were encouraged to maintain a nutrient balance, to eat smaller portions, and to consume less fat, alcohol, and fewer meals outside the home. Dietary recommendations were based on "Food Exchange Lists, Dietary Guidance for People With Diabetes." Current physical activity was assessed and realistic ways of achieving a physical activity goal of 30–40 minutes per day were discussed.
	Minimal intervention	All participants were informed of the importance of maintaining a healthy lifestyle. CG subjects with BMI ≥24 kg/m² were advised to reduce their portion sizes and increase physical activity. Those with BMI <24 kg/m² were told to maintain their current weight. These objectives were repeated at each hospital assessment visit.
EURO-ACTION, 2008[106]	Healthy diet & physical activity counseling	Encouraged to achieve a healthy lifestyle with support from family and health professionals using stages of change and motivational interviewing. Advice provided in terms of food (not nutrients) and patterns of eating and set realistic goals for patients and their families. No supervised exercise classes; physical activity plan developed with goals, step counter used for motivation. For smoking cessation, prepared, set date, and made contingency plans. Workshops focused on lifestyle and risk factors. Goals: not smoking, saturated fat <10% total daily energy, fruits/vegetables >400 g/day, fish >20 g/day, oily fish >3 times/week, alcohol <30 g/day, BMI <25 kg/m², waist circumference <81 cm for women and <95 for men, 30–45 minutes moderate-intensity physical activity 4–5 times/week, blood pressure <140/90 mm Hg (<130/85 mm Hg in diabetics), total cholesterol <5.0 mmol/L, low-density lipoprotein <3.0 mmol/L, blood glucose concentration <6.1 mmol/L (good glycemic control in diabetics); for BMI ≥25 kg/m², reduce weight by 5% in 1 year.
	Usual care	No details provided.
LIHEF, 2002[137]	Healthy diet & physical activity counseling	Individualized counseling focused on changing health behaviors, specifically reducing sodium to <5 g/day, reducing saturated fat consumption, and consuming ≤2 alcoholic beverages per day; increasing physical activity to ≥3 sessions of 30-minute, moderate-intensity activity per week; and smoking cessation. Weight reduction was also emphasized (goal of BMI <25 kg/m²). Participants recorded food consumption in 4-day food diaries. Group sessions concentrated on reducing salt intake and body weight.
	Usual care	Instructed to see their primary care physician according to usual care practices.
HLC, 2011[92]	Healthy diet & physical activity counseling	Pre-course individual session in which personal medical history, eating, and exercise patterns are discussed. Group psychoeducational learning sessions on diet, physical activity, motivation, goal setting, stress, and support to adopt healthier lifestyle choices.
	Waitlist control	Waitlist control. CG was not restricted in their use of usual health care services.
RIS, 1998[112]	Healthy diet & physical activity counseling	Aims to reduce total cholesterol to <6.0 mmol/L, <6.0% in diabetics, and lower diastolic blood pressure to <90 mm Hg. Weekly lessons for 5 weeks for 10–20 patients (and spouses) to change eating habits; basic nutrition, purchase and preparation food book, slide series, textbooks, and food/beverage exhibition. Overweight patients set a weight goal. Restriction of alcohol intake for high consumers; diabetics taught self-monitoring glucose; all provided physical activity information. Followup visit with nurse to discuss results and further changes in dietary habits. Smoking cessation include discussion of smoking habits, symptoms of and diseases secondary to nicotine usage, psychological and social factors, and motivation for quitting.
	Usual care	Usual care. Primary care physician treated hypercholesterolemia, diabetes, and smoking according to normal practice.
ADAPT, 2006[138]	Healthy diet & physical activity counseling	Multifactorial program aimed at reducing need for antihypertension drugs and decrease cardiovascular risk factors; focused on DASH diet for dietary advice: sodium intake <2 g/day; increased intake of fruit, vegetables, and low-fat dairy; reduced intake of total saturated fats, sweets, and sugary drinks; consuming ≥4 fish meals per week; participating in ≥30 minutes of physical activity most days; weight loss (reducing weight by ≥5%); reduced alcohol (consuming ≤2 drinks/day), and smoking cessation. Social support was encouraged by allowing a partner, relative, or friend to accompany participants during group sessions and involving them in grocery shopping, meal preparation, and physical activity. Diet and physical activity calendars were used to track behaviors.
	Usual care (partial attention control)	Usual care; publications from the National Heart Foundation of Australia and the Health Department of Australia; attention control with 4 seminars on topics unrelated to the trial were held as well.

Appendix E. Intervention Descriptions of Included Studies by Intervention Focus and Intensity

Author, Year	Intervention	Description
HTTP, 1993[134]	Healthy diet & physical activity counseling	Intervention objectives are: assumption of greater responsibility for disease management, including blood pressure self-monitoring and treatment decisionmaking; confirming diagnosis of hypertension and treatment using at home blood pressure monitoring; and emphasis on nonpharmacological treatments. First session focuses on group discussions and patients are provided with blood pressure monitors and log books. Second session, blood pressure monitoring and log books are assessed, and strategies for achieving blood pressure control (including dietary and physical activity recommendations) are discussed. The last 2 sessions focus on antihypertension therapy.
	Minimal intervention	Staff and medical doctors at all practices were also trained in blood pressure measurement techniques to increase frequency of blood pressure measurements. Additionally, 20 patients at each site had their medical files marked with a red dot to remind clinic staff to take blood pressure, weight, and medication information at each visit. Control practices continued to treat hypertensive patients without the HTTP program; after the study these practices could initiate the program. In the CG, only the physician and staff training occurred, in the IG, both physician and staff training occurred plus the group HTTP intervention.
Hyman, 2007[135]	Healthy diet & physical activity counseling (IG 1)	Motivational interviewing plus home-based instruction manual to improve adherence to lifestyle behaviors for reducing CVD risk. Primary goals for target areas included: stop smoking, reduce sodium levels to <100 mEq/L/day, and increase physical activity by 1500 steps/day (or >10,000/week); were measured objectively in all areas. Six-month visits included measurements; postcard was mailed to participants to report how their measures compared to goals. IG 1: Simultaneous counseling addressed all 3 behaviors during the 6 months. Counseling interaction and instruction manual.
	Healthy diet & physical activity counseling (IG 2)	Same content as above, but sequential counseling introduced 1 area at a time at each 6-month interaction (all 3 areas addressed over 18-month period, in random order), plus instruction manual.
	Minimal intervention	Brief educational session on 3 target behaviors (smoking cessation, sodium intake reduction, increased physical activity). Postcards mailed after each 6-month measurement to report how measures compared to goals.
Logan Healthy Living, 2009[114]	Healthy diet & physical activity counseling	Telephone counseling focusing on motivational interviewing to promote healthy diet and physical activity. Patients were mailed a workbook and pedometer. Counseling followed the "4A" approach: assessment, advice, assistance, and arranging followup. Advice was consistent with Australian National Guidelines and physical activity goal was 150 minutes/week of moderate-intensity physical activity. Consultations were not tailored to diabetes or hypertension, but healthy diet and physical activity suggested were appropriate for both conditions. Calls were weekly at first and moved to biweekly.
	Minimal intervention	After each assessment, minimal intervention patients received a brief and tailored letter with feedback. They also received generic brochures on a variety of health topics.
RHPP[69]	Healthy diet & physical activity counseling: hospital-based (IG 1)	2 IGs: hospital-based (IG 1) and physician-based (IG 2). Both had initial Health Risk Appraisal with 5 vouchers for free health screenings and health promotion services related to identified risk factors. IG 1 offered health screening and health promotion services through regional hospitals.
	Healthy diet & physical activity counseling: physician-based (IG 2)	IG 2 offered the same services through participating primary care clinics. Seven possible risk factor interventions, ranging from weight management to flu immunizations. Educational mailings on lowering cholesterol were distributed to participating providers; offered education sessions by dieticians covering government/society recommendations (AHA, NHLBI, NCEP) for lowering cholesterol; physician training on lowering cholesterol was offered in the area.
	Usual care	Usual care; not offered vouchers for screening or health education.

Appendix E. Intervention Descriptions of Included Studies by Intervention Focus and Intensity

Author, Year	Intervention	Description
Rodriguez-Cristobal, 2012[172]	Healthy diet & physical activity counseling	With the support of their physicians and psychologists, patients received specific interventions using different measures to help improve their habits. Smoking: motivated to give up smoking and received clear and tailored advice as well as medication when indicated. Physical activity: advice to start, maintain, or increase current level of physical activity. Obesity or overweight: gradual weight loss (methods not reported) and maintaining a healthy diet after healthy weight achieved. Weight objective: BMI 20–25 kg/m^2. Hypertension: dietary and pharmacological treatment according to guidelines. Hypertension objective: physical activity <140/90 mm Hg; diabetics <130/80 mm Hg. Diabetes: dietary or pharmacological treatment according to guidelines. Diabetes objective: HbA1c <7%. Psychologists made phone calls to remind IG of upcoming visits (every 2 months) and to provide encouragement about maintaining lifestyle changes.
	Usual care	Received information about their lifestyle according to current practice guidelines.
Bo, 2007[146]	Healthy diet & physical activity counseling	General healthy lifestyle information from their physicians (see details in CG description), plus the following: 1) an individually-prescribed diet tailored to their current weight and dietary intake; general dietary recommendations about cooking, reducing fat, sugar, and salt intake, and tips for dining out; written recommendations for physical activity; brief written guide on behavioral change; copy of the Food Pyramid; explanations about the benefits of using diet and exercise to control metabolic abnormalities; and individualized diet and physical activity goals; 2) group sessions on 4 different topics: food composition, portion control, strategies for dining out, and physical activity benefits.
	Usual care	General information on the importance of a healthy lifestyle. Physicians gave advice according to their usual practice and had participated in ≥3 meetings on standard practice lifestyle recommendations and the efficacy of preventive lifestyle changes. No written information or recommendations were given.
CouPLES, 2013[67]	Healthy diet & physical activity counseling	Phone intervention targeting diet, physical activity, patient-physician communication, and medication adherence to improve cholesterol control; patients and spouses received information about hypercholesterolemia and an overview of self-management principles; spouses also received an orientation to strategies to support patient goal achievement; patient calls focused on goal setting and problem solving, patients selected their own goals. Patients were able to select 1 of 4 topic modules (diet, physical activity, medication adherence, patient-physician communication): first spouse call focused on learning about the patient's goals and action plans and strategies to help the patient; subsequent followup monitoring of patient progress and modifying or creating new goals and action plans; second spouse call focused on staying informed on patient progress and learning about new goal suggestions to help patients; plus mailed printed materials.
	Minimal intervention	Clinical management of lipid disorders using ATP III guidelines. Reminders for physicians were embedded in 11 emails and electronic medical records. Emails emphasized the use of lipid-lowering medications. Physicians also had access to referral specialty clinics (lipid disorders clinic, risk factor management clinic for high-risk patients)
EDIPS, 2006[177]	Healthy diet & physical activity counseling	Regular counseling using stages of change. Included a dietary assessment using baseline food diary. Stage-specific motivational interviewing was used to develop individual targets for behavior change. Participants were encouraged to eat healthy according to British Diabetic Association recommendations (fat 30% of energy, carbohydrates 50%–55% of energy, polyunsaturated/saturated fats ratio of 1.0, daily dietary fiber 20 g/1000 kcal). Participants were given written nutrition education materials. Level of physical activity was assessed and a graded physical activity plan was tailored to participant's lifestyle (designed to enable 20–30 minutes of aerobic activity 2–3 times/week). Information about exercise facilities was provided and a discount card for public leisure facilities in the city was offered to all participants.
	No advice	No advice.
PHPP, 2007[121]	Healthy diet & physical activity counseling	Team encouraged patients to set their own goals and select lifestyle improvements that they were interested in making; choose and prioritize physical activity to achieve goals; provided advice about how to achieve goals using "stages of change" challenge cards. Problem solving for ways to achieve goals, or discussion about changing goals when appropriate, was part of sessions.
	Usual care	Asked to return to the medical center 1 month after baseline assessments, where they received results and were given instructions on how to enhance physical activity via leaflets only.

Appendix E. Intervention Descriptions of Included Studies by Intervention Focus and Intensity

Author, Year	Intervention	Description
Rodriguez, 2012[113]	Healthy diet & physical activity counseling	Telephone counseling based on transtheoretical model for exercise, diet, and medications, based on patient's current stage of change. Stage of change was evaluated at each session and a computer system was used to deliver standardized interventions; problem solving; tips and information for each behavior; and review of medication log (a calendar tracked medication use).
	Minimal intervention (CG 1)	Nontailored health education telephone calls about hypertension management and other health topics. General information was provided about hypertension, sun safety, flu prevention, sleep hygiene, preventing back injury, and vision/hearing problems.
	Usual care (CG 2)	Participated in in-person assessment visits only.
Hardcastle, 2008[167]	Healthy diet & physical activity counseling	Stage-matched motivational interviewing approach in which the focus on diet or physical activity depended on the participant's priorities and readiness to change.
	Usual care	All patients received a standard leaflet about exercise and nutrition at their baseline assessment.
GOAL, 2009[139]	Healthy diet & physical activity counseling	Initial lifestyle questionnaire followed by physical activity and healthy diet counseling consisting of individual sessions focused on self-awareness, lifestyle education, individual motivation, and goal setting. Patients developed a tailored treatment plan based on goals. Ongoing evaluation of goals by nurse practitioners during sessions; modification of goals, as needed, as well as possible referral to dietician. Diet was assessed via food diaries and physical activity was measured using pedometers.
	Usual care	1 session (10 minutes) to discuss results from screening, followed by usual care.
WISEWOMAN California, 2010[108]	Healthy diet & physical activity counseling	Assessment and counseling for healthy diet and physical activity. Individually tailored; comprised of collaborative goal setting, identifying strategies for overcoming barriers, and outlining small, achievable steps. Emphasis on self-efficacy, self-monitoring, reinforcement, readiness for change, and importance of social support. Delivered in language of choice. Visual aids and hands-on tools used (e.g., food models showing appropriate portions), along with a curriculum binder. Community health workers followed up via telephone in between sessions to encourage healthy behaviors, give referrals to health education classes (e.g., smoking cessation, nutrition, physical activity), and give appointment reminders. Received incentives (e.g., tote bags, water bottles, transportation tokens, grocery store vouchers) during assessments and sessions.
	Usual care	Usual care for elevated blood pressure and cholesterol. May have included brief healthy behavior education, healthy lifestyle handouts (general, related to hypertension/hyperlipidemia), or referral to education classes. Received incentives during assessments.
Wister, 2007[140]	Healthy diet & physical activity counseling	Report card to patient and primary care physician with risk profile and Framingham risk factor. Telephone counseling used staged target levels based on letter grade score for each key lifestyle or Framingham risk factor. Telephone counseling used staged target levels developed for each patient. Smoking was considered the top priority for lifestyle counseling, followed by physical activity, dietary habits, weight management, and stress. A counselor addressed areas in which the grade was lowest first. Comparisons with previous report cards were discussed with the participant to set new goals. Summaries of each counseling session and supporting evidence were mailed to the participants.
	Usual care	Received usual care from their physicians, based on their own determination of the need for visits.
Vitalum, 2011[105]	Healthy diet & physical activity counseling (IG 1)	Four tailored letters based on baseline and followup survey data (variables included current behavior, awareness, age, sex, stage of change, attitude, self-efficacy expectations, and action plans); letters 1 & 3 focused on physical activity (3–6 pages) and 2 & 4 on fruit/vegetable consumption (4–6 pages). Half in each group received pedometers at week 29 (along with instructions to gradually increase their number of steps to 10,000/day), and the remainder received it after the last followup.
	Healthy diet & physical activity counseling (IG 2)	Four telephone calls based on motivational interviewing about physical activity and fruit/vegetable consumption. Half in each group received pedometers at week 29 (along with instructions to gradually increase their number of steps to 10,000/day), and the remainder received it after the last followup.
	Healthy diet & physical activity counseling (IG 3)	Combined methods from IG 1 and 2; 2 tailored print letters and 2 telephone motivational interviews. 1 letter and 1 call focused on physical activity; the other 2 focused on fruit/vegetable consumption. Half in each group received pedometers at week 29 (along with instructions to gradually increase their number of steps to 10,000/day), and the remainder received it after the last followup.
	Usual care	After the intervention periods, received 1 tailored letter addressing physical activity and fruit/vegetable consumption based on participants previous followup questionnaire.

Appendix E. Intervention Descriptions of Included Studies by Intervention Focus and Intensity

Author, Year	Intervention	Description
IMPALA, 2009[133]	Healthy diet & physical activity counseling	To implement a nurse-led cardiovascular risk management program, nurses received a 2-day training focused on 4 strategies: risk assessment, risk communication, use of decision aids, and adapted motivational interviewing. Counseling emphasized resolving ambivalence about behavior change, increasing patient motivation to improve healthy behaviors, self-directed goal setting, and creating concrete action plans. Nurses explained 10-year CVD mortality risk score and used a risk communication tool, which was given to patients. Risk reduction techniques were explained and decision aids were given to patients to review at home. Agenda-setting charts were used to allow patients to guide discussion at each meeting.
	Usual care	Nurses received a 2-hour training on risk assessment. Nurses assessed 10-year CVD mortality risk using table from Dutch guidelines (for those without diabetes) or the UK Prospective Diabetes risk engine (for those with diabetes); patients received usual care after risk assessment step.
Arroll, 1995[128]	Healthy diet & physical activity counseling (IG 1)	Exercise and salt interventions. All participants kept a weekly diary tracking injuries or health problems and medication compliance.
	Healthy diet & physical activity counseling (IG 2)	Exercise: advised to walk briskly for 40 minutes 3 days per week. A plan to build up to this amount of exercise was determined by the patient's doctor.
	Healthy diet & physical activity counseling (IG 3)	Salt: asked to decrease use of high-salt foods and added salt when cooking and eating. Each person received a simple pamphlet, a general article about salt and blood pressure, and an in depth book with information about salt content of common foods.
	Usual care, partial attention control	Usual care; publications from the National Heart Foundation of Australia and the Health Department of Australia; attention control with 4 seminars on topics unrelated to the program were held as well.
Bosworth, 2009[84]	Healthy diet & physical activity counseling (IG 1)	Tailored behavioral self-management intervention. Nurse delivered bimonthly telephone calls. Information presented in an easily understood format with a readability score of 9th grade or less. Factors targeted in calls were: perceived risk for hypertension, memory, literacy, social support, patients' relationships with their healthcare provider, and side effects of medication. Intervention also focused on improving adherence to the DASH diet, weight loss, reduced sodium intake, regular moderate-intensity physical activity, smoking cessation, and moderation of alcohol intake. Each encounter included a core group of modules potentially implemented during each call and additional modules activated at specific intervals.
	Healthy diet & physical activity counseling (IG 2)	Combined intervention. Nurse-led telephone intervention as described above, as well as receipt of a home blood pressure monitor and training on its use. Trial nurse was not aware of home-monitored blood pressure values, but participants asked to maintain and turn in blood pressure logs.
	Usual care	Hypertension treatment from regular provider.
Cochrane, 2012[102]	Healthy diet & physical activity counseling	NHS Health Check plus support for lifestyle change. Lifestyle change based on national Health Trainer motivational interviewing/counseling model. Sessions with lifestyle coach provided opportunity to discuss goals and make a plan. Also, referrals to support sessions for weight management, physical activity, cooking and eating, and positive thinking, as desired by participant. Additional individual support was provided for first 20 weeks of program and ongoing support was available up to 1 year.
	Minimal intervention	NHS Health Check plus usual general practice care, including medication or treatment for elevated blood pressure, cholesterol, and newly diagnosed diabetes and referral to smoking cessation services, but did not receive additional lifestyle support. May have received lifestyle advice from the general practitioner team.

Appendix E. Intervention Descriptions of Included Studies by Intervention Focus and Intensity

Author, Year	Intervention	Description
E-LITE, 2013[87]	Healthy diet & physical activity counseling	Self-management group. IT-assisted self-management lifestyle intervention. Based on social cognitive theory and transtheoretical model of behavior change and focuses on goal setting, skill building, and self monitoring to instill behavior change. Participants attend 1 group session where they were trained to track their weight and physical activity using the AHA online self-management portal and given a scale and pedometer. Introductory session was followed by a 12-week curriculum ("Group Lifestyle Balance") on a DVD developed by DPP (for home use) and access to a study dietitian via secure, online messaging. Participants are given primary goal of 7% weight loss and 150 minutes of moderate physical activity per week, within 5 weeks of initiating intervention. Other goals include total fat reduction (25% of calories from fat) and calorie restriction (reduction of 500 to 1000 calories); lower saturated fat intake; lower cholesterol intake; consume a high plant-based diet (fruits, vegetables, whole grains, low-fat dairy); reduce intake of high glycemic index carbohydrates. After attaining the physical activity goal, participants who wish to be more active (or who have not achieved the weight loss goal) are encouraged to increase their physical activity levels. Three-month intensive phase followed by 12 months of maintenance.
	Usual Care	Primary care physician for usual care.
HIPS, 2012[103]	Healthy diet & physical activity counseling	Physician intervention modeled after SNAP intervention; brief intervention based on the stages of change and 5A models. Physicians were trained in assessing risk factors and motivational interviewing. Patient education resources (waiting room questionnaires, health check visit guides, physician checklists) were available. Patients attended individual counseling sessions if deemed high-risk by the brief intervention. High risk was defined by any 1 of the following: history of diabetes or impaired fasting glucose or glucose tolerance; hypertension; dyslipidemia; BMI >25 kg/m^2, waist circumference >102 cm in males or >88 cm in females; or current smoker. Food diary was assessed and individually-tailored lifestyle goals were developed. Group sessions included health education on self-management strategies and physical activity (20–30 minutes of walking or resistance exercise). Between sessions, patients kept food and exercise diaries, used a pedometer, and participated in home-based exercise.
	Waitlist control	Usual care; after 12 months, control practices offered to join intervention.
HOORN, 2013[132]	Healthy diet & physical activity counseling	Based on the theory of planned behavior and self-regulation; aim of counseling was to increase motivation and ability to change diet, physical activity, and smoking behaviors (patients chose which one[s] they wanted to focus on). Motivational interviewing and problem solving treatment were used to help patients find solutions to overcoming barriers and increase perceived control. In-person counseling sessions (weekly at first, then every 2–3 weeks) were followed by monthly telephone sessions.
	Usual care	Received written information about risk of developing diabetes and CVD and brochures containing health guidelines on physical activity, healthy diet, and smoking cessation. Patients with systolic blood pressure >160 mm HG and/or hypercholesterolemia (>8 mmol/L) were referred to their primary care provider for additional medication. Patients with glucose values >7.0 mmol/L were referred to primary care physician and then excluded from the trial.
Live Well Be Well, 2012[86]	Healthy diet & physical activity counseling	Individually-tailored, phone-based lifestyle program designed for lower socioeconomic status, minority, and low-literacy adults and adapted from interventions with established efficacy. Offered in English and Spanish. Participants had an individual counselor and an introductory session (in-person), personal planning session (in-person), and followup calls and workshops. Program focused on self-monitoring, goal setting, and problem solving, and 2 key social cognitive theory concepts were taught to provide behavior change skills and increase self-efficacy. Six-month active phase was followed by 6-month maintenance phase. Counselor contact occurred mostly at the beginning and decreased over time. Physical activity focus promoted 30 minutes of moderate-intensity activity ≥5 days/week (150 minutes/week). Diet goals were to reduce calorie intake and total fat and increase fiber intake. "Eat Colors" and "Eat Breakfast" were used to enforce these goals. Education about health risks and benefits of healthy behaviors were delivered through written, phone, and in-person methods. Skills building was provided through training on goal setting, self-monitoring, problem solving, and relapse prevention. Motivational interviewing techniques were used during phone calls.
	Waitlist control	Waitlist control; started program after 12 months. During recruitment/enrollment, diabetes prevention materials were distributed.
Melbourne Diabetes Prevention Study (MDPS), 2012[85]	Healthy diet & physical activity counseling	Based on the Life! program; comprised of structured group sessions every 2 weeks for the first 3 months, then the last session 8 months after the first. Sessions focused on problem solving and individually-tailored goals. Goals were based on the Finnish Diabetes Prevention Study: ≤30% calories from fat, ≤10% from saturated fats, ≥15 g/1000 kcal of fiber, ≥30 minutes/day moderate-intensity physical activity, and ≥5% weight reduction.
	Waitlist control	Usual care; offered the intervention after 12 months.

Appendix E. Intervention Descriptions of Included Studies by Intervention Focus and Intensity

Author, Year	Intervention	Description
PRO-FIT, 2012[68]	Healthy diet & physical activity counseling	Developed according to the I-Change model (integrated model for exploring motivational and behavioral change), which targets 3 phases of the behavioral change process: 1) awareness, 2) motivation, and 3) action. The intervention is personalized health counseling and includes use of a Web site on CVD risk communication and how to change these risks; access to online PRO-FIT advice on positive behaviors such as food intake, smoking, and compliance to statin therapy, presented according to the participant's risk profile; and a lifestyle coach who delivers personal feedback and works with participants to make action plans. The goal of the intervention is to help participants adopt a healthier lifestyle with regard to physical activity, diet, smoking, and compliance to statin therapy and to lower the level of low-density lipoprotein cholesterol and other CVD risk factors, through use of online tools and a lifestyle coach.
	Usual care	Usual care (no intervention).
SPRING, 2012[100]	Healthy diet & physical activity counseling	All patients receive counseling on CVD risk from practice nurses trained in motivational interviewing techniques. In the IG, this first meeting was based on self-monitoring results (pedometer, scale, and/or blood pressure device). SCORE risk assessments, present risk factors, and treatment goals were discussed. Participants had followup visits that proactively treated for all present risk factors. The order in which risk factors were treated depended on the preference and state of change of the participant, though quitting smoking was the first goal treated if applicable. Adapted motivational interviewing counseling was used. All treatment had to start within 3 months after initial meeting. All patients were offered self-monitoring tools (scales and pedometers) if applicable. For overweight participants: food diaries, home scales, pedometer, and tracking were used in addition to intensive counseling. For low physical activity participants: pedometers and diaries were used in addition to intensive counseling. For those with hypertension: home blood pressure monitoring was used in addition to intensive counseling.
	Minimal intervention	All patients receive 1 session of counseling on CVD risk from practice nurses trained in motivational interviewing techniques. SCORE risk assessments, present risk factors, and treatment goals were discussed at first visit. After the initial visit, followup visits for the CG followed the Dutch hypertension and hypercholesterolemia guidelines. Standard information leaflets were given to overweight participants, smokers, and low physical activity risk groups at first visit.
Anderson, 1992[70]	Healthy diet counseling: AHA diet (IG 1)	Recommended nutritional targets derived from the AHA Phase II guidelines: 55% carbohydrate energy, 20% protein energy, 25% fat energy, ≤200 mg dietary cholesterol per day, and 15 g fiber. Individually-tailored, preplanned meal patterns with 3 servings fruits/vegetables; 4 starches/breads; 2 low-fat dairy; ≤198.5 g lean meat, poultry, or seafood; no egg yolks; fat servings based on energy content. Optional sweets and alcohol servings available. No additional recommendations on modification of other risk-relevant behaviors (e.g., smoking, exercise). Encouraged to attend small-group educational sessions with spouse/close friend; included demonstrations, problem solving, individual counseling (problems, questions about diet, goals). Home visits by dietitian; also available by telephone.
	Healthy diet counseling: high fiber (IG 2)	Same recommended nutritional targets as IG 1 except 50 g fiber (which was stressed during sessions); same preplanned meal patterns except at least 1 serving of beans and 1 of cereal. All other aspects identical to IG 1.
	Usual care	No details provided.
Moy, 2001[73]	Healthy diet counseling	Individualized instructions to lower fat intake (based on ATP III guidelines), focusing on total fat consumption and daily monitoring (usually a goal of <40 g total fat); taught how to read food labels, use fat counter to monitor and record total daily fat intake; self-monitoring logs. Physicians asked to explicitly not manage dietary interventions as recommended based on results and feedback from baseline screening. At each visit, dietary fat screening instrument used to identify potential problems. Counseling individualized based on initial dietary habits, lifestyles, and progress.
	Usual care	Usual care from primary care physician. Physicians received patient-specific recommendations from results and feedback from the baseline screening for risk factor management on 3 occasions.
DEER, 1998[71]	Healthy diet counseling	NCEP Step 2 diet. Goals: <30% fat, <7% saturated fats, <200 mg cholesterol/day. Sessions included lessons on replacing dietary sources of saturated fat with complex carbohydrates, low-fat dairy foods, and other alternatives, including lean meats. Weight loss not emphasized.
	No advice	CG (no intervention). Asked to maintain usual diet and exercise.

Appendix E. Intervention Descriptions of Included Studies by Intervention Focus and Intensity

Author, Year	Intervention	Description
Delahanty, 2001[72]	Healthy diet counseling	Cholesterol-lowering nutritional counseling and treatment according to NCEP-based protocol. Number of visits each participant received was based on assessment of each's eating habits, lifestyle, capabilities, and motivation for change, in addition to usual care from primary care physicians.
	Usual care	During the 6-month intervention, participants agreed to not use lipid-lowering drugs or to seek additional dietary counseling.
Hyman, 1998[76]	Healthy diet counseling	Patients offered/encouraged to use multimodal counseling options (mailed dietary questionnaire, computer interactive calls, and classes) to make dietary changes to reduce cholesterol levels. Intervention focused on improving practical skills like reading labels, eating out, modifying recipes, and self-monitoring, while being practical for primary care.
	Usual care (waitlist control)	Usual care by primary care physician, hypercholesterolemic patients could be referred to registered dieticians. After trial, offered the series of classes (waitlist control)
Johnston, 1995[77]	Healthy diet counseling (IG 1)	Small-group sessions on source and function of dietary cholesterol, risk associated with high cholesterol intake, debunking of dietary misconceptions, advice for eating out, and benefits of exercise. Partners invited to attend. All patients got basic information (see CG description).
	Healthy diet counseling (IG 2)	Nurse counseling: advised to make changes in food intake to reduce the amount of total and saturated fat; increase amount of dietary fiber and complex carbohydrates. Habitual diet estimated by questionnaire; total score and pattern of individual food sources used to suggest specific changes in food choices.
	Usual care	All patients given simple health questionnaire (basic information on diet and exercise) and verbal advice/pamphlet about diet modification, cooking methods, and physical exercise. No further counseling. Incidental queries from subjects were answered briefly on their return to clinic.
Tomson, 1994[74]	Healthy diet counseling	Counseling intervention aimed at nonpharmacological management of high cholesterol; individualized counseling based on diet history and "step I" or general lipid-lowering advice, low-fat diet, high-fiber diet; spouses were invited to the second session; group session included visiting a grocery store to learn how to identify low-fat and high-fiber foods.
	Usual care	Booklet with diet information was sent with a letter, and dietary recommendations based on the patient's weight was included. For those who were overweight: increase fiber and decrease fat intake to 30% of total daily calories. For those of healthy weight: switch to mono and polyunsaturated fats.
Ammerman, 2003[74]	Healthy diet counseling	Special intervention with 3 components: 1) Food for Heart Program during tailored counseling sessions, 2) referral to local nutritionist if lipids remained elevated at 3-month followup, and 3) reinforcement during the second half of the intervention (phone call, 2 newsletters focusing on seasonal tips for food preparation and strategies to enhance dietary change). Food for Heart Program aimed to reduce consumption of foods high in saturated fat, increase fruit and vegetable intake and complex carbohydrates; individually tailored with goal sheets, pamphlets, and southern-style cookbooks. Participants were also instructed to see their physician if total cholesterol remained high.
	Usual care	Nurses instructed to provide counseling for high cholesterol as usual; participants instructed to see their physician if total cholesterol remained high.
Southeast Cholesterol Project, 1997[81]	Healthy diet counseling	Clinician-directed dietary counseling, including a Dietary Risk Assessment, which assesses sources of fat and cholesterol and enabled individually-tailored counseling via the Food for Heart Program; easy-to-read, culturally-tailored patient education materials; quarterly reinforcement mailing containing recipes and health tips. If low-density lipoprotein levels remained elevated after 4 months, then participants were referred to a dietician or health educator for up to 3 counseling sessions. At 7-months followup, primary care physicians received mailed reminders (based on NCEP guidelines for initiating drug therapy) to consider lipid drug treatment if the patient's low-density lipoprotein levels remained elevated.
	Usual care	No details provided.
Beckmann, 1995[111]	Healthy diet counseling	Instructed to lower sodium intake (e.g., not adding salt at table or while cooking, avoiding sodium-rich foods, processed food; bake own bread; use oil, salt-free margarine; and increase fruits/vegetables); provided with a free 2-week supply of unsalted foods with aim to reduce average daily sodium intake to 30 mmol/day. After, aim of achieving average daily sodium intake of 100 mmol/day; those with elevated BMI or total cholesterol were advised to reduce body weight and reduce saturated and increase intake of polyunsaturated dietary fat.
	Waitlist control	At 12 months, given dietary advice similar to IG.

Appendix E. Intervention Descriptions of Included Studies by Intervention Focus and Intensity

Author, Year	Intervention	Description
Stevens, 2003[82]	Healthy diet counseling	Combined motivational interviewing, problem solving, and social cognitive theory strategies; strategies for overcoming barriers and skills deficits interfering with dietary change or maintenance; opportunities for increasing environmental support; select 1 of 2 goals (reduce dietary fat or increase fruit/vegetable and whole grains); provided feedback on baseline dietary intake. Dietary fat goals were assisted with a computer assessment (30 minutes) and discussion of goals/plans for change (25 minutes) using the Fat and Fiber Behavior Questionnaire, which helped provide tailored strategies. Fruit and vegetable goals focused on barriers, self-efficacy, eating patterns, and stage of change. The second session, 2–3 weeks later, reported progress on current goal and counseled on other goal. Participants made commitments and personally tailored strategies for change, received telephone support after second session.
	Attention control	Attention control on breast self-exams and a 9-minute American Cancer Society video; self-help pamphlets; and barriers-based, problem-solving counseling on interest and motivation for conducting regular breast self-exams. No dietary recommendations.
NFPMP, 2002[79]	Healthy diet counseling	Nutrition information and counseling according to stage of change; practical aspects included reducing saturated fat intake, increasing unsaturated fat intake, and reducing total energy and fat intake. If no progress, intervention stopped. Information package: individualized feedback based on baseline values, educational materials to support aforementioned goals (e.g., short food variation list, menus); if action phase then referral to dietician.
	Usual care	No details provided.
ODES, 1995[80]	Healthy diet counseling	Individualized dietary counseling and education on high-/low-density lipoproteins and weight reduction by dietary change. Recommended against low caloric intake early in day and heavier at dinner; moderate salt restriction in persons with elevated blood pressure; energy restriction in overweight persons; recommended increase in fish, fruits and vegetables, and complex carbohydrates and reduction in sugar and saturated fat. Individualized dietary program of the 5–10 most important points made during counseling session. Target body weight/reduction agreed. Followup dietary advice at 3 and 9 months.
	Waitlist control	Waitlist control offered dietary advice and physical training after 1 year.
Bloemberg, 1991[75]	Healthy diet counseling	Individualized dietary advice based on habitual food intake and the "Guidelines for a Healthy Diet" of the Netherlands Nutrition Council; used computer to generate dietary advice based on actual dietary pattern. Aim of dietary advice to reduce total cholesterol by 1 mmol/L. One week after examination, discussed dietary advice and tried to convince adherence. Telephone calls to inquire about possible problems about dietary advice. Mailers provided information on healthy diet.
	No advice	Did not receive any advice to improve diet during the study period.
Neil, 1995[78]	Healthy diet counseling: dietician (IG 1)	Standard diet history taken and given individual advice on dietary habits and weight. Advised to reduce percentage of total dietary energy from fat to ≤30%; consume ≤10% of energy from saturated, monounsaturated, and polyunsaturated fatty acids; 50%–60% energy derived from carbohydrates, protein 10%–20%; daily intake of <300 mg cholesterol; 35 g fiber. Further advice given during a 10-minute appointment.
	Healthy diet counseling: nurse (IG 2)	Advised to make changes in food intake to reduce the amount of total and saturated fat; increase amount of dietary fiber and complex carbohydrates. Habitual diet estimated by questionnaire; total score and pattern of individual food sources used to suggest specific changes in food choices
	Usual care	Pamphlet containing dietary guidance consistent with advice provided by dietitian. Additional written advice after 2 months.
Watanabe, 2003[97]	Healthy diet counseling	New dietary education. Individualized counseling aimed to reduce total energy intake by modifying dietary intake and adopt habits to prevent diabetes. Program consisted of 1) individual dietary counseling based on questionnaire results, with booklet illustrating recommendations for meals corresponding to the recommended daily allowance for total energy intake at 1 month; and 2) mailed materials at 6 months. Education aimed to reduce late-night total energy intake; keep protein energy at 15%–20%, fat at 20%–25%, and carbohydrates at 55%–60% of total energy intake; optimize intake of whole grains, fruits and vegetables, low-fat milk, beans, fish, meat, eggs, and maintain alcohol intake at an appropriate level by Japanese Diabetes Society and American Diabetes Association recommendations. Mailer included encouragement to improve dietary intake, related information, self-administered checklist corresponding to recommended daily allowances, and information on necessity of blood glucose control.
	Usual care	General oral and written information about results of health examination and questionnaire without detailed explanation; received conventional group counseling with a leaflet with general information for prevention of lifestyle-related disease.

Appendix E. Intervention Descriptions of Included Studies by Intervention Focus and Intensity

Author, Year	Intervention	Description
LIFE, 2010[130]	Physical activity counseling	Home-based lifestyle intervention aimed to stimulate integrated physical activity into immediate environment during daily routines. Prior to randomization, all IG participants attended a group session on healthy aging and benefits of physical activity. Following randomization, IG 1 attended group sessions throughout intervention period. Sessions shared general information about endurance, strength, flexibility, and postural/balance training and to ensure correct performance of exercises. Brochure and pedometer distributed (with training on proper use and heart rate monitoring). An individual session with exercise instructor set up program specific to individual needs, preferences, and experiences. Participants given booklet with exercises targeting strength (using elastic tubes), flexibility, and balance, and asked to choose preferred exercises. Suggested endurance trainings included jogging, cycling, swimming, or other cardiovascular exercises; participants encouraged to exercise at intensity that increased heart rate but still able to talk with their partner. Individual session with exercise psychologist focused on how to integrate exercises into daily life, how to persist, and how to anticipate barriers. Participants asked to keep an activity log and referred to these during "booster" phone calls to discuss program adherence.
	Usual care	Prior to randomization of IG groups, CG volunteers attended a group session on different components of healthy aging (similar to the introductory session offered to IG volunteers, except it excluded the physical activity benefits component). CG volunteers were participating in a "checkup of fitness/health status" program, which involved getting measurements (3 times: pre-, mid-, post-) with no feedback or results until end of study period (after 11 months). Each participant was asked to report changes in lifestyle regarding physical activity, diet, or medication during the program.
Enhanced Fitness Trial, 2012[98]	Physical activity counseling: reduced calls (IG 1)	Reliant on social cognitive theory, the strategy is to enhance self-efficacy for physical activity by integrating self-monitoring, goal setting, reinforcement, modeling, and cognitive function into counseling program. Five-element intervention, including: 1) In-person consultation with health counselor to assess functional status. 2) Primary care physician notified of participant enrollment and endorsed physical activity at next scheduled visit. At 3-month point, participant's physical activity performance was assessed and all those who met >75% of exercise goals (minutes per week) were assigned to IG 1 (reduced calls); those who failed to meet exercise goals (<75%) were allocated to IG 2 (continued care). 3) Health counselor contacted participant for followup counseling by phone, using standardized protocol to reinforce continued physical activity, identify strategies for overcoming barriers, and customize individually-feasible activities. 4) Automated phone calls with recorded messages from the primary care physician. 5) Quarterly tailored progress report, including a graph showing participant change over time and encouragement messages tailored based on participant performance. 6) Referral to local physical activity program (MOVE!).
	Physical activity counseling: continued care (IG 2)	Same as IG 1, with more phone call followup.
	Minimal intervention	Usual care received in primary care clinic plus referral to the MOVE! program (program on physical activity and nutrition that includes self-management programs, classroom sessions, and individualized counseling with goal setting). Participants sent lifestyle questionnaire and could decide whether to enroll in the program.
PAC, 2001[122]	Physical activity counseling	All participants (IG and CG) given brief (2–4 minutes) physical activity counseling during routine visit with primary care provider. Using the 7A shared-care model for physical activity counseling, this brief intervention addressed the first 4 As: Address the subject of physical activity; Ask participants about their physical activity; Advise participants to increase physical activity while personalizing benefits; Agree on 1-month leisure-time physical activity goal. All participants then received a tailored physical activity prescription that included the agreed upon goal. The IG (intensive-counseling group) then received 6 patient-centered physical activity counseling sessions over 3 months from the physical activity counselor, focusing on the other 3 parts of the 7 A model: Assess, Assist, and Arrange. Counseling was highly individualized but always involved encouragement and support, helped participants set a goal and problem solve around potential barriers, and focused on psychological mediators of change.
	Minimal intervention	Brief (2–4 minutes) physical activity counseling intervention with primary care provider. Using the 7A shared-care model for physical activity counseling, this brief intervention addressed the first 4 As: Address the subject of physical activity; Ask participants about their physical activity; Advise participants to increase physical activity while personalizing benefits; Agree on 1-month leisure-time physical activity goal. All participants then received a tailored physical activity prescription that included the agreed upon goal. No further intervention afterward.

Appendix E. Intervention Descriptions of Included Studies by Intervention Focus and Intensity

Author, Year	Intervention	Description
PREPARE Trial, 2009[99]	Physical activity counseling (IG 1)	Single-session group educational program designed to promote increased physical activity (primarily walking) by targeting perceptions and knowledge of impaired glucose tolerance, physical activity self-efficacy, barriers, and self-regulatory skills. Person-centered approach to participant education delivered in groups of 5–10, divided into 4 modules: 1) participant story (participants share their knowledge of impaired glucose tolerance and concerns about program); 2) professional story (overview of healthy glucose metabolism, prediabetes complications and risk factors, calculate risk scores); 3) diet (link between diet and metabolism); 4) physical activity (how physical activity improves glucose control; understand physical activity recommendations; discuss how to incorporate physical activity into daily life, form action plans and set goals; encourage use of physical activity diaries). Only method of goal setting differed between IG 1 and 2. Both groups (IG 1 and 2) had brief 1-on-1 followup counseling with trained educator at 3 and 6 month clinical measurement session. Goal setting: IG 1 (PREPARE group): set physical activity goals based on generic exercise recommendations (i.e., 30 minutes of moderate-intensity exercise on most days of the week). Encouraged to set proximal goals, such as increasing moderate-intensity activity by 5 minutes/day every 2 weeks. Use of action plans and activity logs recommended.
	Physical activity counseling (IG 2)	IG 2-PREPARE and pedometer: received pedometer and trained on its use. Set personalized goals of steps per day based on baseline ambulatory activity levels and step per day categories. Generally recommended to increase by 3,000 steps per day, unless baseline was at ≥9,000 steps, then recommended to sustain. Set proximal goals with timeline. Encouraged to wear pedometer on daily basis and to monitor activity using a log.
	Usual care	Brief information sheet in the mail detailing the likely causes, consequences, symptoms, and timeline associated with impaired glucose tolerance, along with information about how physical activity can be used to treat/control the condition.
Kallings, 2009[141]	Physical activity counseling	Usual care (1 page of physical activity education) plus brief physician message plus individual patient-centered motivational counseling plus physical activity prescription including participant's goals (including specific type of physical activity, frequency, and intensity). Given pedometers and education materials; encouraged to maintain physical activity diary. Participants encouraged to gradually increase levels until they met the recommended ≥30 minutes of moderate-intensity physical activity on most (preferably all) days of the week, including aerobic and strength training and exercises for improved flexibility and balance. Encouraged to reduce sedentary time. Group support session to which patient was encouraged to bring family member or friend; letter with individualized advice from physician; brief phone call.
	Usual care	One page of general information about importance of physical activity for health. Baseline measurement results provided 1–2 months following assessment.
NERS, 2012[109]	Physical activity counseling	IG participated in 16-week tailored exercise program supervised by a qualified exercise professional. IG provided with 1-on-1 initial consultation with exercise professional to complete lifestyle questionnaire, health check, motivational interviewing, and physical activity goal setting using patient-centered approach, and introduction to leisure centers (sport/community centers). IG given option to take part in 1-on-1 exercise instruction or attend group classes at discounted rate (£1 per session). Primary goal was to achieve 30 minutes of moderate physical activity on ≥5 days/week. Exercise professional followed up with IG at specified time points to review goals, provided additional motivational interviewing, and support to encourage attendance and prevent relapse.
	Waitlist control	Usual care and a leaflet highlighting the benefits of exercise, including a Web site address listing locations of local leisure facilities.
PACE, 2005[131]	Physical activity counseling	Participants met with general or nurse practitioner for 10-minute consultation to discuss medical condition(s), offer advice about becoming more physically active, and assess stage of change for physical activity. Provider counseled the patient using the PACE program, the goal of which is to "promote long-term participation in regular physical activity by altering social and psychological factors known to influence physical activity, such as social support, increased self-efficacy, reduced perceived barriers, and increased awareness of the benefits of physical activity." Providers received 1-hour individualized training on PACE approach to increase knowledge and coach on use of PACE materials. PACE physical activity counselors (separate from general/nurse practitioner) provided 2 "booster" phone call consultations (2 and 8 weeks after initial visit), to offer support and resolve possible problems or questions. After initial visit, 1 followup visit with provider (4 weeks), where they focused on stage-specific protocols and checked on participant progress. At 4-week visit, offered new counseling protocol for those who had either progressed or regressed through stages of change.
	Usual care	General practitioners discussed patient's current level of physical activity and, as appropriate, encouraged patient to become more active. Standard text on physical activity promotion was provided.

Appendix E. Intervention Descriptions of Included Studies by Intervention Focus and Intensity

Author, Year	Intervention	Description
Green Prescription Programme, 2003[123]	Physical activity counseling	Primary care clinicians (medical doctors and nurses) received 4 hours of training on how to use motivational interviewing techniques to advise on physical activity and the "green prescription." Following screening, patients given a prompt card with their stage of change, which they gave to their primary care provider (doctor [85%] or nurse [15%]) during their upcoming consultation. The prompt card cues clinician to discuss increasing physical activity and to set appropriate goals with the participant (usually home-based physical activity or walking). Goals are written on a green prescription, given to participant, and faxed to local sports foundation, along with details such as age, weight, health conditions. Exercise specialists from the foundation then call the patient ≥3 times in the next 3 months to encourage and support physical activity through motivational interviewing. Participants receive quarterly newsletters from the sports foundation about physical activity initiatives in the community; interested participants also receive other motivational materials, such as information on specific exercise programs. Clinician staff from general practice are encouraged to provide feedback to the patient during subsequent visits.
	Waitlist control	Usual care.
Moreau 2001[104]	Physical activity counseling	Walking program to reduce blood pressure. IG were given pedometers at baseline and instructed how to wear (belt or waistband, morning to bedtime). After 1–2 week baseline measurement, IG provided a target goal to gradually increase the distance they walked (from 1.4 km over baseline to a 3-km increase in walking by week 3, as recommended by the American College of Sports Medicine and the Centers for Disease Control and Prevention). Walking steps recorded on daily log sheets with other physical activities and turned in every 2 weeks. IG presented to laboratory for measurements at 3 time points: baseline, 12 weeks, and 24 weeks.
	No advice	CG asked not to change daily activity and wore pedometer for 1 week each month to document their walking.

Abbreviations: AHA = American Heart Association; ATP = Adult Treatment Panel; BMI = body mass index; CG = control group; CME = continued medical education; CVD = cardiovascular disease; IG = intervention group; IT = information technology; JNC = Joint National Committee; NCEP = National Cholesterol Education Program; NHLBI = National Heart, Lung, and Blood Institute.

Appendix F Figure 1. Pooled Analysis of Total Cholesterol in All Risk Groups Combined, Sorted by Intervention Intensity

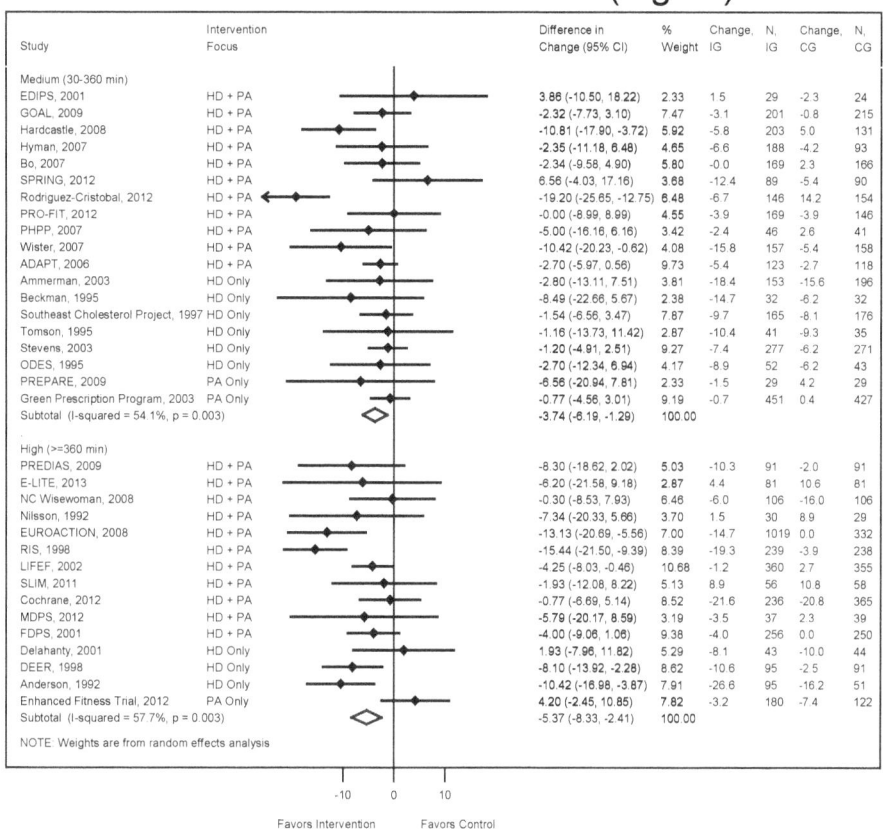

Appendix F Figure 2. Pooled Analysis of Total Cholesterol in All Risk Groups Combined, Sorted by Intervention Intensity and Excluding Physical Activity–Only Interventions

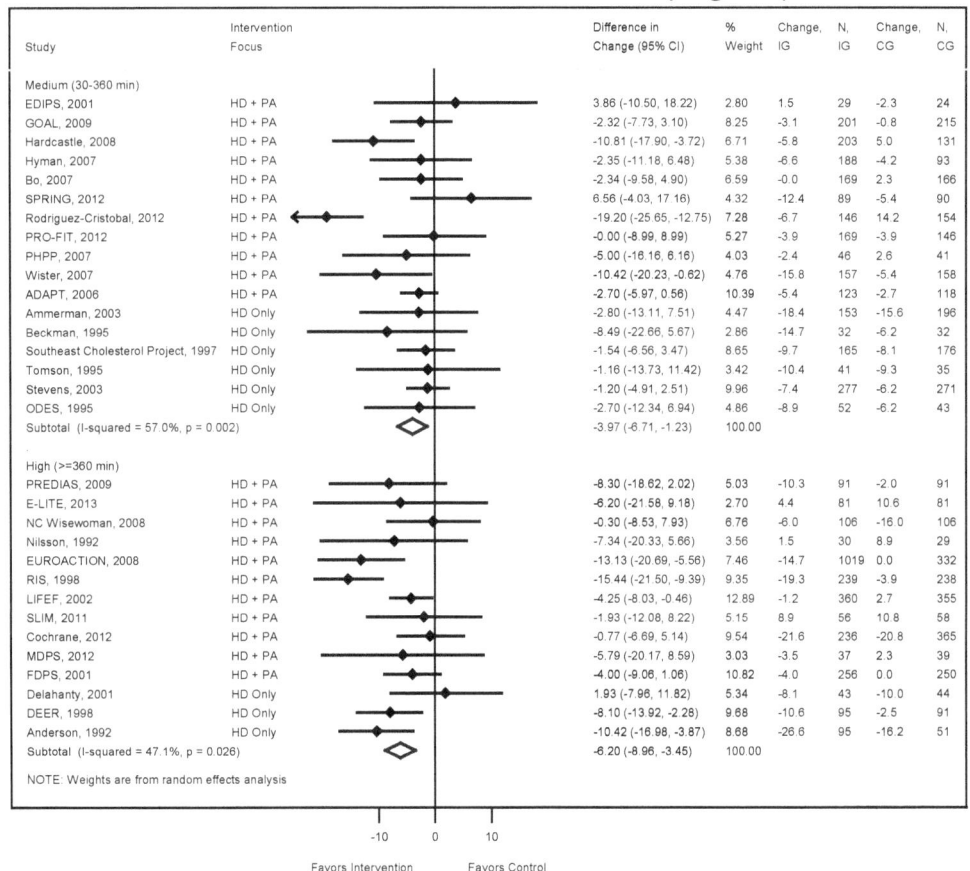

Appendix F Figure 3. Pooled Analysis of Low-Density Lipoprotein Cholesterol in All Risk Groups Combined, Sorted by Intervention Intensity

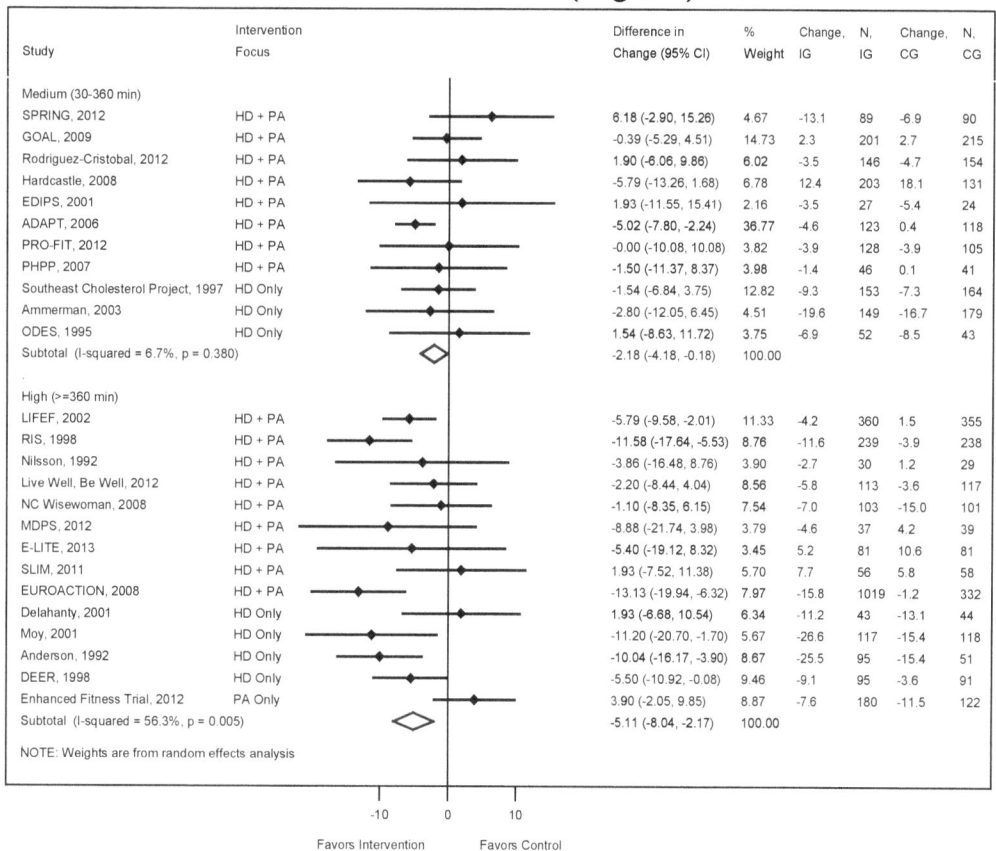

Appendix F Figure 4. Pooled Analysis of Low-Density Lipoprotein Cholesterol in All Risk Groups Combined, Sorted by Intervention Intensity and Excluding Physical Activity–Only Interventions

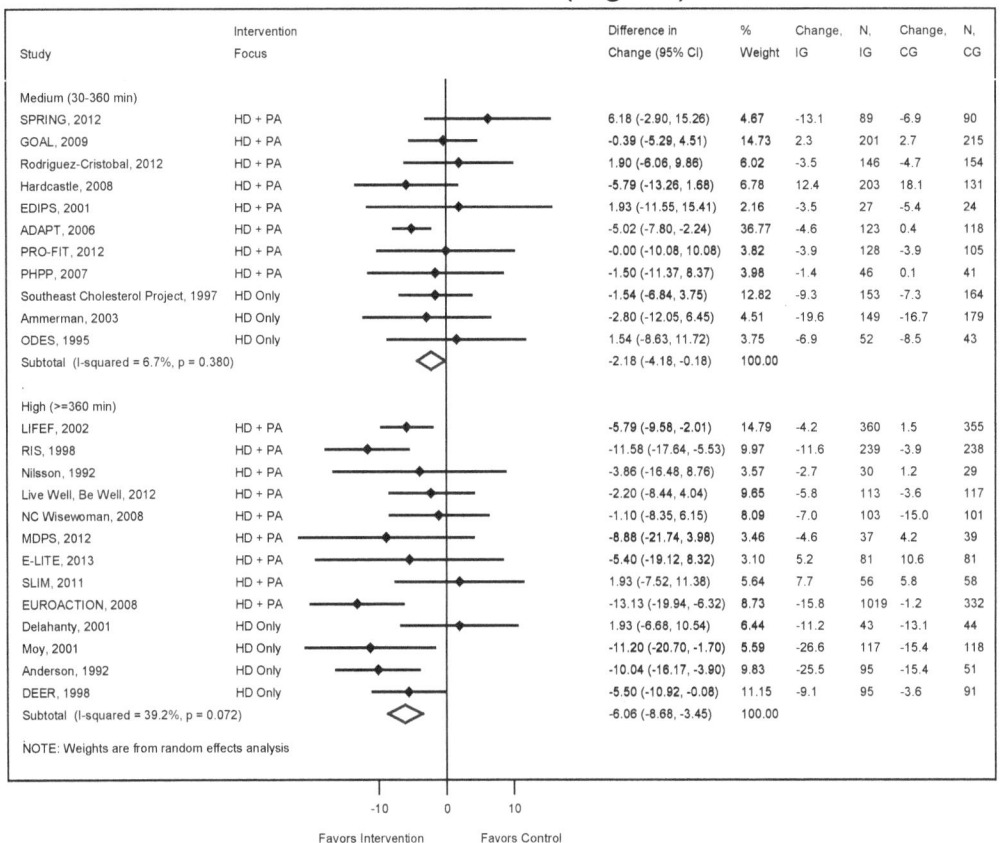

Appendix F Figure 5. Pooled Analysis of Systolic Blood Pressure in All Risk Groups Combined, Sorted by Intervention Intensity

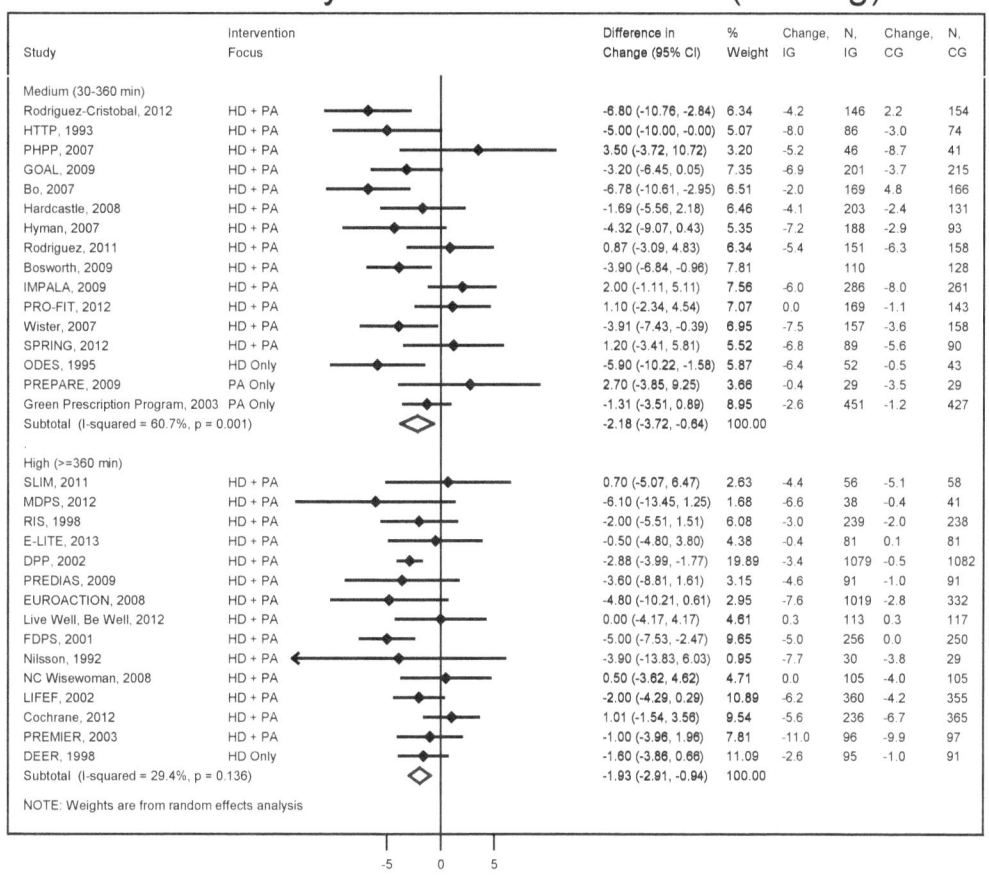

Appendix F Figure 6. Pooled Analysis of Systolic Blood Pressure in All Risk Groups Combined, Sorted by Intervention Intensity and Excluding Physical Activity–Only Interventions

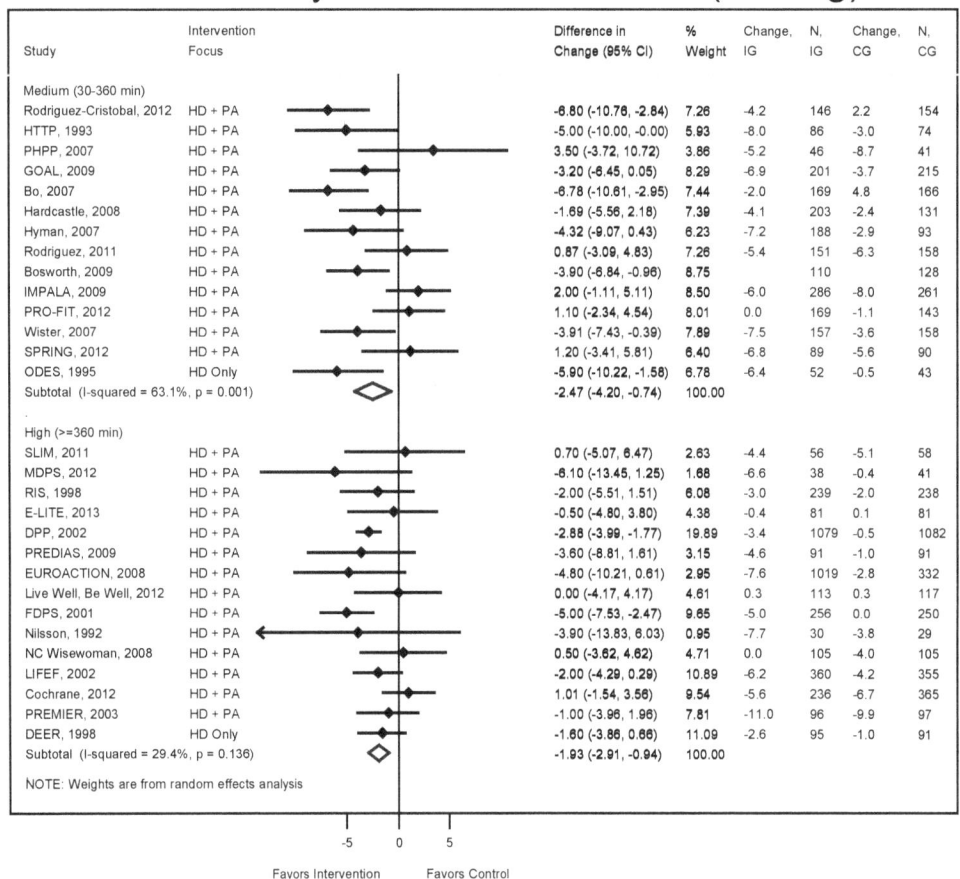

Appendix F Figure 7. Pooled Analysis of Diastolic Blood Pressure in All Risk Groups Combined, Sorted by Intervention Intensity

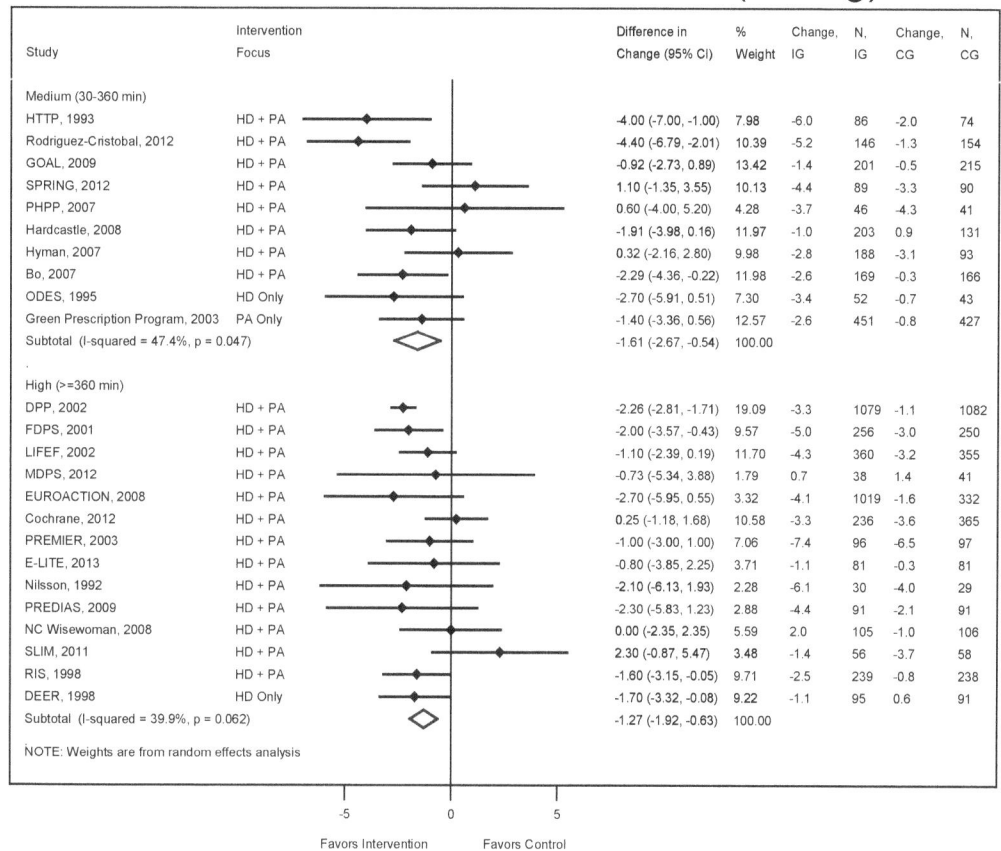

Appendix F Figure 8. Pooled Analysis of Diastolic Blood Pressure in All Risk Groups Combined, Sorted by Intervention Intensity and Excluding Physical Activity–Only Interventions

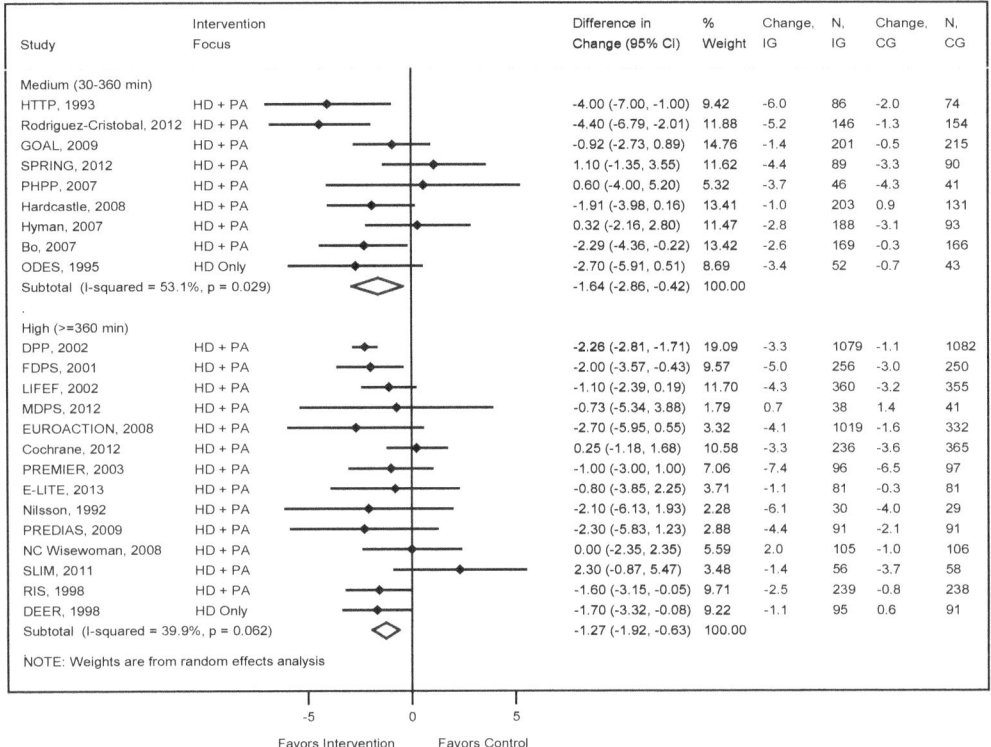

Appendix F Figure 9. Pooled Analysis of Fasting Glucose in All Risk Groups Combined, Sorted by Intervention Intensity

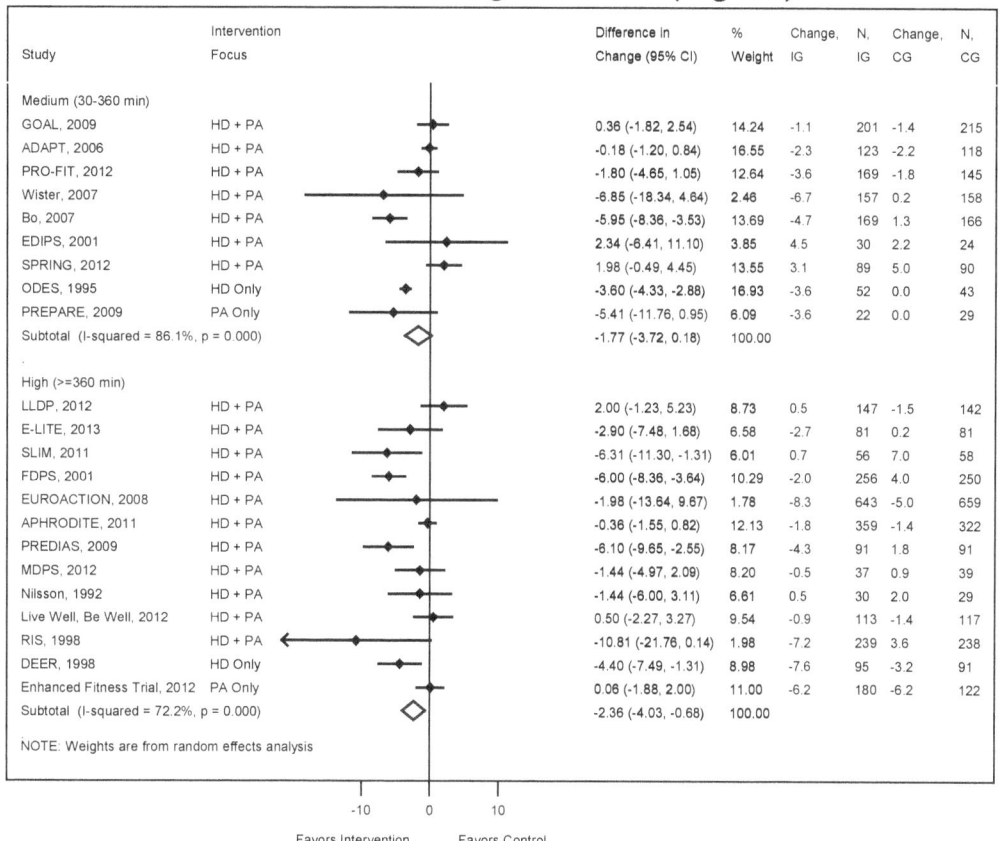

Appendix F Figure 10. Pooled Analysis of Fasting Glucose in All Risk Groups Combined, Sorted by Intervention Intensity and Excluding Physical Activity–Only Interventions

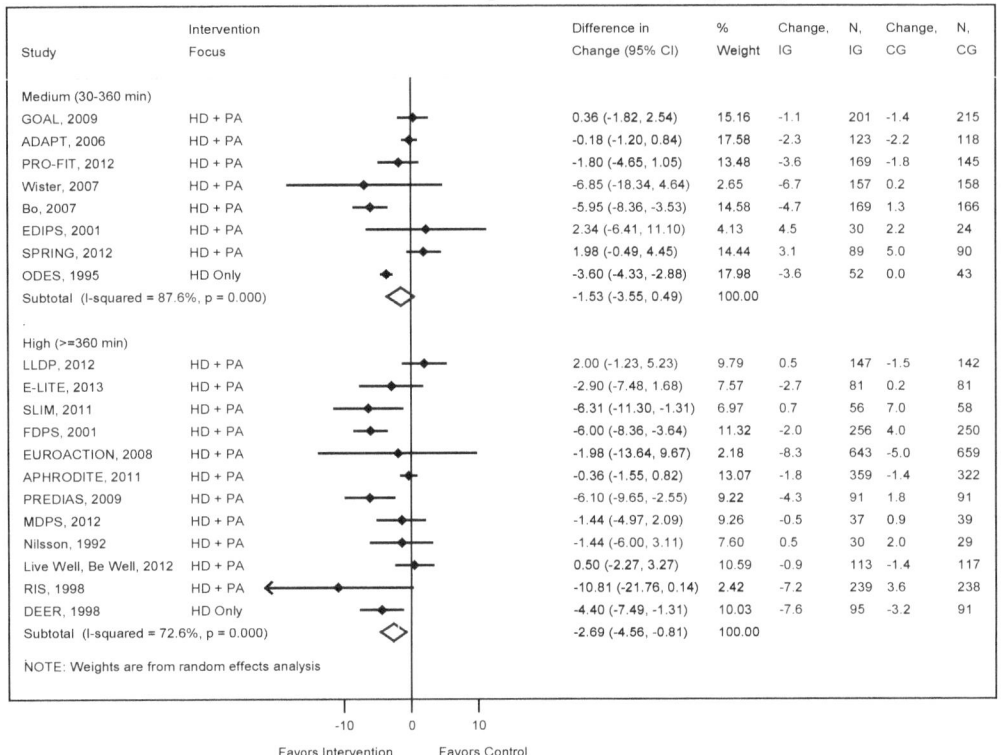

Appendix F Figure 11. Pooled Analysis of Adiposity in All Risk Groups Combined, Sorted by Intervention Intensity

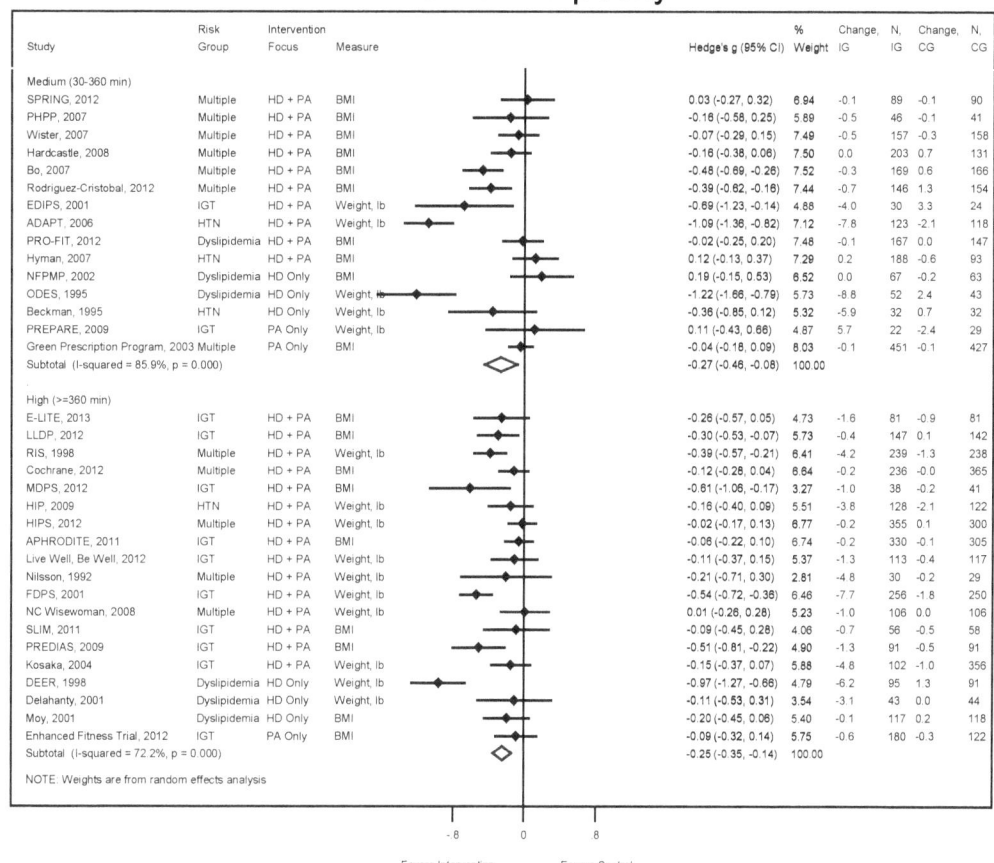

Appendix F Figure 12. Pooled Analysis of Adiposity in All Risk Groups Combined, Sorted by Intervention Intensity and Excluding Physical Activity–Only Interventions

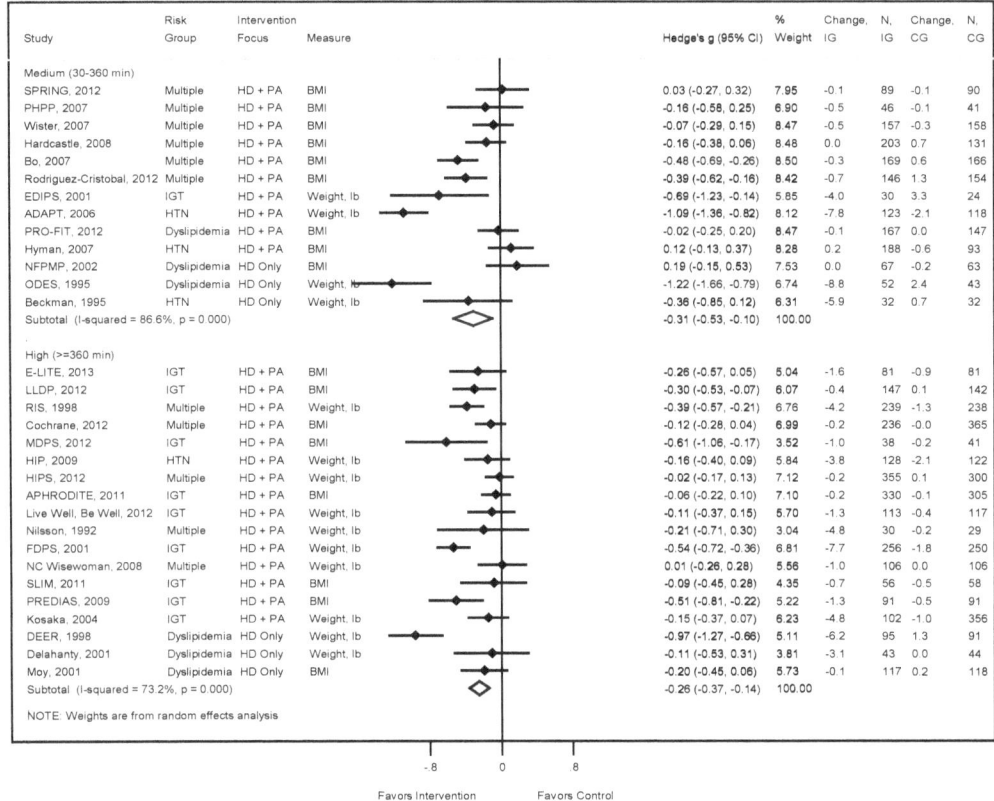

Appendix G Table 1. Health Outcomes (KQ 1 Results): Cardiovascular Disease

Study, Year Quality	N Population Intervention Focus & Intensity	Stroke, MI, TIA	CVD, CVD-Related Mortality, All-Cause Mortality
PREMIER, 2003[116] Good	304 HTN HD+PA, High	N (%) **Stroke, 6 mo:** IG1 0 (0) IG2 0 (0) CG (0.39) **TIA, 6 mo:** IG1 0 (0) IG2 0 (0) CG 1 (0.39) **MI, 6 mo:** IG1 0 (0) IG2 1 (0.40) CG 1 (0.39)	
TONE, 1998[117] Good	975 HTN HD+PA, High	N (%) **Stroke, 29 mo:** IG1 1 (0.3) IG2 0 (0.0) IG3 1 (0.7) CG 2 (0.6) p for IG1+IG3 vs. IG2+CG >0.99 p for IG2+IG3 vs. IG1+CG >0.99 **TIA, 29 mo:** IG1 8 (2.3) IG2 0 (0.0) IG3 1 (0.7) CG 8 (2.3) p for IG1+IG3 vs. IG2+CG=0.80 p for IG2+IG3 vs. IG1+CG=0.37 **MI, 29 mo:** IG1 2 (0.6) IG2 2 (1.4) IG3 2 (1.4) CG 4 (1.2) p for IG1+IG3 vs. IG2+CG >0.99 p for IG2+IG3 vs. IG1+CG >0.99 **Angina, 29 mo:** IG1 10 (2.9) IG2 10 (6.8) IG3 10 (6.8) CG 19 (5.6) p for IG1+IG3 vs. IG2+CG=0.16 p for IG2+IG3 vs. IG1+CG=0.07	N (%) **CHF, 29 mo:** IG1 4 (1.2) IG2 1 (0.7) IG3 0 (0.0) CG 1 (0.3) p for IG1+IG3 vs. IG2+CG >0.99 p for IG2+IG3 vs.IG1+CG >0.99 **Other CVD, 29 mo:** IG1 13 (3.8) IG2 6 (4.1) IG3 8 (5.4) CG 19 (5.6) p for IG1+IG3 vs. IG2+CG=0.44 p for IG2+IG3 vs. IG1+CG >0.99 **Total CVD, 29 mo:** IG1 44 (12.9) IG2 21 (14.3) IG3 23 (15.6) CG 57 (16.7) p for IG1+IG3 vs. IG2+CG=0.24 p for IG2+IG3 vs. IG1+CG=0.35

Appendix G Table 1. Health Outcomes (KQ 1 Results): Cardiovascular Disease

Study, Year Quality	N Population Intervention Focus & Intensity	Stroke, MI, TIA	CVD, CVD-Related Mortality, All-Cause Mortality
DPP, 2002[89] Good	2,161 IFG HD+PA, High		**CVD-related deaths, 3 y (n):** IG 2 CG 4 P=NR **Nonfatal CVD events*, 3 y (%; events per 1,000 p-y):** IG 2.2%; 9.7 CG 1.7%; 7.3 p=NS (exact value NR)
FDPS, 2001[118] Good	522 IFG HD+PA, High		**Death rate per 1,000 p-y, 10.6 y (n):** IG 2.2 (95% CI, 1.0–4.9) CG 3.8 (95% CI, 2.0–7.0) HR=0.57 (95% CI, 0.21–1.58) **CVD event rate per 1,000 p-y, 10.2 y (n):** IG 22.9 (95% CI, 17.7–29.7) CG 22.0 (95% CI, 16.9–28.7) HR=1.04 (95% CI, 0.72–1.51)
RIS, 1998[112] Good	508 Mixed HD+PA, High	N (%) 1 y 3.3 y 6.6 y **MI, fatal and nonfatal:** IG NR 18 (7) NR CG NR 22 (9) NR RR (95% CI) 0.8 (0.5–1.5) NR p NR 0.64 NR **Stroke, fatal and nonfatal:** IG NR 5 (2) 16 (6.3) CG NR 17 (7) 29 (11.4) RR (95% CI) 0.3 (0.11–0.81) 0.53 (0.29–0.97) p NR 0.017 NR **All first events at 6.6 y:** Fatal MI: IG 7 (2.8) CG 10 (3.9) Nonfatal MI: IG 22 (8.7) CG 25 (9.8)	N (%) 1 y 3.3 y 6.6 y **Total mortality:** IG 5 (2.0) 14 (6) 41 (16.2) CG 6 (2.4) 21 (8) 64 (25.1) RR (95% CI) 0.7 (0.4–1.3) 0.62 (0.42–0.92) p NR 0.30 0.021 **CVD mortality:** IG NR 12 (5) 24 (9.5) CG NR 13 (5) 42 (16.5) RR (95% CI) 0.9 (0.4–1.9) 0.56 (0.34–0.92) p NR 0.98 NR **All first cardiovascular events at 6.6 y:** Sudden death: IG 6 (2.4) CG 7 (2.7) All CVD events: IG 63 (24.9) CG 84 (32.9) RR 0.71 (95% CI, 0.51–0.99)

Abbreviations: CG = control group; CHF = congestive heart failure; CI = confidence interval; CVD = cardiovascular disease; DPP = Diabetes Prevention Program; FDPS = Finnish Diabetes Prevention Study; HD = healthy diet; HR = hazard ratio; HTN = hypertension; IFG = impaired fasting glucose; IG = intervention group; MI = myocardial infarction; N = number; NR = not reported; NS = not significant; PA = physical activity; p-y = person-years; RIS = Risk Factor Intervention Study; RR = relative risk; TIA = transischemic attack; TONE = Trial of Non-Pharmacological Interventions in the Elderly.

Appendix G Table 2. Health Outcomes (KQ 1 Results): Self-Reported Quality of Life and Depression Symptoms

Study, Year Quality	N Population Intervention Focus & Intensity	Self-Reported QOL	Self-Reported Depression
DPP, 2002[89] Good	2,161 IFG HD+PA, High	**Mean change on SF-6D (SD)** IG vs. CG at 3.2 y: 0.0084 (0.0041); p<0.05 Physical component summary, IG vs. CG at 3.2 y: 1.57 (0.30); p<0.01 Mental component summary, IG vs. CG at 3.2 y: -0.29 (0.32); p=NR	
HLC, 2011[92] Fair	307 IFG HD+PA, High		**Depression score (DASS-21)** BL 6 mo IG 6.29 (7.28) 5.32 (7.03) CG 6.14 (7.33) 4.87 (6.78) p=NS

Live Well, Be Well, 2012[86]
Good
	230
	IFG
	HD+PA, High
		BL mean (SE), within group change (SE)
		Self-Rated Health
		    BL 6 mo 12 mo
		IG 3.1 (0.1) 0.3 (0.1) 0.1 (0.1)
		CG 2.9 (0.1) 0.1 (0.1) 0.1 (0.1)
		p=0.05 at 6 mo; NS at 12 mo
		Psychological Well-Being II
		    BL 6 mo 12 mo
		IG 3.7 (0.07) 0.01 (0.05) 0.07 (0.06)
		CG 3.75 (0.07) -0.14 (0.05) -0.09 (0.06)
		p=0.05 at 6 mo and p=0.04 at 12 mo compared to CG	

LLDP, 2012[94] Good	312 IFG HD+PA, High		**Depression score** BL 1 yr IG 16.37 (12.3) -1.0 (-3.0 to 1.0) CG 15.20 (10.3) -1.0 (-2.0 to 1.0) Intervention effect (95% CI): 0 (-2.0 to 2.0); p=0.98
Melbourne DPS, 2012[85] Fair	92 IFG HD+PA, High	**Hospital Anxiety & Depression Scale** BL Δ 12 mo p **Depression score** IG 3.16 (2.35) 0.18 (0.34) 0.876 CG 2.91 (2.84) 0.02 (0.27) **Anxiety score** IG 6.08 (3.35) -0.68 (0.38) 0.467 CG 5.15 (3.18) 0.08 (0.34)	

PREDIAS, 2009[95]
Fair
	182
	IFG
	HD+PA, High
		WHO-5 Psychological Well-Being
		    BL 12 mo Change
		IG 15.3 (5.1) 16.7 (4.8) 1.4 (3.9)
		CG 14.3 (4.9) 14.3 (5.1) 0.0 (4.2)
		p=0.101
			Depression score (CES-D), %
			    BL 12 mo Change
			IG 12.0 (9.5) 9.8 (7.5) -2.2 (7.7)
			CG 13.7 (8.2) 11.4 (7.8) -2.3 (6.8)
			p=0.876

Appendix G Table 2. Health Outcomes (KQ 1 Results): Self-Reported Quality of Life and Depression Symptoms

Study, Year Quality	N Population Intervention Focus & Intensity	Self-Reported QOL	Self-Reported Depression
Enhanced Fitness Trial, 2012[98] Fair+	302 IFG PA, High	**SF-36** **General health** BL 3 mo 12 mo IG 61.39 (39.40) 59.84 (42.59) 58.12 (42.29) CG 65.78 (39.52) 66.37 (42.75) 61.68 (41.82) p=0.92 indicating NS differences for group-by-time interactions **Physical function** IG 62.94 (20.97) 63.97 (21.30) 62.52 (21.79) CG 66.88 (20.60) 67.08 (19.86) 66.24 (20.91) p=0.09 indicating NS differences for group-by-time interactions	
Nilsson, 1992[119] Fair	63 Mixed HD+PA, High	Health status, Visual Analogue Scale, mean (SD), at 12 mo IG 72.8 (3.5) CG 54.5 (3.6) p <0.001	
PEGASE, 2008[120] Fair	640 Mixed HD+PA, High	**SF-36** BL 6 mo p **Mental component** IG NR 0.53 NS CG NR 0.69 **Physical component** IG NR 2.57 NR* CG NR -0.5	
WISEWOMAN NC, 2008[110] Fair	236 Mixed HD+PA, High	**SF-8** **Physical component score** BL 6 mo 12 mo IG 49 (0.9) 49 (0.8) 48 (0.8) CG 47 (0.9) 48 (0.8) 48 (0.8) Diff 01.7 (1.1) -0.1 (1.1) p 0.12 0.92 **Mental component score** IG 48 (1.0) 50 (0.8) 50 (0.8) CG 48 (0.9) 50 (0.9) 50 (0.9) Diff -0.6 (1.2) 0.4 (1.2) p 0.60 0.77	
PHPP, 2007[121] Fair	99 Mixed HD+PA, Medium	GHQ-30 score, mean (SD) BL 12 mo IG 4.4 (4.1) 3.1 (3.4) CG 4.0 (3.3) 4.0 (4.2) p=NS	

Appendix G Table 2. Health Outcomes (KQ 1 Results): Self-Reported Quality of Life and Depression Symptoms

Study, Year Quality	N Population Intervention Focus & Intensity	Self-Reported QOL	Self-Reported Depression
PAC, 2011[122] Fair	120 Mixed PA, Medium	**SF-12** BL 13 wk 25 wk **Physical dimension** IG 46.3(6.0) 48.2(6.9) 47.4(6.0) CG 46.0(6.4) 47.1(6.3) 47.1(6.1) **Mental dimension** IG 44.0(5.2) 44.4(5.4) 44.8(6.3) CG 46.0(4.7) 45.2(6.0) 44.8(5.7) p=NS at all time points	

Abbreviations: BL = baseline; CES-D = Center for Epidemiologic Studies Depression Scale; CG = control group; CI = confidence interval; DASS = Depression Anxiety Stress Scale; Diff = difference; DPP = Diabetes Prevention Program; DPS = Diabetes Prevention Study; GHQ = General Health Questionnaire; HD = healthy diet; HLC = healthy lifestyle characteristics; IFG = impaired fasting glucose; IG = intervention group; LLDP = Late Life Depression Prevention; N = number; NR = not reported; NS = not significant; PA = physical activity; PAC = Physical Activity Counselling; PREDIAS = Prevention of Diabetes Self-Management Program; PHPP = Patient-motivated Health Promotion Program; QOL = quality of life; SD = standard deviation; SE = standard error; SF = Short Form; WHO = World Health Organization.

Appendix G Table 3. Behavioral Outcomes (KQ 3 Results): Healthy Diet

Study, Year Quality	N Population Intervention Focus & Intensity	Healthy Diet Behavioral Outcomes		
		BL	6 mo	11 mo
CouPLES, 2013[67] Fair	255 Cholesterol HD+PA, Medium	**Energy, kcal/d** IG 1596 (827) CG 1475 (735) p=0.03 **Total fat, g/d** IG 68.8 (42.7) CG 64.9 (38.1) p=0.02 **Total fat, %** IG 38.2 (7.8) CG 38.4 (7.5) p=0.04 **Saturated fat, g/d** IG 22.5 (14.8) CG 21.3 (12.6) p=0.02 **Saturated fat, %** IG 12.3 (2.9) CG 12.6 (2.7) p=0.09 **Cholesterol, mg/d** IG 210.5 (145.5) CG 211.0 (140.6) p=0.11 **Fiber, g/d** IG 14.8 (6.8) CG 13.9 (6.7) p=0.26	1243 (670) 1245 (588) 49.6 (30.1) 53.1 (28.4) 35.3 (7.0) 38.5 (8.9) 15.8 (10.3) 17.2 (9.6) 11.1 (2.9) 12.5 (3.3) 161.6 (111.1) 182.1 (119.4) 13.4 (6.8) 12.5 (7.7)	1175 (579) 1254 (575) 46.5 (25.6) 54.2 (31.1) 35.4 (7.3) 38.2 (9.1) 15.1 (8.9) 17.4 (9.8) 11.4 (2.8) 12.3 (2.9) 152.1 (97.4) 175.5 (117.1) 13.2 (6.3) 11.9 (5.7)
PRO-FIT, 2012[68] Fair	340 Cholesterol HD+PA, Medium	BL	12 mo	
		Total saturated fat, g/d, mean (SD) IG 15.4 (4.8) CG 14.3 (4.9) Between-group difference at 12 mo: NS (β, -0.61 [-1.35 to 0.14]) **Daily frequency of fruits (servings/d)** IG 1.5 (1.3) CG 1.4 (1.1) Between-group difference at 12 mo: NS (β, 0.05 [-0.12 to 0.22]) **Daily vegetable intake (g/d)** IG 162.1 (75.8) CG 151.2 (77.8) Between-group difference at 12 mo: NS (β, 3.26 [-9.78 to 16.29])	14.0 (5.0) 13.7 (4.6) 1.6 (1.1) 1.4 (1.1) 171.5 (76.6) 163.4 (77.2)	

Appendix G Table 3. Behavioral Outcomes (KQ 3 Results): Healthy Diet

Study, Year Quality	N Population Intervention Focus & Intensity	Healthy Diet Behavioral Outcomes		
		BL	12 mo	Mean difference from BL to 12 mo
Anderson, 1992[70] Fair	177 Cholesterol HD, High	**Energy (kJ), mean (SE)**		
		IG1 8221 (824)	7878 (318)	-343 (280)
		IG2 8678 (335)	8523 (314)	-115 (331)
		CG 9109 (393)	8414 (310)	-695 (364)
		p NSD	NSD	NSD
		% Carbohydrate, mean (SE)		
		IG1 48 (1.3)	53 (1.3)	4.5 (1.2)
		IG2 50 (0.9)	55 (1.0)*	5.3 (1.1)
		CG 48 (1.3)	50 (1.1)	1.4 (1.3)
		p NSD	0.004	NSD
		% Fat, mean (SE)		
		IG1 35 (1.0)	30 (1.1)	-5.0 (1.0)
		IG2 33 (0.9)	27 (0.9)	-5.6 (1.2)
		CG 33 (1.0)	31 (0.8)	-2.0 (1.1)†
		p NSD	0.022	0.040
		% Saturated fatty acid, mean (SE)		
		IG1 11 (0.5)	9 (0.4)	-2.0 (0.4)
		IG2 11 (0.4)	8 (0.4)	-3.0 (0.5)
		CG 11 (0.5)	10 (0.4)	-1.0 (0.5)†
		p NSD	0.001	0.013
		% Monounsaturated fatty acid, mean (SE)		
		IG1 12 (0.5)	11 (0.5)	-2.0 (0.5)
		IG2 12 (0.4)	10 (0.4)	-2.0 (0.5)
		CG 11 (0.4)	11 (0.5)	0.0 (0.5)†
		p NSD	NSD	0.025
		% Polyunsaturated fatty acid, mean (SD)		
		IG1 8 (0.4)	8 (0.4)	0.0 (0.5)
		IG2 8 (0.3)	7 (0.3)	-1.0 (0.4)
		CG 7 (0.4)	7 (0.4)	0.0 (0.4)
		p NSD	NSD	NSD
		% Protein, mean (SD)		
		IG1 16 (0.5)	17 (0.5)	1.0 (0.5)
		IG2 17 (0.5)	18 (0.5)	0.6 (0.6)
		CG 16 (0.5)	18 (0.6)	1.2 (0.7)
		p NSD	NSD	NSD
		Dietary cholesterol, mg, mean (SD)		
		IG1 247 (18)	178 (12)	-69 (18)
		IG2 261 (18)	194 (14)	-67 (18)
		CG 267 (21)	219 (13)	-48 (18)
		p NSD	NSD	NSD
		Fiber, g, mean (SD)		
		IG1 17 (1.1)	20 (1.3)	3.0 (1.3)
		IG2 19 (1.6)‡	25 (1.6)*	5.6 (1.9)*

Appendix G Table 3. Behavioral Outcomes (KQ 3 Results): Healthy Diet

Study, Year Quality	N Population Intervention Focus & Intensity	Healthy Diet Behavioral Outcomes
Ammerman, 2003[74] Keyserling, 1999[173] Fair	468 Cholesterol HD, Medium	CG 17 (1.4) 17 (1.3) 0.1 (1.4) p NSD 0.001 0.40 *p<0.05 vs. CG; †p<0.05 vs. IG1/IG2; ‡p<0.01 vs. CG. BL 12 mo Daily Recommended Allowance total score, mean reduction (SE) IG 23.1 (1.1) 5.4 (0.48) CG 21.9 (1.1) 3.3 (0.43) Difference: p=0.47 2.1 (95% CI, 0.8 to 3.5), p=0.005 Adjusted by age, sex, race, education, CHD, # of risk factors, smoking, and high blood pressure
Bloemberg, 1991[75] Fair	80 Cholesterol HD, Medium	Mean (SD) at BL, mean change from BL (SD) BL 6 mo % Protein energy IG 15.2 (3.0) 0.33 (2.9) CG 13.8 (2.4) 0.57 (1.7) p <0.05 0.66 % Fat energy IG 38.5 (7.1) -5.0 (6.5) CG 38.3 (9.0) -1.5 (5.9) p NSD 0.02 % Saturated fat energy IG 16.5 (3.6) -4.3 (3.9) CG 16.3 (4.7) -0.7 (2.9) p NSD <0.01 % Monounsaturated fatty acid energy IG 14.2 (3.2) -3.0 (3.4) CG 14.0 (3.2) -0.6 (2.6) p NSD <0.01 % Polyunsaturated fatty acid energy IG 6.8 (2.4) 2.8 (3.1) CG 6.6 (2.9) 0.0 (1.5) p NSD <0.01 % Carbohydrate energy IG 38.5 (5.7) 4.4 (6.5) CG 38.5 (8.4) 1.2 (6.1) p NSD 0.03 Cholesterol, mg/mJ IG 33.5 (6.8) -9.7 (8.2) CG 30.7 (9.4) -0.2 (7.2) p NSD <0.01 Fiber, g/mJ IG 2.4 (0.7) 0.6 (0.9) CG 2.5 (0.7) 0.1 (0.8) p NSD <0.01

Appendix G Table 3. Behavioral Outcomes (KQ 3 Results): Healthy Diet

Study, Year Quality	N Population Intervention Focus & Intensity	Healthy Diet Behavioral Outcomes
DEER, 1998[71]	189 Cholesterol HD, High	**Mean change (SD)** BL 12 mo **Caloric intake, kcal/d** IG NR -253.7 (459.2) CG NR -21.9 (426.4) **% Calories from carbohydrates** IG NR 6.8 (8.7) CG NR 0.5 (6.9) **% Calories from fat** IG NR -6.9 (7.8) CG NR -0.5 (6.3) **% Calories from saturated fat** IG NR -2.9 (3.0) CG NR 0.1 (2.6) **% Calories from monounsaturated fatty acid** IG NR -2.5 (3.4) CG NR 0.0 (3.0) **% Calories from polyunsaturated fatty acid** IG NR -1.1 (2.2) CG NR -0.5 (2.1) **Cholesterol, mg/d** IG NR -85.1 (106.8) CG NR 3.9 (105.2)
Delahanty, 2001[72] Good	90 Cholesterol HD, High	**Mean (SD)** 　　　BL　　　　6 mo　　　　12 mo **Kcal** IG 1987 (841) 1679 (796) 1462 (472) CG 1888 (585) 1850 (675) 1675 (522) **% Fat** IG 32 (12) 25 (10)* 26 (10) CG 31 (11) 29 (10) 28 (9) **% Saturated fat** IG 11 (6) 7 (4)† 8 (4) CG 11 (4) 10 (4) 10 (4) **% Monounsaturated fatty acid** IG 12 (5) 9 (4)* 10 (4) CG 12 (5) 11 (4) 10 (4) **% Polyunsaturated fatty acid** IG 6 (4) 7 (4) 5 (3) CG 6 (3) 5 (2) 6 (2) **Cholesterol, mg** IG 235 (191) 165 (132)‡ 166 (154) CG 242 (229) 239 (199) 179 (123)

Appendix G Table 3. Behavioral Outcomes (KQ 3 Results): Healthy Diet

Study, Year Quality	N Population Intervention Focus & Intensity	Healthy Diet Behavioral Outcomes
Hyman, 1998[76] Fair	123 Cholesterol HD, Medium	**Dietary fiber, g** BL 6 mo IG 16(9) 18(8) 16(7) CG 18(10) 16(6) 19(9) *p<0.01 between groups (adjusted for BL & sex); †p<0.001 between groups (adjusted for BL & sex); ‡p<0.05 between groups (adjusted for BL & sex).

Moy, 2001[73] Fair	235 Cholesterol HD, High	**NW Lipid Research Clinic Fat Intake Scale, mean (SD)**
		        BL 6 mo
		IG 22.5 (5.0) 20.4 (NR)
		CG 22.1 (5.2) 20.1 (NR)
		p=0.91
		
		mean (SD), mean change from BL (SD)
		        BL 24 mo
		Total fat, g
		IG 85.1 (42) -14.3 (34)
		CG 85.0 (40) 4.7 (41)
		p=0.0001
		% kcal from total fat
		IG 38.0 (7) -3.9 (8)
		CG 38.3 (8) -0.27 (7)
		p=0.0001
		Saturated fat, g
		IG 30.2 (16) -4.9 (12)
		CG 29.7 (15) 1.9 (16)
		p=0.0002
		% kcal from saturated fat
		IG NR -1.4 (3), p=0.0001 vs. BL
		CG NR -0.0064 (3), p=0.9809
		p NR 0.0005
		Cholesterol, mg
		IG 299.8 (168) -27.3 (122)
		CG 291.8 (140) 19.6 (97)
		p=0.0013
		kcal
		IG 1977 (777) -152.3 (616)
		CG 1978 (752) 114.0 (704)
		p=0.0023

NFPMP, 2002[79]	143 Cholesterol HD, Medium	mean (SD), mean change from BL (SD) BL 6 mo 12 mo **Total energy, MJ/d** IG 9.1 (2.7) -1.4 (1.9) -0.7 (3.0) CG 9.6 (2.6) -0.6 (1.8) -0.9 (2.4) p 0.25 0.01 0.09 (multilevel analysis, p=0.00) **% Fat** IG 42.1 (6.3) -7.9 (6.5) -5.6 (6.9)

Appendix G Table 3. Behavioral Outcomes (KQ 3 Results): Healthy Diet

Study, Year Quality	N Population Intervention Focus & Intensity	Healthy Diet Behavioral Outcomes
ODES, 1995[80] Fair	98 Cholesterol HD, Medium	CG 42.6 (5.2) -2.2 (4.9) -2.0 (6.7) p 0.64 0.00 0.00 (multilevel analysis, p=0.00) **% Saturated fat** IG 15.2 (2.6) -3.4 (2.7) -2.6 (2.7) CG 15.5 (2.3) -0.8 (2.2) -0.9 (2.6) p 0.42 0.00 0.00 (multilevel analysis, p=0.00) **% Monounsaturated fatty acid** IG 14.6 (3.3) -3.4 (3.3) -1.9 (4.1) CG 14.9 (2.6) -0.7 (2.4) -0.3 (3.3) p 0.53 0.00 0.01 (multilevel analysis, p=0.00) **% Unsaturated fat** IG 9.4 (3.0) -1.0 (3.1) -1.0 (2.7) CG 9.3 (3.0) -0.8 (3.0) -0.7 (3.7) p 0.79 0.37 0.73 (multilevel analysis, p=0.73) **Cholesterol, mg** IG 239.1 (91.5) -62 (68.9) -46.4 (77.1) CG 254.8 (90.8) -22.8 (66.4) -33.4 (83.1) p 0.31 0.00 0.02 (multilevel analysis, p=0.03) mean (SE), mean change from BL (SE) change at 12 mo **Total energy intake, kJ/d** IG NR -2268 (356) CG NR -589 (450) Net difference (SE): -1679 (450) p NSD <0.05 **% Fat energy** IG NR -5.5 (0.8) CG NR -0.6 (0.7) Net difference (SE): -4.9 (1.1) p NSD <0.05 **% Saturated fat, g/d** IG NR -14.0 (1.8) CG NR -1.9 (2.0) p NSD <0.05 **Energy, mJ/d** IG 11.0 (3.5) -2.2 (2.6) CG 10.3 (3.2) -0.5 (3.1) p NSD <0.01
Southeast Cholesterol Project, 1997[81] Fair	372 Cholesterol HD, Medium	Dietary Recommended Allowance score, adjusted mean (SE) from BL 　　　BL　　change 12 mo　Diff (95% CI)　　p IG　22.0 (0.55)　-5.3 (0.55)　3.3 (1.8 to 4.9)　p<0.001 CG　22.0 (0.54)　-2.0 (0.54)

Appendix G Table 3. Behavioral Outcomes (KQ 3 Results): Healthy Diet

Study, Year Quality	N Population Intervention Focus & Intensity	Healthy Diet Behavioral Outcomes
Stevens, 2003[82] Fair	616 Cholesterol HD Medium	mean (SD) BL 12 mo **% Fat energy** IG 40.60 (7.25) 34.86 (6.56) CG 39.41 (6.27) 38.61 (6.57) Difference: -3.75; p<0.001 **Number of fruit/vegetable servings** IG 3.09 (1.76) 4.33 (1.90) CG 3.21 (1.97) 3.40 (1.90) Difference: 0.93; p<0.001 **Kristal fat behavior score** IG 1.97 (0.45) 1.70 (0.28) CG 1.87 (0.37) 1.91 (0.28) Difference: -0.20; p<0.001 **% Saturated fat energy** IG 14.0 12.4 CG 13.6 13.2 p NR <0.001 **% Polyunsaturated fat energy** IG 8.3 6.7 CG 8.1 7.5 p NR <0.001 **% Monounsaturated fat energy** IG 15.2 13.1 CG 14.8 14.0 p NR <0.001
ADAPT, 2006[138] Fair	241 HTN HD+PA, Medium	Mean (95% CI) BL 12 mo 36 mo **Energy, MJ** IG 8.04 (7.61–8.47) 6.74 (6.38–7.11) 7.65 (7.21–8.09) CG 7.91 (7.45–8.37) 7.08 (6.64–7.53) 7.44 (7.02–7.85) **Fat, % energy** IG 28.9 (27.8–29.9) 25.3 (24.2–26.4)‡ 27.9 (26.4–29.4) CG 28.8 (27.6–30.1) 28.5 (27.2–29.8) 29.1 (27.5–30.6) **Saturated fat, % energy** IG 12.3 (11.3–13.3) 9.4 (8.9–10.0)‡ 10.8 (10.1–11.5)† CG 12.0 (11.0–13.1) 11.4 (10.4–12.4) 11.4 (10.6–12.1) **Polyunsaturated fat, % energy** IG 4.6 (4.2–4.9) 4.4 (4.0–4.7) 4.6 (4.2–4.9) CG 4.8 (4.4–5.2) 4.6 (4.2–5.0) 4.5 (4.1–4.8) **Monounsaturated fat, % energy** IG 10.6 (9.7–11.6) 8.7 (8.2–9.2)‡ 9.9 (9.3–10.5) CG 10.7 (9.8–11.7) 10.8 (9.9–11.7) 10.5 (9.8–11.2)

Appendix G Table 3. Behavioral Outcomes (KQ 3 Results): Healthy Diet

Study, Year Quality	N Population Intervention Focus & Intensity	Healthy Diet Behavioral Outcomes
		Cholesterol, mg/d IG 292.7 (263.2–322.2) 250.4 (223.5–277.3) 279.7 (249.5–309.9) CG 278.8 (254.8–302.9) 251.2 (225.5–277.0) 265.2 (242.0–288.5) **Fiber, g/d** IG 24.0 (22.6–25.3) 26.3 (24.6–28.0)* 24.2 (22.7–25.6) CG 24.1 (22.8–22.5) 24.2 (22.5–25.8) 24.1 (22.8–25.5) **Protein, % energy** IG 19.5 (18.9–20.1) 22.4 (21.7–23.2)† 20.8 (20.1–21.5) CG 20.2 (19.4–20.7) 21.1 (20.3–21.9) 21.1 (20.3–21.8) **Carbohydrates, % energy** IG 44.3 (43.0–45.6) 45.7 (44.3–47.0)* 45.0 (43.6–46.4) CG 44.4 (42.9–45.9) 43.9 (42.4–45.4) 45.3 (43.8–46.7) **Sodium, g/d** IG 2.7 (2.5–2.8) 2.3 (2.2–2.5)* 2.5 (2.3–2.6) CG 2.8 (2.6–2.9) 2.6 (2.4–2.8) 2.7 (2.5–2.8) *Servings per week* **Low-fat dairy** IG 5.8 (5.0–6.7) 7.4 (6.5–8.3) CG 7.0 (6.0–8.0) 7.1 (5.8–8.0) **Fish** IG 2.7 (2.2–3.2) 5.1 (4.5–5.7) CG 2.7 (2.2–3.2) 3.3 (2.8–3.8) **Meat** IG 3.6 (3.1–4.1) 2.7 (2.2–3.2) CG 3.4 (2.8–3.9) 2.9 (2.4–3.4) **Fruit** IG 11.9 (10.5–13.3) 12.6 (11.2–14.0) CG 13.3 (11.9–14.7) 12.6 (11.2–14.0) **Vegetables** IG 18.2 (16.8–19.6) 23.1 (21.0–24.5) CG 18.9 (17.5–20.3) 19.6 (18.2–21.0) Between group p-values compared with BL: *p<0.05; †p<0.01; ‡p<0.001. At 36 mo there was a significant between-group difference in consumption of vegetables (p=0.003) & fish (p=0.007). Greater intake of fruit was NS (p=0.138). 65% of CG and 83% of IG ate ≥2 fish servings/week (p=0.001); 37% of CG and 46% of IG ate ≥5 servings of fruit & vegetables/day (p=0.147).
Arroll, 1995[128] Fair	208 HTN HD+PA, Medium	**Salt frequency, mean score (SE)** BL 6 mo IG1 21.3 (1.3) 14.3 (1.0) IG2 22.0 (1.3) 20.6 (1.0) IG3 22.3 (1.3) 15.2 (1.1) CG 21.2 (1.3) 20.3 (1.1) p=NR; text states it is statistically significant for IG1 and IG3. **24-hr urinary sodium excretion, mmol/24-hr, median value (SE)** IG1 NR 105.5 (NR)

Appendix G Table 3. Behavioral Outcomes (KQ 3 Results): Healthy Diet

Study, Year Quality	N Population Intervention Focus & Intensity	Healthy Diet Behavioral Outcomes
HIP, 2009[136] Fair	574 HTN HD+PA, High (Pt, MD+Pt); Medium (MD only)	IG2 NR 124 (NR) IG3 NR 107 (NR) CG NR 120 (NR) p=NR; text states it is statistically significant for IG1 and IG3. BL Δ at 6 mo (SD) Δ at 18 mo (SD) **Total energy, kcal** IG1 1594 (643) -72.2 (464) -73 (543) IG2 1780 (826) -287.4 (660) -260.8 (741) CG1 1725 (763) -170.6 (554) -119.1 (698) CG2 1664 (843) -249.8 (586) -158.8 (535) *Patient intervention vs. control: p<0.05 at 6 mo **Fruit/vegetable servings per day** IG1 1.33 (0.99) 0.59 (1.27) 0.41 (1.13) IG2 1.42 (1.13) 0.92 (1.34) 0.55 (1.13) CG1 1.28 (0.90) 0.04 (0.81) 0.01 (0.90) CG2 1.23 (0.88) 0.09 (0.72) -0.03 (0.87) MDI main effect 6 mo, p=0.02; 18 mo, p=0.53 PTI main effect 6mo, p<0.0001; 18 mo p<0.0001 **Dairy servings per day** IG1 0.94 (0.89) 0.06 (0.67) 0.08 (0.51) IG2 0.95 (0.81) 0.21 (0.75) -0.01 (0.79) CG1 0.94 (0.90) -0.01 (0.72) -0.03 (0.80) CG2 0.89 (0.89) 0.01 (0.56) -0.00 (0.61) MDI main effect 6 mo, p=0.17; 18 mo p=0.57 PTI main effect 6 mo, p= 0.01; 18 mo p=0.56 Slightly different numbers are reported in Lin 2013 **Total fat, % kcal** IG1 38.4 (8.1) -2.3 (8.5) -1.7 (7.7) IG2 37.3 (6.8) -4.3 (7.1) -2.8 (7.8) CG1 38.1 (8.0) 0.6 (7.0) 0.8 (8.0) CG2 39.8 (8.3) -1.2 (6.7) -1.1 (6.6) MDI main effect at 6 mo, p =0.002;18 mo p=0.02 PTI main effect at 6 mo, p<0.0001; 18 mo p<0.0001 Slightly different numbers are reported in Lin 2013 **Saturated fat, % kcal** IG1 10.9 (2.7) -1.0 (2.7) -0.9 (2.1) IG2 10.5 (2.4) -1.3 (2.1) -1.0 (2.2) CG1 10.6 (2.5) 0.2 (2.3) 0.1 (2.3) CG2 11.0 (2.3) -0.2 (2.0) -0.2 (2.0) MDI main effect at 6 mo, p=0.07; 18 mo p=0.28 PTI main effect at 6 mo, p<0.0001; 18 mo p <0.0001 grams reported in Lin 2013 **Carbohydrates, % kcal** IG1 46.8 (9.0) 0.9 (7.4) 1.1 (7.9)

Appendix G Table 3. Behavioral Outcomes (KQ 3 Results): Healthy Diet

Study, Year Quality	N Population Intervention Focus & Intensity	Healthy Diet Behavioral Outcomes
		IG2 48.8 (8.4) 4.7 (8.4) 3.0 (8.6) CG1 48.6 (9.5) -0.4 (7.8) -0.9 (8.3) CG2 48.2 (10.3) 2.5 (10.2) 2.2 (9.9) *Patient intervention vs. control: p<0.05 at 6 and 18 mo **Physician intervention vs. control: p<0.001 at 6 and 18 mo **Protein, % kcal** IG1 14.7 (2.9) 0.2 (2.5) 0.2 (3.1) IG2 14.5 (2.4) 0.8 (2.5) 0.3 (3.0) CG1 14.6 (3.0) 0.02 (3.2) 0.1 (2.5) CG2 14.2 (3.0) 0.8 (3.0) 0.01 (3.8) *Patient intervention vs. control: p<0.05 at 6 mo **Cholesterol, mg** IG1 196 (104) -4.7 (76.1) -5.9 (115) IG2 217 (135) -49.8 (111) -43.5 (115) CG1 209 (129) -16.5 (67.8) -8.5 (96.6) CG2 198 (138) -30.2 (116) -26.9 (99.5) *Patient intervention vs. control: p<0.001 at 6 mo **Fiber, g** IG1 15.9 (8.2) -0.7 (5.6) -0.5 (6.7) IG2 16.4 (8.4) 2.0 (7.4) 0.6 (7.3) CG1 17.2 (9.0) -1.8 (7.5) -0.9 (9.9) CG2 16.3 (9.4) 0.3 (8.7) 0.2 (8.6) *Patient intervention vs. control: p<0.001 at 6 mo **Urinary sodium, mmol/24-hr** IG1 150.9 (68.0) -13.1 (62.2) -24.0 (85.2) IG2 170.3 (76.2) -31.4 (79.7) -28.0 (76.6) CG1 174.7 (77.0) -22.8 (71.2) -8.3 (84.1) CG2 175.2 (82.9) -23.6 (75.2) -1.4 (69.9) MDI main effect at 6 mo, p=0.62; 18 mo p=0.03 PTI main effect at 6 mo, p=0.14; 18 mo p=0.32
Hyman, 2007[135] Fair	281 HTN HD+PA, Medium	**24-hr urine sodium level** BL 6 mo 18mo IG1 185.8 (77.9) 169.2 (104.4) 195.3 (110.0) IG2 200.7 (88.2) 200.4 (94.8) 208.6 (101.2) CG 189.0 (71.0) 189.3 (92.1) 189.8 (90.5) p* 0.39 0.14 0.49
LIHEF, 2002[137] Fair	715 HTN HD+PA, High	Mean (SD) at BL, mean (SD) change from BL at 12 & 24 mo BL 12 mo 24 mo p (between) **Energy, kcal** IG 1897 (572) -125 (467) -157 (477) @12 mo, 0.137 CG 1896 (572) -72 (395) -92 (395) @24 mo, 0.092 **Fat, % of total energy** IG 33.5 (6.0) -1.9 (6.5) -2.9 (6.4) @12 mo, 0.001 CG 33.4 (6.4) -0.1 (5.8) -0.1 (7.0) @24 mo, <0.0005

Appendix G Table 3. Behavioral Outcomes (KQ 3 Results): Healthy Diet

Study, Year Quality	N Population Intervention Focus & Intensity	Healthy Diet Behavioral Outcomes
Migneault, 2012[126] Fair	337 HTN HD+PA, High	**Saturated fat, % of total energy** IG 13.6 (3.1) -1.3 (3.3) @12 mo, <0.0005 CG 13.6 (3.2) -0.1 (2.8) @24 mo, <0.0005 **Monounsaturated fatty acid, % of total energy** IG 11.8 (2.5) -0.5 (2.7) @12 mo, 0.054 CG 11.7 (2.8) -0.1 (2.8) @24 mo, <0.008 **Polyunsaturated fatty acid, % of total energy** IG 5.5 (1.5) -0.1 (1.6) @12 mo, 0.512 CG 5.3 (1.5) 0.0 (1.7) @24 mo, <0.105 **Cholesterol, mg** IG 264 (118) -36 (115) @12 mo, 0.01 CG 260 (117) -13 (99) @24 mo, <0.0005 **Fiber, g/d** IG 22.8 (8.6) -0.1 (7.7) 0.8 (7.3) @12 mo, 0.349 CG 22.9 (8.4) -0.7 (6.7) -1.4 (6.9) @24 mo, <0.001 **24-hr urinary sodium, mmol** IG 146 (57) -11 (62) -7 (58) @12 mo, 0.483 CG 142 (56) -10 (53) -2 (63) @24 mo, 0.856 **Composite diet quality score** BL mean (SD) Change @ 8 mo IG 53.9 (17.6) 2.8 CG 55.8 (17.0) -0.74 p<0.03
PREMIER, 2003[116] Good	304 HTN HD+PA, High	**Fruits/vegetables, servings/d** BL mean (SD) Change IG1 4.7 (2.3) 0.6 (2.5) IG2 4.8 (2.4) 3.2 (3.8) CG 4.1 (2.1) 0.5 (2.6) p=NR **Dairy, servings/d** IG1 1.8 (1.3) -0.3 (1.2) IG2 1.9 (1.6) 0.4 (1.7) CG 1.5 (1.2) 0.1 (1.8) p=NR **Urinary sodium, mmol/24-h** IG1 166.9 (70.6) -40.6 (62.6) IG2 175.8 (72.1) -35.5 (70.7) CG 176.3 (65.8) -21.3 (72.1) p=NR **Saturated fat, % of kcal** IG1 10.8 (3.4) -1.8 (4.2) IG2 11.1 (3.2) -3.3 (4.4) CG 11.3 (3.3) -1.1 (3.3) p=NR

Appendix G Table 3. Behavioral Outcomes (KQ 3 Results): Healthy Diet

Study, Year Quality	N Population Intervention Focus & Intensity	Healthy Diet Behavioral Outcomes
TONE, 1998[117] Good	975 HTN HD+PA, High	**24-hr urinary sodium excretion, mmol/24-hr, all participants** N BL* Within-group Δ* Btwn-group Δ** Subgroup p† IG1 319 144 (53) -45 (55.8) -40 (-48 to -32); p<0.001 NA CG 320 145 (55) -5 (50.0)
Vitalum[105] Fair	1,629 HTN HD+PA, Medium (IG2 and 3), Low (IG1)	Mean (SD) (raw, unadjusted data); self-reported on 16-item short questionnaire **Fruit intake (servings/d)** BL 25 wks 47 wks 73 wks IG1 (mail) 2.16 (1.69) 2.90 (1.76) 3.02 (2.22) 2.68 (1.81) IG2 (phone) 2.04 (1.55) 2.90 (1.65) 2.78 (2.12) 2.30 (1.58) IG3 (combo) 2.04 (1.63) 2.59 (1.69) 2.70 (2.09) 2.28 (1.59) CG 2.10 (1.69) 2.57 (1.64) 2.36 (1.87) 2.09 (1.58) p (see note in text) **Vegetable intake (g/d)** IG1 (mail) 166 (88) 191 (81) 205 (96) 187 (92) IG2 (phone) 164 (81) 190 (75) 183 (86) 175 (88) IG3 (combo) 163 (81) 181 (79) 188 (86) 174 (85) CG 167 (80) 183 (80) 176 (83) 164 (81) p (see note in text)
Arroll, 1995[128] Fair	208 HTN HD+PA, Medium	**Salt frequency, mean score (SE)** BL 6mo IG1 21.3 (1.3) 14.3 (1.0) IG2 22.0 (1.3) 20.6 (1.0) IG3 22.3 (1.3) 15.2 (1.1) CG 21.2 (1.3) 20.3 (1.1) p=NR; text states it is statistically significant for IG1 and IG3 **24-hr urinary sodium excretion, mmol/24-hr, median value (SE)** IG1 NR 105.5 (NR) IG2 NR 124 (NR) IG3 NR 107 (NR) CG NR 120 (NR) p=NR; text states it is statistically significant for IG1 and IG3
Beckman, 1995[111] Fair	64 HTN HD+PA, Medium	**Urinary sodium, mmol/24-hr, mean (SE)** BL 6 mo 12 mo mean change IG 195 (12) 116 (11) 123 (7) 72 CG 177 (10) 175 (14) 167 (9) Mean difference: 44; p<0.001
TONE, 1998[117] Good	975 HTN HD, High	**24-hr urinary sodium excretion, mmol/24-hr** BL* Within-group Δ* Btwn-group Δ** Subgroup p† IG1 144 (53) -45 (55.8) -40 (-48 to -32); p<0.001 NA CG 145 (55) -5 (50.0) *Mean (SD); **Mean (95% CI)

Appendix G Table 3. Behavioral Outcomes (KQ 3 Results): Healthy Diet

Study, Year Quality	N Population Intervention Focus & Intensity	Healthy Diet Behavioral Outcomes
Arroll, 1995[128] Fair	208 HTN PA, Medium	Salt frequency, mean score (SE) BL 6 mo IG1 21.3 (1.3) 14.3 (1.0) IG2 22.0 (1.3) 20.6 (1.0) IG3 22.3 (1.3) 15.2 (1.1) CG 21.2 (1.3) 20.3 (1.1) p=NR; text states it is statistically significant for IG1 and IG3 24-hr urinary sodium excretion, mmol/24-hr, median value (SE) IG1 NR 105.5 (NR) IG2 NR 124 (NR) IG3 NR 107 (NR) CG NR 120 (NR) p=NR; text states it is statistically significant for IG1 and IG3
Moreau, 2001[104] Fair	24 HTN PA, Medium	Average caloric intake IG 1826 ± 140 kcal CG 1855 ± 338 kcal
APHRODITE, 2011[88] Fair	925 IFG HD+PA, High	mean (SD) BL Δ 6 mo Δ 18 mo Kcal/d IG 2047 (622) -262 (390) -278* (466) CG 1979 (576) -198 (387) -197 (449) p=0.11 Total fat intake, % of energy IG 35.0 (6.2) -0.3 (6.0) -0.5 (6.2) CG 34.4 (6.1) 0.5 (5.4) 0.5 (6.4) p=0.13 Total saturated fat, % of energy IG 11.8 (2.7) -0.2 (2.4) -0.3 (2.5) CG 11.8 (2.5) 0.3 (2.0) 0.2 (2.3) p=0.03 Fiber intake, g/MJ IG 3.5 (1.0) -0.3 (0.8) -0.1 (0.8) CG 3.5 (1.0) -0.4 (0.7) -0.3 (0.8) p=0.01
DPP, 2002[89] Good	2,161 IFG HD+PA, High	Mean change from baseline to 1 yr Energy, kcal Mean change (SE) IG -450 (26) CG -249 (27) p<0.001 Fat, % calories Mean change (SE) IG -6.6 (0.2) CG -0.8 (0.2) p<0.001

Appendix G Table 3. Behavioral Outcomes (KQ 3 Results): Healthy Diet

Study, Year Quality	N Population Intervention Focus & Intensity	Healthy Diet Behavioral Outcomes
		Median change from baseline to 1 yr **Energy intake, kJ/d** IG -452 CG -250 $p<0.003$ (adjusted for sex and ethnicity) **% Energy from fat** IG -6.6 CG -0.8 $p<0.003$ (adjusted for sex and ethnicity) **% Energy from saturated fat** IG -2.8 CG -0.4 $p<0.003$ **% Energy from polyunsaturated fat** IG -1.0 CG 0.0 $p<0.003$ **% Energy from carbohydrates** IG 5.4 CG 0.1 $p<0.003$ **Fiber intake, g/d** IG 0.3 CG -0.6 $p<0.003$ **Fruit intake, servings/d** IG 1.6 CG -0.08 $p<0.003$ **Vegetable intake, servings/d** IG 1.1 CG -0.09 p=NS **Fish intake, servings/d** IG 0.0 CG 0.0 p=NS **Red meat intake, servings/d** IG -2.3 CG -0.5 $p<0.003$ **Dairy intake, servings/d** IG -2.1 CG -1.3

Appendix G Table 3. Behavioral Outcomes (KQ 3 Results): Healthy Diet

Study, Year Quality	N Population Intervention Focus & Intensity	Healthy Diet Behavioral Outcomes
EDIPS, 2001[90] Fair	78 IFG HD+PA, Medium	p<0.003 **Sweets intake, servings/d** IG -4.9 CG -3.0 p<0.003 Mean (SD) BL 6 mo Diff btwn groups (95% CI) p **Energy, kJ/d** IG 8317 (2464) 7485 (2390) -862 (-2002 to 279) NS CG 8942 (2298) 8972 (2977) **Total fat, g/d** IG 85.4 (29.0) 68.7 (30.0)* -21.8 (-37.8 to -5.8) 0.008 CG 84.7 (23.4) 89.8 (34.3) **Monounsaturated fat, g/d** IG 26.4 (10.1) 21.2 (10.1)* -6.8 (-12.6 to -1.01) 0.022 CG 27.1 (8.5) 28.8 (11.6) **Polyunsaturated fat, g/d** IG 15.6 (6.8) 12.7 (7.2) -5.0 (-9.8, -0.19) 0.042 CG 13.5 (6.1) 15.6 (9.3) **Saturated fat, g/d** IG 27.9 (10.3) 23.9 (13.1) -3.1 (-9.6, 3.4) NS CG 32.2 (11.8) 31.1 (15.1) **Sucrose, g/d** IG 1.3 (2.5) 2.2 (5.4) -0.6 (-3.3, 2.1) NS CG 0.91 (1.9) 2.5 (4.3) **Fiber, g/d** IG 20.0 (6.6) 20.2 (7.5) 1.0 (-1.9, 3.9) NS CG 19.8 (8.2) 19.0 (7.3)
EDIPS-Newcastle, 2009[91] Fair	102 IFG HD+PA, High	N (%) of participants with sustained benefit change **Energy intake from fat†** IG 21 (41) CG 21 (41) p=NR **Energy intake from carbohydrates†** IG 15 (29) CG 16 (31) p=NR †Based on annual 3-day food diaries. No significant difference in mean values for % carbohydrate, fat, and fiber intake between IG and CG at BL or annual followup in any year.
FDPS, 2001[118] Good	522 IFG HD+PA, High	Success in achieving intervention goals at year 1, % of participants **Fat intake <30% of energy** IG 47 CG 26

Appendix G Table 3. Behavioral Outcomes (KQ 3 Results): Healthy Diet

Study, Year Quality	N Population Intervention Focus & Intensity	Healthy Diet Behavioral Outcomes
		p=0.001 **Saturated fat intake <10% of energy** IG 26 CG 11 p=0.001 **Fiber intake ≥15 g/1000 kcal** IG 25 CG 12 p=0.001 Self-reported change in dietary habits during year 1, % **Decreased consumption of fat** IG 87 CG 70 p=0.001 **Increased consumption of vegetables** IG 72 CG 62 p=0.01 **Decreased consumption of sugar** IG 55 CG 40 p=0.001 **Decreased consumption of salt** IG 59 CG 50 p=0.03 Mean change (SD) from BL BL 1 year p 3 years p **Energy intake, kcal/d** IG 1771 (520) -247 (438) 0.0001 -204 (489) 0.0067 CG 1744 (527) -108 (464) -97 (458) **% Energy from carbohydrates** IG 43.6 (7.5) 3.3 (8.1) 0.0023 3.3 (8.0) 0.0070 CG 43.2 (6.7) 1.7 (7.3) 2.0 (7.6) **% Energy from fat** IG 36.0 (6.7) -3.4 (8.2) 0.0002 -4.7 (7.7) <0.0001 CG 37.1 (6.5) -2.1 (7.6) -3.2 (7.5) **% Energy from saturated fat** IG 16.2 (4.0) -2.7 (4.6) <0.0001 -3.2 (4.5) <0.0001 CG 17.0 (4.3) -1.2 (5.1) -1.9 (4.9) **Energy from monounsaturated fat** IG 12.9 (2.8) -0.8 (3.8) 0.0257 -1.0 (3.6) 0.0453 CG 13.0 (2.9) -0.4 (3.4) -0.6 (3.5)

Appendix G Table 3. Behavioral Outcomes (KQ 3 Results): Healthy Diet

Study, Year Quality	N Population Intervention Focus & Intensity	Healthy Diet Behavioral Outcomes
		% Energy from polyunsaturated fat
		IG 5.7 (1.7) −0.0 (2.1) 0.5020 0.0 (2.4) 0.0872
		CG 5.8 (2.2) −0.2 (2.5) −0.4 (2.3)
		Cholesterol intake, mg
		IG 312 (137) −69 (138) 0.0005 −63 (167) 0.0586
		CG 304 (130) −28 (148) −31 (155)
		Fiber, g
		IG 20 (7) 1 (7) 0.1146 1 (8) 0.4393
		CG 20 (8) 0 (7) 1 (7)
		% of participants reaching dietary goals during year 1
		Fat intake goal <30% of energy
		IG 37
		CG 20
		p <0.0001
		Saturated fat intake goal of <10% of energy
		IG 21
		CG 9
		p <0.0001
		Fiber density goal of ≥15 g/1000kcal
		IG 37
		CG 23
		p<0.0006
		Mean (SD) BL Early FU‡ Late FU‡ p§
		Total energy (kJ)
		IG 7415 (2177) 6624 (1704) 6778 (1746) 0.06
		CG 7302 (2206) 6942 (1863) 6875 (1788)
		% Fat
		IG 36.0 (6.7) 31.9 (5.7) 32.7 (6.3) 0.0009
		CG 37.1 (6.5) 33.9 (6.1) 34.7 (5.9)
		% Saturated fat
		IG 16.2 (4.0) 11.8 (3.5) 12.2 (3.7) <0.0001
		CG 17.0 (4.3) 13.7 (3.7) 14.0 (3.5)
		% Carbohydrates (g also reported)
		IG 43.6 (7.5) 47.6 (6.9) 46.9 (7.3) 0.08
		CG 43.2 (6.7) 46.2 (6.8) 45.7 (6.9)
		% Protein
		IG 17.6 (3.4) 18.7 (3.1) 18.8 (3.2) 0.0019
		CG 17.6 (3.4) 18.3 (3.1) 17.9 (3.1)
		Total fiber, g (g/MJ also reported)
		IG 20 (7) 21 (7) 21 (8) 0.10
		CG 20 (8) 20 (6) 20 (7)

Appendix G Table 3. Behavioral Outcomes (KQ 3 Results): Healthy Diet

Study, Year Quality	N Population Intervention Focus & Intensity	Healthy Diet Behavioral Outcomes
HLC, 2011[92] Fair	307 IFG HD+PA, High	**Healthy eating, based on the 16-item Food Choices Questionnaire, mean (SD)** BL 6 mo IG 3.14 (0.33) 3.33 (0.27) CG 3.11 (0.34) 3.12 (0.34) time X group p<0.001
Live Well, Be Well, 2012[86] Good	238 IFG HD+PA, High	BL mean (SE), within group change (SE) BL 6 mo 12 mo **Total calories, kcal/d** IG 1870.5 (78.1) -264.3 (50.6) -301.6 (64.7) CG 1915.1 (81.0) -216.6 (69.2) -245.9 (52.7) Between group comparison of change: NS at either timepoint **Total Fat, g/d** IG 71.5 (3.6) -12.95 (2.4) -14.4 (2.9) CG 67.9 (3.1) -5.3 (3.1) -7.8 (2.4) Between group comparison of change: p=0.05 at 6 mo; NS at 12 mo (p=0.08) **Dietary fiber, g/d** IG 17.8 (0.9) -1.1 (0.7) -1.97 (0.8) CG 19.7 (1.1) -1.3 (0.8) -1.8 (0.7) Between group comparison of change: NS at either time point **Daily frequency of fruits/vegetables** IG 3.0 (0.2) 0.3 (0.2) 0.1 (0.1) CG 3.1 (0.2) -0.3 (0.2) -0.3 (0.1) Between group comparison of change: p=0.02 at 6 mo; p=0.04 at 12 mo

Appendix G Table 3. Behavioral Outcomes (KQ 3 Results): Healthy Diet

Study, Year Quality	N Population Intervention Focus & Intensity	Healthy Diet Behavioral Outcomes
LLDP[94] Good	312 IFG HD+PA, High	BL, mean (SD)　　　1-year change (median, 95% CI) **kcal/d** IG　1546.78 (604.9)　　-21.8 (-103.6 to 55.3) CG　1531.56 (593.7)　　3.8 (-57.3 to 70.2) Intervention effect (95% CI): -30.1 (-141.2 to 76.9); p=0.57 **Energy from fat, %** IG　26.49 (6.0)　　-2.02 (-3.77, -0.29) CG　25.82 (6.4)　　-0.42 (-1.38, 1.57) Intervention effect (95% CI): -1.77 (-3.48 to -0.08); p=0.04 **Energy from saturated fat, %** IG　8.50 (2.6)　　-0.65 (-1.03, -0.27) CG　8.17 (2.7)　　-0.43 (-0.75, 0.36) Intervention effect (95% CI): -0.59 (-1.28 to 0.07); p=0.08 **Energy from carbohydrates, %** IG　55.36 (7.8)　　1.20 (-0.18 to 3.54) CG　55.92 (8.5)　　0.41 (-0.94 to 2.14) Intervention effect (95% CI): 1.73 (-0.23 to 3.76); p=0.08 **Energy from protein, %** IG　17.59 (5.8)　　0.61 (-0.62 to 1.60) CG　17.49 (4.7)　　-0.11 (-0.79 to 0.88) Intervention effect (95% CI): 0.02 (-1.15 to 1.22); p=0.97 **Total fiber, g/d** IG　15.74 (8.2)　　3.13 (0.88 to 4.46) CG　15.71 (7.0)　　0.48 (-2.10 to 2.12) Intervention effect (95% CI): 1.98 (-0.16 to 4.01); p=0.07
Melbourne DPS, 2012[85] Fair	92 IFG HD+PA, High	Mean (SD); change in mean (SE) 　　　BL　　　Δ 12 mo　　p (btwn group) **Total fat, %** IG　36.3 (4.45)　-2.01 (0.83)　　0.290 CG　36.2 (4.51)　-0.42 (0.77) **Saturated fat, %** IG　14.6 (3.25)　-1.64 (0.51)　　0.088* CG　14.0 (2.93)　0.29 (0.38) **Fiber, g/d** IG　13.6 (2.97)　1.95 (0.58)　　0.030 CG　13.5 (3.32)　0.51 (0.47) *After adjusting for BL characteristics, p=0.003
SLIM[49] Fair	147 IFG HD+PA, High	**Energy intake (MJ/d)** 　　　BL　　　　　　1-year IG　9.1 (0.4)　7.9 (0.3)　　7.94 (0.35) CG　8.5 (0.3)　8.2 (0.3)　　8.28 (0.38) 1-year p=0.02; 2-year group X time interaction p= 0.13 **Carbohydrates (energy %)** IG　42.2 (1.0)　46.9 (1.1)　　47.4 (0.9) CG　43.2 (0.9)　43.9 (1.0)　　43.7 (0.9)

Appendix G Table 3. Behavioral Outcomes (KQ 3 Results): Healthy Diet

Study, Year Quality	N Population Intervention Focus & Intensity	Healthy Diet Behavioral Outcomes
Watanabe, 2003[97] Fair	173 IFG HD, Low	1-year p <0.01; 2-year group X time interaction p<0.01 **Fat (energy %)** IG 36.2 (0.9) 31.2 (1.0) 31.8 (0.8) CG 35.7 (0.9) 34.7 (0.8) 35.6 (0.6) 1-year p<0.01; 2-year group X time interaction p<0.01 **Saturated fat (energy %)** IG 14.0 (0.4) 11.2 (0.4) 11.1 (0.4) CG 13.9 (0.4) 13.3 (0.5) 14.1 (0.3) 1-year p <0.01; 2-year group X time interaction p<0.01 **Monounsaturated fat (energy %)** IG 12.9 (0.4) 10.8 (0.4) NR CG 12.8 (0.4) 12.4 (0.4) NR 1-year p <0.01 **Polyunsaturated fat (energy %)** IG 6.7 (0.4) 6.9 (0.4) NR CG 6.5 (0.3) 6.5 (0.3) NR 1-year p=NS **Cholesterol (mg/MJ)** IG 25.7 (1.4) 22.5 (1.2) 22.5 (1.1) CG 27.5 (1.6) 26.1 (1.3) 26.0 (1.8) 1-year p=NS; 2-year p=NS **Protein (energy %)** IG 15.7 (0.4) 17.4 (0.5) 17.5 (0.4) CG 16.0 (0.4) 16.3 (0.5) 16.1 (0.4) 1-year p=0.06; 2-year p=0.07 **Fiber (g/MJ)** IG 2.8 (0.1) 3.3 (0.1) 3.1 (0.1) CG 2.6 (0.1) 2.8 (0.1) 2.7 (0.1) 1-year p=0.03; 2-year p=0.07 Absolute value of the "over/underintake fraction" for total energy intake (%), mean (SD), mean change from BL (SD) IG 21.6 (15.0) -1.8 (1.5) CG 19.9 (14.9) 4.0 (1.4) p NSD adjusted mean difference between groups: -6.0 (-9.8 to -2.2); p=0.002
Bo, 2007[146] Fair	375 Mixed HD+PA, Medium	BL 12 mo Difference 95% CI **kcal/d** IG 1978.6 (692.5) 1904.0 (631.6) -74.6 (-153.3 to 41.4) CG 1993 (633.8) 2018.8 (583.1) 25.8 (-43.7 to 95.2) p=0.06 **Total energy from fat, %** IG 35.3 (5.2) 32.7 (6.5) -2.64 (-3.52 to -1.76) CG 35.0 (5.8) 35.0 (6.8) -0.02 (-1.30 to 1.25) p<0.001

Appendix G Table 3. Behavioral Outcomes (KQ 3 Results): Healthy Diet

Study, Year Quality	N Population Intervention Focus & Intensity	Healthy Diet Behavioral Outcomes
Cochrane, 2012[102] Fair	601 Mixed HD+PA, High	**Total energy from saturated fat, %** IG 12.3 (2.6) 10.3 (3.7) -1.97 (-2.53 to -1.41) CG 12.0 (2.6) 11.8 (3.3) -0.17 (-0.72 to 0.38) p<0.001 **Total energy from polyunsaturated fat** IG 4.3 (1.3) 5.3 (1.8) 0.99 (0.73 to 1.25) CG 4.1 (1.2) 4.1 (1.5) 0.04 (0.32 to 0.24) p<0.001 **Total energy from carbohydrates** IG 48.2 (7.1) 50.3 (7.7) 2.14 (1.02 to 3.26) CG 48.7 (7.0) 47.8 (8.2) -0.89 (-2.33 to 0.55) p=0.001 **Total energy from protein** IG 16.5 (2.3) 16.6 (5.6) 0.09 (-0.80 to 0.98) CG 16.3 (2.4) 16.1 (4.7) -0.21 (-0.89 to 0.47) p=0.06 **Total energy from fiber, %** IG 19.2 (6.4) 20.9 (6.6) 1.70 (1.11 to 2.29) CG 19.4 (7.8) 19.6 (7.9) 0.17 (-0.30 to 0.64) p<0.001

EUROACTION, 2008[106] Fair	2,384 Mixed HD+PA, High	Mean diet score from Primary Prevention Toolkit
		  BL 12 mo
		IG 2.2 2.45
		CG 2.1 2.4
		"No significant difference between groups on any of the measures."
		Number of participants (%)
		  BL 12 mo
		Oily fish (≥3 times/week)
		IG 55/1094 (5) 113/1019 (11)
		CG 10/331 (3) 60/1004 (6)
		Difference (95% CI): 6.7 (-4.1 to 17.6); p=0.13
		Note: in text, difference (95% CI): 2.2% (-1.7 to 6.2); p=0.20 (unclear which groups)
		Fish (≥20 g/d)
		IG 680/1096 (62) 841/1018 (83)
		CG 217/331 (66) 666/1003 (66)
		Difference (95% CI): 16.8 (-1.7 to 35.2); p=0.07
		Note: in text, difference (95% CI): 16.5% (-0.1 to 33.1); p=0.051 (unclear which groups)
		Fruits/vegetables (≥400 g/d)
		IG 548/1093 (50) 799/1019 (78)
		CG 117/331 (35) 388/1001 (39)
		Difference (95% CI): 39.7 (18.1 to 61.3); p=0.005
		Note: in text, difference (95% CI): 23.6% (9.1 to 38.2); p=0.009 (unclear which groups)

Appendix G Table 3. Behavioral Outcomes (KQ 3 Results): Healthy Diet

Study, Year Quality	N Population Intervention Focus & Intensity	Healthy Diet Behavioral Outcomes

GOAL, 2009[139] Good	457 Mixed HD+PA, Medium	Mean (95% CI) for BL, mean change at 12 mo and 36 mo, based on self-reported FFQ
		
		    BL Δ at 12 mo (CI)
		Energy, kcal
		IG 2052 (1955 to 2149) −179 (−248 to −109)
		CG 2047 (1956 to 2139) −175 (−246 to 105)
		p* 0.97
		
		    BL Δ at 36 mo (SD)
		Energy, kJ/d
		IG 8521 (2600) −587 (2059)
		CG 8455 (2753) −523 (2114)
		p 0.737
		
		    BL Δ at 12 mo (CI) Δ at 36 mo (SD)
		Fat, %
		IG 35.3 (34.4 to 36.2) −2.6 (−3.5 to −1.7) −1.2 (5.7)
		CG 34.6 (33.6 to 35.5) −1.9 (−2.8 to −1.0) −0.7 (5.8)
		p 0.56 0.797
		Saturated fat, %
		IG 12.9 (125 to 13.4) −1.6 (−2.0 to −1.2) −0.9 (2.9)
		CG 12.5 (12.1 to 13.0) −1.0 (−1.4 to −0.6) −0.4 (2.7)
		p 0.16 0.164
		Protein, %
		IG 15.4 (15.1 to 158.8) 0.6 (0.3 to 1.0) 0 (2.2)
		CG 15.5 (15.1 to 15.8) 0.5 (0.2 to 0.9) 0 (2.6)
		p 0.68 0.452
		Carbohydrates, %
		IG 44.6 (43.6 to 45.5) 2.0 (1.2 to 2.9) 1.4 (6.1)
		CG 45.3 (44.3 to 46.3) 1.3 (0.3 to 2.2) 1.1 (6.3)
		p 0.43 0.945
		Cholesterol, mg
		IG 188.6 (177.6 to 200.0) −27.4 (−37.0 to −17.8) −11.9 (66.8)
		CG 185.8 (174.3 to 197.3) −21.9 (−31.3 to −12.4) −11.0 (69.1)
		p 0.49 0.939
		Vegetables, g
		IG 145.2 (120.3 to 140.7) 16.1 (6.3 to 25.9) 11.7 (74.1)
		CG 158.6 (125.4 to 148.5) 13.6 (1.9 to 25.2) 18.2 (86.7)
		p 0.87 0.556
		Fruit, g
		IG 130.5 (103.8 to 136.4) 85.1 (65.5 to 104.7) 84.0 (174.9)
		CG 137.0 (109.1 to 144.6) 64.1 (43.2 to 84.9) 63.0 (165.9)
		p 0.27 0.468
		
		*p values corrected for BL values.
		Maintenance of change, BL to 3 yr (ANOVA).
		No significant difference between groups for changes from BL to year 1, year 1 to year 3, and BL to year 3 on any dietary intake measure.

Appendix G Table 3. Behavioral Outcomes (KQ 3 Results): Healthy Diet

Study, Year Quality	N Population Intervention Focus & Intensity	Healthy Diet Behavioral Outcomes

Hardcastle, 2008[167] Fair	334 Mixed HD+PA, Medium	**Fat intake (%/d)**
		    BL 6 mo difference in mean (SEM)
		IG 23.85 (0.55) -0.92
		CG 23.72 (0.67) -2.92
		95% CI (-3.46 to -0.55); p<0.01
		    BL mean (SD) 18 mo mean (SD)
		Fat intake (%/d)
		IG 23.87 (7.67) 22.97 (7.26)
		CG 23.89 (7.70) 20.41 (5.96)
		Time x Group: p<0.05
		Fruit/vegetable portions per day
		IG 6.41 (0.31) 1.05 (0.30)
		CG 6.88 (0.39) 0.73 (0.44)
		95% CI (-1.36 to 0.72); p=NS
		Fruit/vegetable portions per day: ITT
		IG 6.31 (4.02) 6.30 (3.76)
		CG 6.94 (4.48) 6.23 (3.58)
		Time x Group: NS. F statistic: 0.78; effect size: 0.005.

HIPS, 2012[103] Fair	814 Mixed HD+PA	**Fruit/vegetable portions per day at 12 mo, mean (95% CI)** BL 6 mo 12 mo IG 4.73 (NR) 5.58 (5.33 to 5.83) 4.85 (4.56 to 5.14) CG 4.67 (NR) 4.99 (4.70 to 5.28) 4.52 (4.23 to 4.81) p NR 0.002 0.1
HOORN, 2013[132] Fair	622 Mixed HD+PA, Medium	**Fruit/d, mean (SD)** BL 6 mo 12 mo IG 1.1 (0.9) 1.1 (0.9) 1.1 (0.9) CG 1.1 (0.8) 1.3 (1.0) 1.2 (0.9) Difference -0.2 (-0.3 to 0.0) -0.1 (-0.2 to 0.0) OR (95% CI) NR NR **Meeting reccomended fruit intake*, n (%)** IG 63 (20.1) 57 (18.2) 58 (18.5) CG 67 (21.8) 70 (22.7) 68 (22.1) Difference NR NR OR (95% CI)† 1.6 (0.9 to 2.6) 1.4 (0.9 to 2.4) **Vegetable intake, g/d, mean (SD)** IG 148 (69.5) 161 (126.6) 156 (74.6) CG 150 (70.4) 151 (68.5) 157 (89.9) Difference 9.2 (-7.3 to 25.7) -0.4 (-12.7 to 11.9) OR (95% CI) NR NR **Meeting reccomended vegetable intake, n (%)** IG 72 (22.9) 55 (17.5) 62 (19.7) CG 63 (20.5) 57 (18.5) 56 (18.2) Difference NR NR OR (95% CI)† 1.1 (0.7 to 1.7) 0.9 (0.6 to 1.5)

Appendix G Table 3. Behavioral Outcomes (KQ 3 Results): Healthy Diet

Study, Year Quality	N Population Intervention Focus & Intensity	Healthy Diet Behavioral Outcomes
IMPALA, 2009[133] Fair	615 Mixed HD+PA, Medium	Mean (SD) BL 12 mo p **Fat score** IG 16.6 (5.7) 14.4 (5.4) 0.034 CG 17.2 (5.3) 15.4 (5.4) **Met recommended fat intake*, n (%)** IG 123 (41) 140 (56) 0.06 CG 3 (33) 111 (47) **Fruit, pieces per week** IG 12.1 (9.2) 13.7 (9.8) 0.70 CG 13.1 (10.5) 14.1 (11.0) **Met recommended fruit intake (200 g/d), n (%)** IG 117 (39) 114 (45) 0.91 CG 121 (43) 108 (46) **Vegetables, # tbsp** IG 23.7 (11.2) 25.5 (12.7) 0.09 CG 22.7 (12.9) 23.4 (13.3) **Met recommended vegetable intake (200 g/d), n (%)** IG 95 (32) 93 (39) 0.045 CG 79 (29) 65 (30)
Inter99, 2008[107] Fair	4,053 Mixed HD+PA, High	**Intake of saturated fat (% energy) in men (95% CI)** BL 1 Year 3 Year 5 Year IG 12.8 (12.4 to 13.4) 11.4 (10.9 to 13.4) 11.5 (11.0 to 12.1) 11.8 (11.2 to 12.3) CG 12.8 (12.0 to 13.6) 12.5 (11.6 to 13.4) 11.6 (10.7 to 12.6) 12.3 (11.4 to 13.3) p for 1 y=0.002; p for 3 y=0.63; p for 5 y=0.10 Net change between groups at 1 y in saturated fat intake: -1.13%; p=0.003 Net change between groups at 5 y in saturated fat intake: -0.68%; p=0.10 **Intake of saturated fat (% energy), women (95% CI)** IG 11.5 (11.1 to 11.9) 9.9 (9.5 to 10.4) 9.9 (9.4 to 10.4) 10.0 (9.6 to 10.5) CG 11.5 (10.7 to 12.2) 9.7 (8.9 to 10.5) 10.3 (9.4 to 11.1) 10.2 (9.3 to 11.1) p for 1 y=0.65; p for 3 y=0.26; p for 5 y=0.59 Net change between groups at 1 y in fruit intake, g/d: -50; p=0.03 (increase lower in IG) **Unsaturated/saturated fat ratio (95% CI)** IG 1.34 (1.30 to 1.38) 1.47 (1.43 to 1.51) 1.46 (1.42 to 1.50) 1.50 (1.46 to 1.54) CG 1.37 (1.31 to 1.43) 1.40 (1.32 to 1.48) 1.48 (1.40 to 1.56) 1.44 (1.36 to 1.52) p for 1 y=0.01; p for 3 y=0.74; p for 5 y=0.01 Net change between groups at 5 y in unsaturated/saturated; fat ratio: 0.09; p=0.01 *reported in text; not extrapolated **Fish intake, g/d (95% CI)** IG 31.9 (29.1 to 34.7) 33.9 (30.9 to 36.9) 31.8 (28.9 to 34.9) 33.8 (30.7 to 36.7) CG 33.5 (27.7 to 37.3) 32.2 (26.8 to 37.5) 31.8 (26.4 to 37.2) 29.1 (23.4 to 34.6) p for 1 y=0.34; p for 3 y=0.86; p for 5 y=0.05 Net change between groups at 5 y in fish intake (g/d): 5.4; p=0.05

Appendix G Table 3. Behavioral Outcomes (KQ 3 Results): Healthy Diet

Study, Year Quality	N Population Intervention Focus & Intensity	Healthy Diet Behavioral Outcomes
Logan Healthy Living, 2009[114] Fair	434 Mixed HD+PA, Medium	mean (SE) BL change 12 mo change 18 mo **Fat, % total calories** IG 36.8 (5.0) -1.98 (0.29) -2.39 (0.29) CG 36.9 (5.5) -0.83 (0.31) -1.07 (0.31) 12-mo difference between groups: -1.17; p= 0.007 (95% CI, -2.00 to -0.35) 18-mo difference between groups: -1.33; p= 0.002 (95% CI, -2.16 to -0.50) **Saturated fat, % total calories** IG 14.5 (3.3) -1.57 (0.25) -1.58 (0.22) CG 14.2 (3.3) -0.60 (0.26) -0.52 (0.23) 12-mo difference between groups: -0.97; p=0.007 (95% CI, -1.68 to -0.26) 18-mo difference between groups: -1.06, p= 0.001 (95% CI, -1.70 to -0.43) **Vegetable servings per day** IG 3.0 (1.7) 1.05 (0.24) 0.77 (0.21) CG 3.0 (1.7) 0.34 (0.25) 0.18 (0.21) 12-mo difference between groups: 0.71; p=0.04 (95% CI, 0.04 to 1.39) 18-mo difference between groups: 0.59; p=0.051 (95% CI, -0.01 to 1.17) **Fiber intake, g/d** IG 22.4 (7.8) 1.83 (0.46) 1.55 (0.43) CG 21.6 (8.1) -0.40 (0.48) -0.38 (0.45) 12-mo difference between groups: 2.23; p<0.001 (95 CI, 0.93 to 3.52) 18-mo difference between groups 0.22; p=0.002 (95% CI, 0.72 to 3.15) **Fruit servings per day** IG 1.6 (1.0) 0.50 (0.06) 0.47 (0.06) CG 1.5 (1.3) 0.20 (0.06) 0.24 (0.06) 12-mo difference between groups: 0.30; p<0.001 (95% CI, 0.12 to 0.47) 18-mo difference between groups: 0.22, p=0.010 (95% CI, 0.05 to 0.40)
Nilsson, 1992[119] Fair	63 Mixed HD+PA, High	mean (SD) BL 12 mo **Energy, kcal** IG 1937 (534) 1704 (384) CG 1987 (396) 1893 (424) **Protein, g/d** IG 76.8 (17.9) 71.6 (16.5) CG 76.9 (15.6) 75.2 (19.3) **Carbohydrates, g/d** IG 224.0 (55.6) 218.1 (53.2) CG 227.5 (43.8) 226.0 (57.1) **Fat, g/d** IG 72.8 (30.2) 53.6 (17.3) CG 77.6 (23.2) 71.1 (23.4) **Fiber, g/d** IG 16.2 (6.6) 21.3 (10.8) CG 16.1 (3.1) 15.9 (4.4)

Appendix G Table 3. Behavioral Outcomes (KQ 3 Results): Healthy Diet

Study, Year Quality	N Population Intervention Focus & Intensity	Healthy Diet Behavioral Outcomes
PHPP, 2007[121] Fair	99 Mixed HD+PA, Medium	**Saturated fat, g/d** IG 28.5 (14.4) 18.8 (7.5) CG 30.6 (11.2) 27.4 (10.9) **Monounsaturated fat, g/d** IG 24.3 (10.6) 18.3 (6.6) CG 26.0 (8.2) 24.1 (8.3) **Polyunsaturated fat, g/d** IG 12.3 (6.1) 8.9 (3.2) CG 13.8 (5.0) 11.8 (3.8) **Cholesterol, mg/d** IG 270.8 (114.8) 186.8 (85.7) CG 300.2 (97.5) 256.9 (141.9) **Polyunsaturated/saturated fat ratio** IG 0.48 (0.26) 0.50 (0.16) CG 0.38 (0.09) 0.45 (0.20)
WISEWOMAN NC, 2008[110] Fair	236 Mixed HD+PA, Medium	**Mean energy intake per day, kcal (SD)** BL 12 mo IG 1931 (482) 1868 (510) CG 1859 (417) 1815 (484) p=NS **Number of meals per day with vegetable servings ≥2, n (%)** IG 34 (73.9) 40 (87.0) CG 29 (70.7) 30 (73.2) **Number of meals per day with vegetable servings ≥1, n (%)** IG 12 (26.1) 6 (13.0) CG 12 (29.3) 11 (26.8) Adjusted OR (adjusted for age, sex, and disease) at 12 mo: 3.8 (95% CI, 1.0 to 14.0); p<0.05

Wister, 2007[140] Good	315 Mixed HD+PA, Medium	Mean (SE)
		    BL 6 mo 12 mo
		Dietary Risk Assessment, total score†
		IG 34.2 (1.0) 29.6 (0.9) 29.5 (1.0)
		CG 34.2 (1.0) 33.8 (0.9) 32.9 (1.0)
		Difference -4.1 (0.9) -3.4 (1.0)
		p <0.0001 <0.0001
		†Comparison adjusted for age, race, education, BMI, marital status, smoking, and known CHD
		Adjusted change (95% CI)
		    BL 12 mo
		Nutrition level
		IG NR 0.30 (0.13 to 0.47)
		CG NR -0.05 (-0.22 to 0.12)
		p<0.01

Abbreviations: AHA = American Heart Association; BL = baseline; CG = control group; CHD = congenital heart defect; CI = confidence interval; DRA = daily recommended allowance; FFQ = Food Frequency Questionnaire; F/U = followup; HBP = high blood pressure; HTN = hypertension; IFG = impaired fasting

Appendix G Table 3. Behavioral Outcomes (KQ 3 Results): Healthy Diet

glucose; IG = intervention group; MDI = medical doctor intervention; n = sample; N = study population; NR = not reported; NS = not significant; NSD = no significant difference; OR = odds ratio; PTI = patient intervention; SD = standard deviation; SE = standard error; SEM = standard error of the mean.

Appendix G Table 4. Behavioral Outcomes (KQ 3 Results): Physical Activity

Study, Year Quality	N Population Intervention Focus & Intensity	Physical Activity Behavioral Outcomes

CouPLES, 2013[67] Fair	255 Cholesterol HD+PA, Medium	**Frequency of moderate PA/wk**
		     BL 6 mo 11 mo
		 IG 8.3 10.5 10.1
		 CG 8.3 8.9 8.4
		 p=0.06; incidence rate ratio: 1.2 (95% CI, 1.0 to 1.5)
		 Duration of moderate intensity PA/week (hr)
		     BL 6 mo 11 mo
		 IG 6.9 7.5 7.3
		 CG 6.9 6.7 6.6
		 p=0.37; incidence rate ratio: 1.1 (95% CI, 0.9 to 1.4)

PRO-FIT, 2012[68] Fair	340 Cholesterol HD+PA, Medium	**MVPA (min/wk), mean (SD)** BL 12 mo IG 422.0 (3.1) 501.0 (3.3) CG 363.1 (3.5) 428.0 (3.7) Difference between groups at 12 mo: NS (β, 1.11 [95% CI, -0.12 to 0.33])
RHPP Trial, 1993[69] Fair	1,197 Cholesterol HD+PA, Medium	**PA, min/wk, mean (SD)** BL 6 mo IG 413.16 (300.72) 451.48 (367.13) CG 497.91 (432.85) 440.95 (357.81) p=NS
Anderson, 1992[70] Fair	177 Cholesterol HD, High	**Exercise, total energy (kJ*kg/lb*d), mean (SD), mean change from BL (SD)** BL 12 mo IG1 155.5 (22.5) -5.73 (19.0) IG2 155.0 (27.2) -0.08 (16.9) CG 148.4 (11.5) 13.7 (28.2) p=NR
Delahanty, 2001[72] Good	90 Cholesterol HD, High	**Activity (min/wk), mean (SD)** BL 6 mo 12 mo IG 119 (126) 144 (130) 148 (102) CG 92 (97) 108 (109) 135 (185) p=NS
NFPMP, 2002[79]	143 Cholesterol HD, Medium	BL only **No exercise, %** IG 20 CG 13 **Exercise <3 times/wk, %** IG 37 CG 30 **Exercise 3 times/wk, %** IG 18 CG 26 **Exercise >3 times/wk, %** IG 25 CG 31 Note: No significant changes in physical activity (p>0.85)
ADAPT, 2006[138]	241	At least moderate-intensity exercise (hr/wk), mean (95% CI) at BL & 36 mo, mean

Appendix G Table 4. Behavioral Outcomes (KQ 3 Results): Physical Activity

Study, Year Quality	N Population Intervention Focus & Intensity	Physical Activity Behavioral Outcomes
Arroll, 1995[128] Fair	HTN HD+PA Medium	change (95% CI) at 12 mo followup (min/wk) BL 12 mo 36 mo IG 2.7 (2.3 to 3.1) 41 (19 to 63) 3.8 (3.3 to 4.3) CG 2.7 (2.5 to 3.1) 0 (-2 to 41) 3.1 (2.7 to 3.6) p† 0.185 0.007

HIP, 2009[136] Fair	208 HTN HD+PA, Medium	Moderate exercise, kJ/kg/d (SE)
		      BL 6 mo
		 IG1 15.7 (3.9) 43.5 (7.0)
		 IG2 15.1 (4.0) 53.4 (7.1)
		 IG3 10.6 (4.0) 38.0 (7.1)
		 CG 13.5 (4.0) 21.0 (7.2)
		 Total exercise, kJ/d (SE)
		      BL 6 mo
		 IG1 145.2 (2.7) 161.4 (4.6)
		 IG2 145.2 (2.8) 169.2 (4.7)
		 IG3 143.0 (2.8) 157.9 (4.7)
		 CG 145.5 (2.8) 152.5 (4.7)
		 p=NR; text states only significant for IG1 and IG2

Hyman, 2007[135] Fair	574 HTN HD+PA, High (Pt, MD&Pt); Medium (MD only)	Moderate to vigorous activity, min/wk BL Δ @ 6 mo (SD) Δ at 18mo (SD) IG1 37.9 (89.1) 6.2 (103.2) -21.5 (138.8) IG2 28.8 (106.7) 28.4 (134.9) -0.7 (112.3) CG1 43.9 (122.5) -15.7 (122.0) -13.0 (145.7) CG2 36.4 (127.1) 18.5 (287.8) 5.0 (95.1) MDI main effect at 6 mo, p=0.15; at 18 mo, p= 0.07 PTI main effect at 6 mo, p=0.07; at 18 mo, p=0.10
LIHEF, 2002[137] Fair	281 HTN HD+PA, Medium	Pedometer steps per day BL 6 mo 18mo IG1 3624.4(2917.5) 4149.4(3446.8) 3751.4 (2697.0) IG2 3306.0(2785.3) 3715.0(4025.6) 3744.9 (5515.7) CG 3933.0(3363.6) 3852.0(3675.6) 3648.5 (4285.0) p* 0.41 0.78 0.99
Migneault, 2012[126] Fair	715 HTN HD+PA, High	Moderate PA ≥3 time/wk for 30 min (self-reported), % BL 12 mo 24 mo p* IG 51 34.7 34.1 NR CG 51 24.0 22.8 Difference at 12 mo: 10.7 (95% CI, 1.2 to 20.3) Difference at 24 mo: 11.3 (95% CI, 1.8 to 20.8) *NR, but text states that the change at 12 & 24 mo was significant between groups
	337 HTN HD+PA, High	Moderate or greater PA (min/wk), mean (SD) BL Change @ 8 mo IG 162.4 (169.0) -3.44 CG 126.3 (144.3) 2.77 p=NS (NR) >150 min/wk of moderate or greater PA (%) IG 38.5 -2

Appendix G Table 4. Behavioral Outcomes (KQ 3 Results): Physical Activity

Study, Year Quality	N Population Intervention Focus & Intensity	Physical Activity Behavioral Outcomes
PREMIER, 2003[116] Good	304 HTN HD+PA, High	CG 26.2 5 p=NS (p NR) 12-mo outcomes in figure only, text states no statistically significant effects at 12 mo Total energy expenditure, kcal/d IG 3234.7 (860.7) 43.8 CG 3188.5 (820.3) -36.2 p<0.05
Rodriguez, 2012[113] Fair (poor for diet)	533 HTN HD+PA, Medium	Fitness (HR at stage 2 or last available at stage 1), mean (SD), at 6 mo BL Change IG1 128.4 (12.7) -6.8 (10.3) IG2 128.5 (14.1) -7.4 (10.3) CG 130.5 (13.6) -6.1 (9.4) p=NR

Vitalum[105] Fair	1,629 HTN HD+PA, Medium (IG 2&3); Low (IG1)	7-day PA recall (continuous score), mean (SD), hr/wk
		          BL 6 mo 12 mo
		IG 5.26 (7.55) 4.58 (4.43) 4.25 (5.91)
		CG1 4.45 (6.22) 4.84 (7.00) 4.38 (6.40)
		CG2 4.95 (6.39) 4.32 (3.98) 5.47 (7.50)
		p=NR, text states no significant difference between 3 groups
		
		PA, hr/wk, mean (SD)
		         BL 25 wk 47 wk 73 wk
		IG1 4.86 (3.98) 6.92(5.40) 6.85(5.22) 5.73(4.70)
		IG2 4.84 (3.96) 6.75 (5.17) 5.67 (4.43) 5.58 (4.49)
		IG3 4.31 (3.73) 6.69 (5.19) 6.13 (4.40) 5.91 (4.55)
		CG 5.61 (3.63) 5.92 (4.70) 5.32 (4.53) 5.37 (4.53)
		p (see text)

Arroll, 1995[128] Fair	208 HTN HD+PA, Medium	Moderate exercise, kJ/kg/d (SE) BL 6 mo IG1 15.7 (3.9) 43.5 (7.0) IG2 15.1 (4.0) 53.4 (7.1) IG3 10.6 (4.0) 38.0 (7.1) CG 13.5 (4.0) 21.0 (7.2) Total exercise, kJ/d (SE) IG1 145.2 (2.7) 161.4 (4.6) IG2 145.2 (2.8) 169.2 (4.7) IG3 143.0 (2.8) 157.9 (4.7) CG 145.5 (2.8) 152.5 (4.7) p=NR, text states only significant for IG1 and IG2

Appendix G Table 4. Behavioral Outcomes (KQ 3 Results): Physical Activity

Study, Year Quality	N Population Intervention Focus & Intensity	Physical Activity Behavioral Outcomes

Arroll, 1995[128]
Fair
	208
	HTN
	PA, Medium
		Moderate exercise, kJ/kg/d (SE)
		    BL 6 mo
		IG1 15.7 (3.9) 43.5 (7.0)
		IG2 15.1 (4.0) 53.4 (7.1)
		IG3 10.6 (4.0) 38.0 (7.1)
		CG 13.5 (4.0) 21.0 (7.2)
		Total exercise, kJ/d (SE)
		    BL 6 mo
		IG1 145.2 (2.7) 161.4 (4.6)
		IG2 145.2 (2.8) 169.2 (4.7)
		IG3 143.0 (2.8) 157.9 (4.7)
		CG 145.5 (2.8) 152.5 (4.7)
		p=NR, text states only significant for IG1 and IG2

Moreau, 2001[104] Fair	24 HTN PA, Medium	**Pedometer step counts, km/d-1 (SD)** BL Δ at 24 wk IG 3.4 (±0.3) 2.9 (±0.2) CG 4.7 (±0.4) -0.3 (±0.3) p <0.05 <0.05
APHRODITE, 2011[88] Fair	925 IFG HD+PA, High	**Total activity, min/wk, mean (SD)** BL Δ 6 mo Δ 18 mo IG 1502 (914) 248 (949) -84 (1023) CG 1629 (1005) 31 (1014) -290 (994) p=0.02 **Average- to high-intensity activity, min/wk, mean (SD)** IG 658 (564) -1 (461) 70 (562) CG 649 (521) 28 (494) 29 (512) p=0.34
DPP, 2002[89] Good	2,161 IFG HD+PA, High	**Mean change in PA from BL, MET-hr/wk** 1 y 2 y 3 y 4 y IG 7.2 5.9 5.3 7.7 CG 0.9 1.4 0.3 1.8 p<0.001 ("over time")

EDIPS, 2001[90]
Fair
	78
	IFG
	HD+PA, Medium
		Vigorous activity >3 times/wk, n (%)
		    BL 6 mo
		IG 5 (14.3) 14 (41.2)
		CG 6 (18.8) 5 (15.6)
		Difference between groups: 30.1 (95% CI, 4.3 to 52.7); p=0.02
		    BL 24 mo p
		Regular activity ≥1 time/wk, % (N)
		IG 25.0 (7) 57.1 (16) <0.02
		CG 50.0 (12) 45.8 (11)
		Regular, vigorous PA ≥1 time/wk; BL is n (%), all others are % change from BL (95% CI)
		    BL 6 mo 12 mo 24 mo
		IG 8 (24.2) 33.3 (13 to 50) 34.3 (16 to 49) 32.1 (12 to 48)
		CG 17 (53.1) -3.1 (-14 to 8.5) 7.1 (-8 to 21) -4.2 (-23 to 14)
		p 0.017 0.030 0.020 0.030

Appendix G Table 4. Behavioral Outcomes (KQ 3 Results): Physical Activity

Study, Year Quality	N Population Intervention Focus & Intensity	Physical Activity Behavioral Outcomes
EDIPS-Newcastle, 2009[91] Fair	102 IFG HD+PA, High	N (%) of participants with sustained benefit change **Physical activity score†** IG 18 (35) CG 19 (37) †Based on annual 3-day PA diaries; scores were calculated (using MET) based on reported activity No significant difference between IG and CG at BL or annual F/U in any year

FDPS, 2001[118] Good	522 IFG HD+PA, High	Self-reported change in exercise during year 1, %
		Increased exercise*
		IG 36
		CG 16
		p=0.001
		Meeting goal of exercise >4 hr/wk
		IG 86
		CG 71
		p=0.001
		*Subjects reported exercise in terms of a shift to a higher category among 4 levels of activity
		    BL 1 Year p 3 Year p
		Median change (IQR) from BL in total LTPA, min/wk
		IG 339 (193 to 545) 16 (-126 to 115) 0.9045 50 (-126 to 115) 0.2415
		CG 329 (173 to 586) 21 (-133 to 138) 23 (-142 to 171)
		Median change (IQR) from BL in moderate to vigorous LTPA, min/wk
		IG 156 (62 to 288) 49 (-41 to 140) 0.0073 61 (-33 to 168) 0.0057
		CG 169 (65 to 352) 14 (-47 to 90) 6 (-91 to 104)
		    BL Early FU‡ Late FU‡ p§
		Median change (IQR) in total activity (hr/wk)
		IG 5.7 (3.2 to 9.1) 6.3 (3.8 to 9.9) 6.2 (3.5 to 9.5) 0.54
		CG 5.5 (3.0 to 9.7) 5.9 (3.1 to 9.4) 5.7 (3.3 to 9.3)
		Median change (IQR) in moderate to vigorous activity (hr/wk)
		IG 1.8 (0.6 to 3.8) 3.5 (1.5 to 5.5) 3.1 (1.5 to 5.1) 0.15
		CG 1.6 (0.4 to 4.2) 2.8 (1.3 to 4.8) 2.8 (1.4 to 5.4)
		†1–3 y after intervention phase; ‡4–9 y after intervention phase; §Adjusted for BL & sex at late FU

HLC, 2011[92] Fair	307 IFG HD+PA, High	**PA, min/wk, mean (SD)** BL 6 mo IG 413.16 (300.72) 451.48 (367.13) CG 497.91 (432.85) 440.95 (357.81) p=NS
Live Well, Be Well, 2012[86] Good	238 IFG HD+PA, High	BL mean (SE), within-group change (SE) BL 6 mo 12 mo **PA, hr/wk** IG 8.0 (0.6) 0.7 (0.6) 0.7 (0.7) CG 7.0 (0.5) 0.4 (0.6) 1.1 (0.6) Between-group comparison of change NS at either time point

Appendix G Table 4. Behavioral Outcomes (KQ 3 Results): Physical Activity

Study, Year Quality	N Population Intervention Focus & Intensity	Physical Activity Behavioral Outcomes
LLDP[94] Good	312 IFG HD+PA, High	**PA, MET-hr/wk** IG 25.6 (2.1) 3.0 (2.2) 2.2 (2.1) CG 23.6 (2.2) 0.4 (2.0) 6.4 (2.8) Between-group comparison of change NS **Walking, hr/wk** IG 4.4 (0.4) 0.4 (0.4) 0.6 (0.5) CG 3.9 (0.4) 0.3 (0.4) 0.6 (0.5) Between-group comparison of change NS
Melbourne DPS, 2012[85] Fair	92 IFG HD+PA, High	**Leisure time PA, min/wk** BL, mean (SD) 1-year change (median, 95% CI) IG 247.50 (164.1) 5.8 (-12.8 to 21.7) CG 251.08 (158.4) 3.3 (-20.7 to 18.3) Intervention effect: 3.33 (95% CI, -26.7 to 33.3); p=0.82
PREDIAS, 2009[95] Fair	182 IFG HD+PA, High	Achieved goal of ≥30 min/d moderate PA, n (%), at 12 mo IG 4 (10.8) CG 4 (9.5) p=NR

SLIM[149] Fair	147 IFG HD+PA, High	**Physical exercise, min/wk, mean (SD)**
		       BL 12 mo Change
		IG 104.2 (80.24) 150.8 (75.18) 46.6 (95.5)
		CG 96.9 (76.3) 114.0 (72.6) 17.9 (63.8)
		Between-group p=0.034
		Active days/wk, mean (SD)
		     BL 3 y Change
		IG 2.9 (2.4) 3.8 (2.5) 0.9 (2.8)
		CG 3.0 (2.6) 2.5 (2.7) -0.55 (3.31)
		p=NR
		VO$_2$max, L/min, mean (SD)
		     BL 1 y 2 y End
		IG 2.18 (0.59) 2.38 (0.63) 2.39 (0.62) 2.35 (0.63)
		CG 2.06 (0.57) 2.14 (0.60) 2.04 (0.59) 2.08 (0.61)
		Group x time p=0.04

Enhanced Fitness Trial, 2012[98] Fair	302 IFG PA, High	**Endurance, min/wk, mean (SD)**
		     BL 3 mo 12 mo
		IG 73.39 (±119.81) 124.30 (±127.15) 133.60 (±136.47)
		CG 115.29 (±183.66) 92.87 (±115.01) 112.62 (±135.45)
		p<0.001 for group x time interaction, indicating between-group differences
		Strength, min/wk, mean (SD)
		IG 19.19 (±74.97) 20.92 (±33.46) 28.44 (±57.62)
		CG 25.11 (±75.68) 27.42 (±68.69) 40.15 (±93.35)
		p=0.11, indicating no significant differences for group x time interactions
		% Meeting goal of 150 min/wk
		     BL 12 mo
		IG 16% 42%
		CG 31% 31%

Appendix G Table 4. Behavioral Outcomes (KQ 3 Results): Physical Activity

Study, Year Quality	N Population Intervention Focus & Intensity	Physical Activity Behavioral Outcomes
Prepare Trial, 2009[99] Fair	98 IFG PA, Medium	OR, 1.65 (95% CI, 1.08 to 2.53) **Cardiorespiratory fitness on SF-36, 6-min walk test, average (SD)** 　　　　BL　　　　3 mo　　　　　　6 mo　　　　　　12 mo IG　　495.7 (±119.9)　516.5 (±128.2)　518.3 (±127.4) CG　500.9 (±109.3)　526.4 (±113.9)　517.2 (±129.1) p=0.81 for group x time interactions **Ambulatory activity, mean (SD), change (95% CI) at F/U** 　　　BL　　　　　　　6 mo　　　　　　　　　12 mo IG1　6560 (4,424)　　870 (-54 to 1,793)　　549 (-290 to 1,390) IG2　6600 (2,402)　　2093 (944 to 3,242)　1039 (135 to 1,943) CG　6873 (3,537)　　-152 (-778 to 573)　　-940 (-1,574 to -307) 　　　　　　　　　　　6 mo　　　　　p　　　12 mo　　　　　　　p IG1 vs. CG　968 (-297 to 2,234)　0.132　1,401 (417 to 2,385)　0.06 IG2 vs. CG　2,207 (989 to 3,246)　0.001　1,902 (954 to 2,859)　<0.001 **Self-reported walking activity (MET-min/wk), mean (SD), change (95% CI) at F/U** 　　　BL　　　　　　　6 mo　　　　　　　　　12 mo IG1　891 (297 to 2,079)　154 (-582 to 889)　　421 (-224 to 1,067) IG2　1,386 (594 to 2,772)　1,083 (517 to 1,649)　708 (72 to 1,344) CG　801 (292 to 2,161)　123 (-619 to 864)　　-361 (-849 to 127) Change from BL; adjusted intervention effect 　　　　　　　　　　6 mo　　　　　p　　　　12 mo　　　　　p IG1 vs. CG　-23 (-889 to 842)　0.957　764 (14 to 1,515)　0.046 IG2 vs. CG　1,031 (206 to 1,755)　0.015　1,150 (428 to 1,872)　0.002 **Total moderate to vigorous PA (MET-min/wk), mean (SD), change (95% CI) at F/U** 　　　BL　　　　　　　6 mo　　　　　　　　　12 mo IG1　2,359 (947 to 3,989)　1,533 (-254 to 3,320)　1,459 (327 to 2,571) IG2　3,480 (1,524 to 6,339)　3,830 (1,637 to 6,024)　1,589 (48 to 3,130) CG　2,335 (923 to 3,921)　340 (-1,048 to 1,729)　-1,377 (-2,852 to 98) Change from BL; adjusted intervention effect 　　　　　　　　　　6 mo　　　　　p　　　12 mo　　　　　　p IG1 vs. CG　928 (-2,008 to 3,242)　0.468　2,364 (513 to 4,214)　0.13 IG2 vs. CG　3,557 (1,126 to 5,987)　0.005　3,060 (1,301 to 4,819)　0.001
Bo, 2007[146] Fair	375 Mixed HD+PA, Medium	**PA (MET-hr/wk)** 　　　BL　　　　　　12 mo　　　Difference (95% CI) IG　18.9 (13.3)　　23.6 (17.7)　　4.73 (2.91 to 6.55) CG　18.1 (16.0)　　17.8 (15.2)　　-0.26 (-0.92 to 0.40) p<0.001
Cochrane, 2012[102] Fair	601 Mixed HD+PA, High	**Mean PA score from Primary Prevention Toolkit** 　　　BL　　　12 mo IG　2.67　　2.81 CG　2.65　　2.8 p NR for difference between groups at 12 mo ("no significant difference between groups on any of the measures")

Appendix G Table 4. Behavioral Outcomes (KQ 3 Results): Physical Activity

Study, Year Quality	N Population Intervention Focus & Intensity	Physical Activity Behavioral Outcomes
Edelman, 2006[129] Fair	154 Mixed HD+PA, High	**Days per week of exercise** BL 12 mo IG 1.6 3.7 CG 1.4 2.4 p=0.002
EUROACTION, 2008[106] Fair	2,384 Mixed HD+PA, High	BL 12 mo **Physical activity (≥30 min ≥4 times/wk), N (%)** IG 313/1080 (29) 512/1018 (50) CG 107/331 (32) 222/1003 (22) Difference: 29.4% (95% CI, 10.7 to 48.0); p=0.01 **Physical activity, %, change from BL to 12 mo (compared with CG subsample)** IG 23.5 CG -10.2 Difference: 32.9% (95% CI, 11.8 to 53.9); p=0.01

GOAL, 2009[139] Good	457 Mixed HD+PA, Medium	Mean (95% CI) for BL, mean change (95% CI) at 12 mo, mean change (SD) at 36 mo, based on self-reported SQUASH questionnaire
		
		 Total PA (min/wk)
		      BL Δ at 12 mo Δ at 36 mo
		 IG 2304 (2095 to 2513) -126 (-304 to 53) -167 (1321)
		 CG 2026 (1867 to 2185) -68 (-225 to 89) -92 (1218)
		 p 0.52 0.387
		 Moderate- to high-intensity PA (min/wk)
		 IG 596 (496 to 695) 97 (1 to 194)
		 CG 720 (616 to 823) -22 (-112 to 68)
		 p 0.24
		 % Meeting Dutch national reccomendations for 150 min/wk of PA
		      BL 3 y
		 IG 68.6 73.8
		 CG 71.4 73.9
		 p=0.28
		 % Meeting ACSM guidelines for 60 min/wk of vigorous PA
		 IG 53.4 64.1
		 CG 50.4 61.3
		 p=0.99
		 Other nonsignificant PA measures reported for 12 and 36 mo: low-intensity (<4 METs); leisure time PA total; leisure time PA for individual activities. Two significant PA findings: At 12 mo, IG had significantly greater improvements in walking than CG (p=0.05) At 36 mo, IG had significantly more moderate-intensity sport min/wk than CG (p=0.042)

Hardcastle, 2008[167] Fair	334 Mixed HD+PA, Medium	6-mo difference in mean (SEM) BL **Overall PA (MET-min/wk)** IG 2039 (204) 245 (104) CG 2320 (294) -122 (158) 95% CI, -739 to 4.70; p≤0.05 **Vigorous PA (MET-min/wk)** IG 679 (114) 149 (64) CG 752 (151) 50 (109)

Appendix G Table 4. Behavioral Outcomes (KQ 3 Results): Physical Activity

Study, Year Quality	N Population Intervention Focus & Intensity	Physical Activity Behavioral Outcomes
HIPS, 2012[103] Fair	814 Mixed HD+PA, High	95% CI, -348 to 150; p=NS **Moderate PA (MET-min/wk)** IG 437 (82) 89 (72) CG 554 (107) -29 (97) 95% CI, -358 to 121; p=NS **Walking (MET-min/wk)** IG 1089 (97) 198 (63) CG 1244 (141) -145 (109) 95% CI, -592 to -94; p<0.01 Mean (SD) for outcome measure (ITT analyses) BL 18 mo **Total MET-min/wk** IG 1854 (2175) 3154 (3394) CG 2278 (2820) 3272 (3875) Time x group p=NS **Vigorous PA (MET-min/wk)** IG 590 (1294) 1061 (2120) CG 747 (1672) 972 (2023) Time x group p=NS **Moderate PA (MET-min/wk)** IG 441 (1091) 862 (1526) CG 576 (1159) 1086 (1670) Time x group p=NS **Walking (MET-min/wk)** IG 996 (1117) 1265 (1352) CG 1243 (1433) 1327 (1642) Time x group p<0.01

HOORN, 2013[132] Fair	622 Mixed HD+PA, Medium	**Physical Activity Score at 12 mo, mean (95% CI)**
		     BL 6 mo 12 mo
		IG 3.71 (NR) 4.59 (4.30 to 4.88) 4.60 (4.33 to 4.87)
		CG 3.38 (NR) 3.89 (3.56 to 4.22) 4.09 (3.80 to 4.38)
		p 0.002 0.01
		Median (Q1;Q3); based on SQUASH questionnaire*
		        BL 6 mo 12 mo
		Moderate activities
		IG 56 (19;150) 47 (21;120) 52 (21;138)
		CG 47 (19;120) 47 (19;121) 56 (26;126)
		Difference (95% CI)† -9.5 (-22.3 to 3.2) -9.4 (-22.0 to 3.2)
		OR (95% CI)† NR NR
		Vigorous activities
		IG 0 (0;17) 0 (0;17) 0 (0;17)
		CG 0 (0;17) 6 (0;17) 0 (0;17)
		Difference (95% CI)† -0.8 (-3.3 to 1.8) -0.1 (-3.3 to 3.1)
		OR (95% CI)† NR NR

Appendix G Table 4. Behavioral Outcomes (KQ 3 Results): Physical Activity

Study, Year Quality	N Population Intervention Focus & Intensity	Physical Activity Behavioral Outcomes

IMPALA, 2009[133] Fair	615 Mixed HD+PA, High	**Met recommendations, n (%)**
		          BL 12 mo
		IG 201 (64.0) 161 (51.3) 162 (51.6)
		CG 184 (59.7) 167 (54.2) 160 (51.9)
		Difference NR NR
		OR (95% CI)† 0.7 (0.5 to 1.1) 0.9 (0.6 to 1.4)
		†Adjusted for BL values
		Moderate or vigorous PA on modified CHAMPS questionnaire
		          BL 12 mo p
		Min/wk, mean (SD) 0.74
		IG 405 (343) 460 (362)
		CG 447 (345) 449 (365)
		Met recommendations for PA*, n (%) 0.97
		IG 183 (60) 163 (65)
		CG 181 (64) 153 (65)
		*≥30 min of moderate-intensity activity ≥5 days per week

Inter99, 2008[107] Fair	4,053 Mixed HD+PA, High	**PA in men, min/wk** BL, mean (SE) 12 mo 36 mo IG 286 (3.1) +11* NR** CG 304 (9.1) NR** NR** *p<0.05 for within-group change over time; **p=NS for within-group change over time; p NR for between-group comparisons **PA in women, min/wk** IG 291 (3.0) NR** NR** CG 327 (9.3) NR** NR** **p=NS for within-group change over time; p NR for between-group comparisons

Logan Healthy Living, 2009[114] Fair	434 Mixed HD+PA, Medium	Adjusted* mean (SE)
		       BL Δ 12 mo Δ 18 mo
		Moderate to vigorous PA, min/wk
		IG 142.5 (22.2) 71.2 (14.3) 62.19 (14.20)
		CG 142.4 (197.3) 84.5 (14.9) 74.73 (14.91)
		12-mo difference between groups: -11.14 (95% CI, -51.56 to 29.28); p=0.589
		18-mo difference between groups: -12.54 (95% CI, 52.95 to 27.88); p=0.543
		Moderate to vigorous PA, sessions/wk
		IG 2.9 (3.6) 2.6 (0.4) 2.24 (0.33)
		CG 2.9 (3.8) 2.3 (0.4) 2.13 (0.35)
		12-mo difference between groups: 0.39 (95% CI, -0.55 to 1.33); p=0.491
		18-mo difference between groups: 0.11 (95% CI, -0.83 to 1.05); p= 0.815
		% meeting PA guidelines (≥150 min, ≥5 sessions/wk)
		      BL 12 mo
		IG 57 (25.0) 103 (45.1)
		CG 52 (25.7) 77 (37.3)
		OR, 1.50 (95% CI, 0.73 to 3.03)

Appendix G Table 4. Behavioral Outcomes (KQ 3 Results): Physical Activity

Study, Year Quality	N Population Intervention Focus & Intensity	Physical Activity Behavioral Outcomes
PHPP, 2007[121] Fair	99 Mixed HD+PA, Medium	**Mean # of steps/d (SD)** BL 12 mo IG 7345 (3890) 10373 (4089)* CG 7196 (3682) 6815 (3421) *p<0.001
SPRING, 2012[100] Fair	201 Mixed HD+PA, Medium	**Physically inactive participants, % (95% CI)** BL Δ 12 mo IG 23 -11.8 (-20.6 to -5.5) CG 28 -4.5 (-11.2 to -1.3) Difference between groups: 7.3 (95% CI, -0.8 to 15.4) p=0.54
WISEWOMAN California, 2010[108] Fair	1,093 Mixed HD+PA, Medium	**Self-reported moderate level of exercise, n (%)** BL 12 mo p† IG 309 (71) 365 (84) <0.001 CG 328 (75) 335 (77) 0.57 **Self-reported vigorous level of exercise, n (%)** IG 57 (13) 143 (33) <0.001 CG 69 (16) 75 (17) 0.58 Moderate activity defined as walking or running; vigorous as participating in exercise or sports †p-values are within group; between group p-values NR
WISEWOMAN NC, 2008[110] Fair	236 Mixed HD+PA, Medium	Mean (SE) BL 6 mo 12 mo **Physical activity, moderate, min/d†** IG 11.6 (1.3) 12.5 (1.0) 13.2 (1.1) CG 13.0 (1.2) 11.3 (1.1) 10.5 (1.1) Difference 1.2 (1.5) 2.7 (1.5) p 0.43 0.08 **Physical activity assessment (self-reported), moderate** IG 13.3 (0.4) 14.5 (0.3) 14.0 (0.4) CG 13.4 (0.4) 13.4 (0.3) 12.9 (0.3) Difference 1.1 (0.5) 1.1 (0.5) p 0.013 0.027 **Physical activity assessment (self-reported), vigorous** IG 8.8 (0.4) 9.5 (0.3) 9.0 (0.3) CG 9.1 (0.4) 8.7 (0.3) 8.5 (0.3) Difference 0.8 (0.4) 0.6 (0.5) p 0.05 0.23 **Physical activity assessment (self-reported), all activity** IG 29.4 (0.8) 31.2 (0.7) 30.0 (0.7) CG 29.2 (0.8) 29.4 (0.6) 28.4 (0.6) Difference -4.1 (0.9) -3.4 (1.0) p 0.04 0.12

Appendix G Table 4. Behavioral Outcomes (KQ 3 Results): Physical Activity

Study, Year Quality	N Population Intervention Focus & Intensity	Physical Activity Behavioral Outcomes
Wister, 2007[140] Good	315 Mixed HD+PA, Medium	Adjusted change (95% CI) in physical activity 　　　BL　　12 mo IG　NR　0.17 (-0.06 to 0.40) CG　NR　0.16 (-0.08 to 0.40) p=NR, NS
Green Prescription Programme (Walk to Heart, Health, & Activity Study), 2003[123] Fair	878 Mixed HD+PA, Medium	BL (SD)　Δ at 12 mo (95% CI)　Difference between groups (95% CI)　p Total energy expenditure (kcal/kg/wk) IG 237.5 (42.2)　9.76 (5.85 to 13.68)　9.38 (3.96 to 14.81)　0.001 CG 235.7 (45.3)　0.37 (-3.39 to 4.14)　(975 kcal/wk) Leisure PA (kcal/kg/wk) IG 6.0 (12.2)　4.32 (3.26 to 5.38)　2.67 (0.48 to 4.86)　0.02 CG 6.5 (11.1)　1.29 (0.11 to 2.47)　(247 kcal/wk) Moderate or vigorous exercise (min/wk) IG 11.3 (21.7)　54.6 (41.4 to 68.4)　33.6 (2.4 to 64.2)　0.04 CG 12.0 (20.5)　16.8 (6.0 to 32.4) % meeting recommended PA levels (2.5 hr/wk of moderate to vigorous PA) IG 66/451 (14.6%) CG 21/427 (4.9%) p=0.003
NERS, 2012[109] Fair (poor for quality of life)	2,160 Mixed PA, Medium	Total exercise (min), median (IQR), at 12 mo IG 200 (60 to 435) CG 165 (50 to 370) Text states "of borderline statistical significance"; p=NR
PAC, 2011[122] Fair	120 Mixed PA, Medium	BL　　　　13 wk　　　　25 wk　　　Adjusted mean Δ (BL to 13wk) Activity counts/min IG 213.1 (79.8)　209.5 (85.8)　199.4 (76.6) CG 231.5 (71.3)　218.6 (68.2)　208.6 (64.2) Moderate activity, min/d (%) IG 13.36 (4.90)　12.28 (4.39)　12.08 (4.42) CG 15.67 (5.11)　14.11 (4.16)　13.63 (3.62) Vigorous activity, min/d (%) IG 3.98 (2.64)　3.80 (2.74)　3.56 (2.44) CG 3.88 (2.31)　3.88 (2.23)　3.54 (2.06) NS for all accelerometer measures VO$_2$ peak, LO$_2$min-1 IG 2.3 (0.7)　2.4 (0.8)　2.4 (0.8)　0.079 (-0.02 to 0.17) CG 2.2 (0.7)　2.3 (0.7)　2.3 (0.7)　0.128 (0.01 to 0.24)
PACE, 2005[131] Fair	771 Mixed PA, Medium	Self-reported PA on SQUASH Questionnaire 　　　BL　　6 mo　　12 mo Median amount of at least moderate PA, min, overall IG 240　360　350 CG 30　410　390 Median amount of at least moderate PA, min, leisure time IG 215　300　295 CG 240　300　325

Appendix G Table 4. Behavioral Outcomes (KQ 3 Results): Physical Activity

Study, Year Quality	N Population Intervention Focus & Intensity	Physical Activity Behavioral Outcomes
Kallings, 2009[141] Good	101 Mixed PA, Medium	**Increase of ≥3,000 steps/d** IG 32% CG 14% $p<0.05$ BL 6 mo **Moderate-intensity PA ≥30 min 5 times/wk** IG 17% 38% CG 7% 17% $p<0.05$ **Vigorous-intensity PA ≥20 min 3 times/wk** IG 11% 21% CG 7% 7% $p<0.05$ **Moderate- to high-intensity muscle strengthening ≥2 times/wk** IG 2% 21% CG 6% 9% $p=0.09$
LIFE, 2010[130] Fair	186 Mixed PA, Medium	BL BL to 6 mo Δ 6 to 11 mo Δ BL to 11 mo Δ **VO$_2$max (mL/kg/min)** IG1 22.0 (±0.66) +2.3 +0.7 +3.0 CG 22.3 (±0.63) +0.9 +1.1 +2.0 p NS <0.05 NS NS **F static strength, peak torque in a knee-joint angle of 120°** IG1 137.7±5.8 +4.3 +2.8 +7.1 CG 137.3±5.4 +1.5 +0.0 +1.5 p NS NS NS NS **F dynamic strength, peak torque of 6 contractions at 240°** IG1 70.0±2.9 +1.2 +0.4 +1.6 CG 68.6±2.8 -0.6 +0.6 +0.0 p NS NS NS NS Other strength endurance tests: arm curl test, IG significantly greater than CG from 6 mo to 11 mo and from BL to 11 mo; chair stand test, IG significantly greater than CG from BL to 6 mo, 6 to 11 mo, and BL to 11 mo; vertical jump, IG significantly greater than CG from BL to 11 mo

Abbreviations: ACSM = American College of Sports Medicine; BL = baseline; CG = control group; CI = confidence interval; F/U = followup; HR = heart rate; HTN = hypertension; IG = intervention group; IFG = impaired fasting glucose; IQR = interquartile range; ITT = intention to treat; LTPA = leisure time physical activity; MDI = medical doctor intervention; MET = metabolic equivalent; MVPA = moderate to vigorous physical activity; n = sample; N = study population; NR = not reported; NS = not significant; OR = odds ratio; PA = physical activity; PTI = patient intervention; SD = standard deviation; SE = standard error; SEM = standard error of the mean.

www.ingramcontent.com/pod-product-compliance
Lightning Source LLC
Chambersburg PA
CBHW081721170526
45167CB00009B/3652